T0293377

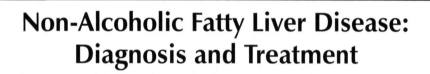

# Non-Alcoholic Fatty Liver Disease:
## Diagnosis and Treatment

# Non-Alcoholic Fatty Liver Disease: Diagnosis and Treatment

Editor: Heidi Hamlin

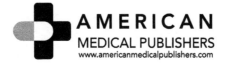

**AMERICAN**
MEDICAL PUBLISHERS
www.americanmedicalpublishers.com

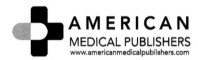

Cataloging-in-Publication Data

Non-alcoholic fatty liver disease : diagnosis and treatment / edited by Heidi Hamlin.
    p. cm.
Includes bibliographical references and index.
ISBN 978-1-63927-756-8
1. Fatty liver. 2. Fatty liver--Diagnosis. 3. Fatty liver--Treatment. 4. Liver--Diseases.
5. Fatty degeneration. 6. Hepatitis. I. Hamlin, Heidi.
RC848.F3 N663 2023
616.362--dc23

American Medical Publishers,
41 Flatbush Avenue,
1st Floor, New York,
NY 11217, USA

ISBN 978-1-63927-756-8 (Hardback)

# Contents

# Preface

Non-alcoholic fatty liver disease (NAFLD) refers to a heterogeneous condition with an extensive range of clinical presentations and disease severity. People who suffer from this disease are observed to consume little or no alcohol, and have excessive fat stored in their liver cells. Damage to the liver under this condition is caused by the generation of oxidative metabolites and by the translocation of gut-derived endotoxin. These processes result in cellular injury and stimulation of the inflammatory responses facilitated by a range of molecules. The injury develops with impairment in tissue regeneration and extracellular matrix turnover which results in causing cirrhosis and fibrogenesis. Some of the major risk factors for this disease are obesity, insulin resistance and diabetes. This book explores all the important translational and clinical researches on non-alcoholic fatty liver disease in the modern day. It presents researches and studies performed by experts across the globe. The extensive content of this book provides the readers with a thorough understanding of the subject.

The information contained in this book is the result of intensive hard work done by researchers in this field. All due efforts have been made to make this book serve as a complete guiding source for students and researchers. The topics in this book have been comprehensively explained to help readers understand the growing trends in the field.

I would like to thank the entire group of writers who made sincere efforts in this book and my family who supported me in my efforts of working on this book. I take this opportunity to thank all those who have been a guiding force throughout my life.

**Editor**

# The Vicious Circle of Hepatic Glucagon Resistance in Non-Alcoholic Fatty Liver Disease

**Katrine D. Galsgaard** [1,2]

[1]   Department of Biomedical Sciences, Faculty of Health and Medical Sciences, University of Copenhagen, 2200 Copenhagen, Denmark; katrine@sund.ku.dk;

[2]   Novo Nordisk Foundation Center for Basic Metabolic Research, Faculty of Health and Sciences, University of Copenhagen, 2200 Copenhagen, Denmark

**Abstract:** A key criterion for the most common chronic liver disease—non-alcoholic fatty liver disease (NAFLD)—is an intrahepatic fat content above 5% in individuals who are not using steatogenic agents or having significant alcohol intake. Subjects with NAFLD have increased plasma concentrations of glucagon, and emerging evidence indicates that subjects with NAFLD may show hepatic glucagon resistance. For many years, glucagon has been thought of as the counterregulatory hormone to insulin with a primary function of increasing blood glucose concentrations and protecting against hypoglycemia. However, in recent years, glucagon has re-emerged as an important regulator of other metabolic processes including lipid and amino acid/protein metabolism. This review discusses the evidence that in NAFLD, hepatic glucagon resistance may result in a dysregulated lipid and amino acid/protein metabolism, leading to excess accumulation of fat, hyperglucagonemia, and increased oxidative stress contributing to the worsening/progression of NAFLD.

**Keywords:** autophagy; amino acids; glucagon; NAFLD; the liver–alpha cell axis

## 1. Processing and Secretion of Glucagon

Glucagon is encoded by the preproglucagon gene (GCG) [1], expressed in alpha cells, enteroendocrine L-cells, and the brain [2]. In alpha cells, GCG is processed by prohormone convertase (PC) 2 yielding glucagon [3], whereas in L-cells, GCG is processed by PC1/3, yielding glucagon-like peptide (GLP)-1, GLP-2, glicentin, and oxyntomodulin [4]. However, recent evidence suggests that the processing is not as tissue-specific as previously thought, since PC1/3 may also be active in alpha cells, giving rise to pancreatic GLP-1 [5–8], and PC2 might act in L-cells to create gut-derived glucagon [9–11]. It is a matter of debate whether this only occurs as a consequence of metabolic alterations, such as pancreatectomy [9,10] and bariatric surgery [11], resulting in gut-derived glucagon, or glucagon receptor inhibition [12] and streptozotocin treatment [13], resulting in pancreatic-derived GLP-1. Pancreatic GLP-1 has been suggested to be part of heathy physiology by contributing to a local incretin axis [14–16]. In the measurement of glucagon, analytical challenges due to cross-reactivity with other GCG-derived peptides have been an issue [17,18], and using liquid chromatography–mass spectrometry, glucagon secretion was not found to be increased after bypass surgery [19]. Upon secretion, glucagon binds to its receptor, the glucagon receptor, and regulates hepatic glucose, lipid, and amino acid/protein metabolism [20].

## 2. The Glucagon Receptor as a Target in the Treatment of Type 2 Diabetes, Obesity, and NAFLD

In recent years, the glucagon receptor has emerged as a target in the treatment of type 2 diabetes [21–24], obesity, and non-alcoholic fatty liver disease (NAFLD) [25–27]. An international consensus panel recently proposed that NAFLD should be renamed to metabolic-associated fatty liver disease (MAFLD) [28]. The criteria for MAFLD are evidence of hepatic steatosis in addition to either overweight/obesity, the presence of type 2 diabetes, or evidence of metabolic dysfunction [28]. Glucagon receptor signaling increases hepatic glucose production and a majority of subjects with type 2 diabetes show increased plasma concentrations of glucagon (hyperglucagonemia) [29,30]. Hyperglucagonemia is now known to be at least partly responsible for diabetic hyperglycemia [31,32], and therefore, clinical trials using glucagon receptor antagonists (GRAs) have been conducted in subjects with type 2 diabetes. GRA treatment improves diabetic hyperglycemia [21–24], but disturbing adverse effects including increased plasma concentrations of low-density lipoprotein and liver enzymes (aspartate- and alanine-transaminase) and hepatic fat accumulation halted further development of GRAs [33,34]. However, based on the observed changes in lipid metabolism and the possibility that glucagon may decrease food intake [35,36] and increase energy expenditure [37–40] (possibly through the sympathetic nervous system [41] or other indirect effects [42]), the focus has now shifted from glucagon receptor inhibition to glucagon receptor activation.

Glucagon analogs and agonists are being investigated as potential agents in NAFLD treatment partly due to glucagon's regulatory effects on hepatic lipid metabolism, where glucagon increases hepatic lipolysis and fatty acid oxidation [43,44] while decreasing lipogenesis [45] and the secretion of triglycerides and very-low-density lipoprotein [46–48]. Consistent with this, subjects with endogenous glucagon deficiency (pancreatectomized subjects) [49] and diabetic (db/db) mice treated with glucagon receptor antisense oligonucleotide [50] have increased hepatic fat. Furthermore, glucagon has a lipid-mobilizing effect and decreases plasma concentrations of cholesterol [51–55], non-esterified fatty acids [44], triglycerides [52,56,57], and very-low-density lipoprotein [47], suggesting that glucagon may improve dyslipidemia.

To counteract the hyperglycemic effect of glucagon, glucagon receptor agonists are being combined with agonists of either one or both of the receptors for the incretin hormones: GLP-1 and glucose-dependent insulinotropic polypeptide [58–60]. Glucagon/GLP-1 co-agonists reversed obesity in diet-induced obese mice, decreased body weight to a larger degree than GLP-1 agonist comparators [61], and appear to increase energy expenditure [62]. Glucagon/GLP-1 co-agonists also improve NAFLD [63] and show promising results in models of non-alcoholic steatohepatitis, a subtype of NAFLD which potentially can progress to liver fibrosis, cirrhosis, and hepatocellular carcinoma [64], by decreasing inflammation and fibrosis while increasing mitochondrial β-oxidation, thus reducing hepatic steatosis [65]. Improvement of NAFLD has also been observed in obese or overweight individuals with type 2 diabetes treated with a glucagon/GLP-1 co-agonist [66]. Glucagon's effect on energy expenditure and satiety may be translatable to humans, since glucagon/GLP-1 and glucagon infusions, but not the GLP-1 infusion, increased energy expenditure to a similar degree in overweight subjects without diabetes [67], and a glucagon/GLP-1 infusion decreased food intake [68]. In another human study, glucagon infusion decreased food intake but had no effect on energy expenditure, possibly due the low dose used compared to other studies [69]. The effect on energy expenditure may thus be mediated by indirect effects, possibly by glucagon acting on the GLP-1 receptor, which can be activated by high concentrations of glucagon [70,71], whereas the hepatic effects of the co-agonists may be ascribed to direct glucagon receptor activation since it, unlike the GLP-1 receptor [72], is expressed in the liver.

## 3. The Liver–Alpha Cell Axis May be Impaired in NAFLD

The rationale for the use of GRAs and glucagon agonists in the treatment of patients with type 2 diabetes (55–68% of whom have liver steatosis [73]) and obesity is based on glucagon's effects on hepatic glucose and lipid metabolism, respectively. However, glucagon is also a key regulator of amino acid/protein metabolism [74–78], and glucagon has been suggested to be even more important for amino acid/protein metabolism than glucose metabolism [79]. Glucagon is part of an endocrine feedback loop (the liver–alpha cell axis), in which amino acids control glucagon secretion and the proliferation of alpha cells, while glucagon in turn controls hepatic amino acid metabolism and ureagenesis [80–85].

During conditions of disrupted glucagon signaling, glucagon's effect on amino acid metabolism is impaired and as a consequence, hyperaminoacidemia develops, which in turn results in hyperglucagonemia [80,82–84,86,87]. In line with this, the hyperglucagonemia observed in most subjects with type 2 diabetes is associated with hyperaminoacidemia. Especially, elevated plasma levels of alanine seem to mark a disturbed liver–alpha cell axis [85,88–90], and alanine also appears to be a potent glucagonotropic amino acid [91]. Importantly, hyperglucagonemia seems to be associated with a fatty liver rather than with diabetes per se [92], and plasma concentrations of glucagon and non-branched-chain amino acids are characteristically increased in subjects with increased liver fat (as reflected by elevated HOMA-IR levels) [85]. Furthermore, ureagenesis is impaired in subjects with NAFLD and non-alcoholic steatohepatitis [93,94] as well as in mice with impaired glucagon receptor signaling and obese Zucker rats with hepatic steatosis [89]. Impaired liver function thus mimics the conditions of experimental glucagon deficiency (e.g., brought about by GRAs [87]), leading to the suggestion that subjects with impaired liver function due to steatosis also show glucagon resistance [95,96]. Interestingly, subjects with NAFLD appear to exhibit resistance towards glucagon-stimulated amino acid metabolism but not towards glucagon-stimulated glucose metabolism, since the hyperglycemic effect of glucagon was preserved in a pancreatic clamp study carried out in individuals with biopsy-verified NAFLD versus lean controls, whereas the effect on amino acid turnover and ureagenesis was attenuated [97]. This is consistent with the fact that the biochemical pathway of glucagon-stimulated glycogenolysis is separate from that involved in ureagenesis, whereas gluconeogenesis is closely associated with amino acid turnover and ureagenesis [98]. Considering that glucagon mainly promotes hepatic glucose production via glycogenolysis [99], this may explain why sensitivity to glucagon's hyperglycemic effect can be preserved while its hypoaminoacidemic effect is impaired. In contrast, rats with high-fat-diet–induced hepatic steatosis showed a reduction in glucagon-stimulated hepatic glucose production, most likely due to reduced glycogenolysis [100], and this state of glucagon resistance could be reversed by exercise training, which resulted in a reduction in hepatic liver triglycerides [100]. Studies by the same group also showed that hepatic triglyceride accumulation (induced by a high-fat diet) reduced hepatic glucagon receptor density and glucagon-mediated signal transduction [101,102]. Whether this applies to human liver steatosis is unknown.

## 4. Hepatic Glucagon Resistance May Impair Autophagy Resulting in Increased Oxidative Stress

Exogenous glucagon stimulates hepatic autophagy [103–106], and during conditions of increased endogenous glucagon secretion, such as starvation [107], hypoglycemia [108], and type 1 diabetes [109], the number of hepatic lysosomes is increased. By stimulating autophagic protein degradation, glucagon may provide substrates for gluconeogenesis and ketogenesis and thus, sustain nutrient and energy homeostasis during starvation [110,111]. Autophagy also functions to remove damaged and non-functional organelles [112], and the autophagic degradation of mitochondria (mitophagy), which may be induced by glucagon [113], is important for maintaining mitochondrial turnover. Impaired mitophagy thus leads to the accumulation of dysfunctional mitochondria generating reactive oxygen species, resulting in oxidative stress and inflammation [114]. Autophagy is, furthermore, an important regulator of lipid metabolism and lipophagy; in other words, the degradation of triglycerides into free fatty acids in autolysosomes functions to regulate intracellular lipid stores and energy homeostasis by utilization of the released free fatty acids in mitochondrial β-oxidation [115]. Inhibition of autophagy in cultured hepatocytes and mouse livers increased triglyceride storage in lipid droplets and decreased β-oxidation and very-low-density lipoprotein secretion [116], processes which are influenced in the opposite direction by glucagon [43,44,56]. The hepatic lipolytic effect of glucagon could therefore potentially be partly mediated by lipophagy. The process of autophagy has been shown to be impaired in obesity and NAFLD [117], and hepatic resistance to glucagon in subjects with NAFLD may therefore partly explain the impaired autophagy. Amino acids, especially glutamine, leucine, and arginine, are potent activators of the mammalian target of the rapamycin complex 1 [118], which suppress autophagy [119]. The hyperaminoacidemia observed in NAFLD may therefore further impair hepatic autophagy. In NAFLD, impaired hepatic autophagy would result in the worsening/progression of NAFLD by increasing oxidative stress and lipid accumulation, and increased glucagon signaling could potentially improve NAFLD by increasing the autophagic removal of damaged organelles and lipid droplets. Whether the stimulatory effect of glucagon on hepatic autophagy is a contributing factor to the reversal of NAFLD observed by glucagon agonist treatment is currently unknown; however, the possibility provides a new perspective on the role of tri- and dual-agonists in the treatment of NAFLD.

In summary, hepatic glucagon resistance may result in a dysregulated lipid and amino acid/protein metabolism and possibly impaired autophagy, leading to excess accumulation of fat, increased oxidative stress, and hyperaminoacidemia, resulting in hyperglucagonemia and hyperglycemia. Hepatic glucagon resistance in NAFLD would thus result in the creation of a vicious circle and contribute to the worsening/progression of NAFLD (Figure 1 and Table 1). However, the majority of studies investigating these aspects of NAFLD have been performed on cells and rodents, some with contrasting findings. Further studies translating these observations to humans are thus warranted. Recognizing that glucagon's primary role may not reside in glucose metabolism alone, but also includes important aspects of lipid and amino acid/protein metabolism, is becoming increasingly important in view of the current development of glucagon-based therapeutics for the treatment of NAFLD and obesity.

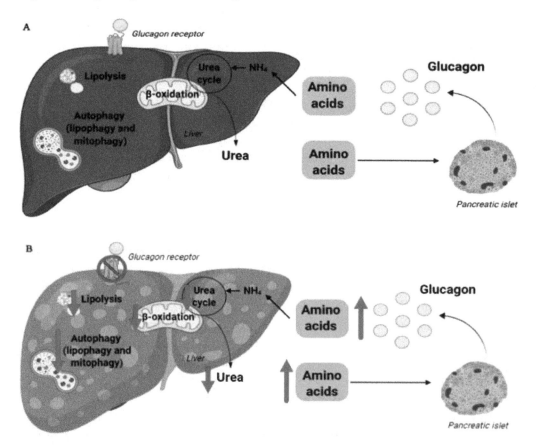

**Figure 1.** (**A**) Glucagon is secreted from the pancreatic alpha-cell and binds to its hepatic receptor. This results in increased hepatic amino acid uptake and metabolism (ureagenesis). Hepatic glucagon signaling also increases lipolysis and ß-oxidation and may increase hepatic autophagy. (**B**) During conditions of disrupted glucagon signaling, hepatic amino acid metabolism and ureagenesis is halted, as is hepatic lipolysis, ß-oxidation, and autophagy. This results in the accumulation of hepatic fat and damaged organelles, inducing oxidative stress and increased plasma amino acids, leading to hyperglucagonemia. This figure was created using BioRender.

**Table 1.** The molecular mechanisms that may be impaired by hepatic glucagon resistance inhibition and the pathologies that are involved.

|  | Metabolic Process | Pathology |
|---|---|---|
| Amino acid/protein metabolism | Amino acid transport Amino acid catabolism Ureagenesis | Hyperaminoacidemia Hyperglucagonemia Hyperammonemia |
| Autophagy | Lipophagy Mitophagy | Increased hepatic fat Increased oxidative stress |
| Lipid metabolism | β-oxidation Lipolysis | Increased hepatic fat Dyslipidemia |

**Acknowledgments:** I am ever grateful for the support, guidance, and inspiration granted by Jens Juul Holst, Nicolai J. Wewer Albrechtsen, Gerald Shulman and Kitt Falk Petersen. Department of Biomedical Sciences, Faculty of Health and Medical Sciences, University of Copenhagen, Copenhagen, Denmark; Department of Internal Medicine, Yale School of Medicine, New Haven, CT 06520-8020, USA.

## References

1.  Bell, G.I.; Sanchez-Pescador, R.; Laybourn, P.J.; Najarian, R.C. Exon duplication and divergence in the human preproglucagon gene. *Nature* **1983**, *304*, 368–371. [CrossRef]
2.  Drucker, D.J. Glucagon and the Glucagon-like Peptides. *Pancreas* **1990**, *5*, 484–488. [CrossRef]
3.  Rouille, Y.; Westermark, G.; Martin, S.K.; Steiner, D.F. Proglucagon is processed to glucagon by prohormone convertase PC2 in alpha TC1-6 cells. *Proc. Natl. Acad. Sci. USA* **1994**, *91*, 3242–3246. [CrossRef]
4.  Rouillé, Y.; Martin, S.; Steiner, D.F. Differential Processing of Proglucagon by the Subtilisin-like Prohormone Convertases PC2 and PC3 to Generate either Glucagon or Glucagon-like Peptide. *J. Biol. Chem.* **1995**, *270*, 26488–26496. [CrossRef] [PubMed]
5.  Kilimnik, G.; Kim, A.; Steiner, N.F.; Friedman, T.C.; Hara, M. Intraislet production of GLP-1 by activation of prohormone convertase 1/3 in pancreatic α-cells in mouse models of β-cell regeneration. *Islets* **2010**, *2*, 149–155. [CrossRef] [PubMed]
6.  Whalley, N.M.; Pritchard, L.E.; Smith, D.M.; White, A. Processing of proglucagon to GLP-1 in pancreatic α-cells: Is this a paracrine mechanism enabling GLP-1 to act on β-cells? *J. Endocrinol.* **2011**, *211*, 99–106. [CrossRef] [PubMed]
7.  Marchetti, P.; Lupi, R.; Bugliani, M.; Kirkpatrick, C.L.; Sebastiani, G.D.; Grieco, F.A.; Del Guerra, S.; D'Aleo, V.; Piro, S.; Marselli, L.; et al. A local glucagon-like peptide 1 (GLP-1) system in human pancreatic islets. *Diabetologia* **2012**, *55*, 3262–3272. [CrossRef]
8.  Taylor, S.W.; Nikoulina, S.E.; Andon, N.L.; Lowe, C. Peptidomic Profiling of Secreted Products from Pancreatic Islet Culture Results in a Higher Yield of Full-length Peptide Hormones than Found using Cell Lysis Procedures. *J. Proteome Res.* **2013**, *12*, 3610–3619. [CrossRef]
9.  Holst, J.J.; Pedersen, J.H.; Baldissera, F.; Stadil, F. Circulating glucagon after total pancreatectomy in man. *Diabetologia* **1983**, *25*, 396–399. [CrossRef]
10. Lund, A.; Bagger, J.I.; Albrechtsen, N.J.W.; Christensen, M.; Grøndahl, M.; Hartmann, B.; Mathiesen, E.R.; Hansen, C.P.; Storkholm, J.H.; Van Hall, G.; et al. Evidence of Extrapancreatic Glucagon Secretion in Man. *Diabetes* **2015**, *65*, 585–597. [CrossRef]
11. Jorsal, T.; Albrechtsen, N.J.W.; Christensen, M.M.; Mortensen, B.; Wandall, E.; Langholz, E.; Friis, S.; Worm, D.; Ørskov, C.; Støving, R.K.; et al. Investigating Intestinal Glucagon After Roux-en-Y Gastric Bypass Surgery. *J. Clin. Endocrinol. Metab.* **2019**, *104*, 6403–6416. [CrossRef] [PubMed]
12. Gelling, R.W.; Du, X.Q.; Dichmann, D.S.; Romer, J.; Huang, H.; Cui, L.; Obici, S.; Tang, B.; Holst, J.J.; Fledelius, C.; et al. Lower blood glucose, hyperglucagonemia, and pancreatic cell hyperplasia in glucagon receptor knockout mice. *Proc. Natl. Acad. Sci. USA* **2003**, *100*, 1438–1443. [CrossRef] [PubMed]
13. Nie, Y.; Nakashima, M.; Brubaker, P.L.; Li, Q.-L.; Perfetti, R.; Jansen, E.; Zambre, Y.; Pipeleers, D.; Friedman, T.C. Regulation of pancreatic PC1 and PC2 associated with increased glucagon-like peptide 1 in diabetic rats. *J. Clin. Investig.* **2000**, *105*, 955–965. [CrossRef]

14. Chambers, A.P.; Sorrell, J.E.; Haller, A.; Roelofs, K.; Hutch, C.R.; Kim, K.-S.; Gutierrez-Aguilar, R.; Li, B.; Drucker, D.J.; D'Alessio, D.A.; et al. The Role of Pancreatic Preproglucagon in Glucose Homeostasis in Mice. *Cell Metab.* **2017**, *25*, 927–934.e3. [CrossRef] [PubMed]

15. Campbell, S.A.; Golec, D.P.; Hubert, M.; Johnson, J.; Salamon, N.; Barr, A.; Macdonald, P.E.; Philippaert, K.; Light, P.E. Human islets contain a subpopulation of glucagon-like peptide-1 secreting α cells that is increased in type 2 diabetes. *Mol. Metab.* **2020**, *39*, 101014. [CrossRef]

16. Fava, G.E.; Dong, E.W.; Wu, H. Intra-islet glucagon-like peptide 1. *J. Diabetes Its Complicat.* **2016**, *30*, 1651–1658. [CrossRef]

17. Albrechtsen, N.J.W.; Hartmann, B.; Veedfald, S.; Windeløv, J.A.; Plamboeck, A.; Bojsen-Møller, K.N.; Idorn, T.; Feldt-Rasmussen, B.; Knop, F.K.; Vilsbøll, T.; et al. Hyperglucagonaemia analysed by glucagon sandwich ELISA: Nonspecific interference or truly elevated levels? *Diabetologia* **2014**, *57*, 1919–1926. [CrossRef]

18. Albrechtsen, N.J.W.; Veedfald, S.; Plamboeck, A.; Deacon, C.F.; Hartmann, B.; Knop, F.K.; Vilsboll, T.; Holst, J.J. Inability of Some Commercial Assays to Measure Suppression of Glucagon Secretion. *J. Diabetes Res.* **2015**, *2016*, 1–5. [CrossRef]

19. Roberts, G.P.; Kay, R.G.; Howard, J.; Hardwick, R.H.; Reimann, F.; Gribble, F.M. Gastrectomy with Roux-en-Y reconstruction as a lean model of bariatric surgery. *Surg. Obes. Relat. Dis.* **2018**, *14*, 562–568. [CrossRef]

20. Müller, T.D.; Finan, B.; Clemmensen, C.; DiMarchi, R.D.; Tschöp, M.H. The New Biology and Pharmacology of Glucagon. *Physiol. Rev.* **2017**, *97*, 721–766. [CrossRef]

21. Kelly, R.P.; Garhyan, P.; Raddad, E.; Fu, H.; Lim, C.N.; Prince, M.J.; Pinaire, J.A.; Loh, M.T.; Deeg, M.A. Short-term administration of the glucagon receptor antagonist LY2409021 lowers blood glucose in healthy people and in those with type 2 diabetes. *Diabetes Obes. Metab.* **2015**, *17*, 414–422. [CrossRef] [PubMed]

22. Kazda, C.M.; Ding, Y.; Kelly, R.P.; Garhyan, P.; Shi, C.; Lim, C.N.; Fu, H.; Watson, D.E.; Lewin, A.J.; Landschulz, W.H.; et al. Evaluation of Efficacy and Safety of the Glucagon Receptor Antagonist LY2409021 in Patients With Type 2 Diabetes: 12- and 24-Week Phase 2 Studies. *Diabetes Care* **2015**, *39*, 1241–1249. [CrossRef]

23. Kazierad, D.J.; Bergman, A.; Tan, B.; Erion, D.M.; Somayaji, V.; Lee, D.S.; Rolph, T. Effects of multiple ascending doses of the glucagon receptor antagonist PF-06291874 in patients with type 2 diabetes mellitus. *Diabetes Obes. Metab.* **2016**, *18*, 795–802. [CrossRef] [PubMed]

24. Vajda, E.G.; Logan, D.; Lasseter, K.; Armas, D.; Plotkin, D.J.; Pipkin, J.; Li, Y.-X.; Zhou, R.; Klein, D.; Wei, X.; et al. Pharmacokinetics and pharmacodynamics of single and multiple doses of the glucagon receptor antagonist LGD-6972 in healthy subjects and subjects with type 2 diabetes mellitus. *Diabetes Obes. Metab.* **2016**, *19*, 24–32. [CrossRef] [PubMed]

25. Henderson, S.J.; Konkar, A.; Hornigold, D.C.; Trevaskis, J.L.; Jackson, R.; Fredin, M.F.; Jansson-Löfmark, R.; Naylor, J.; Rossi, A.; Bednarek, M.A.; et al. Robust anti-obesity and metabolic effects of a dual GLP-1/glucagon receptor peptide agonist in rodents and non-human primates. *Diabetes Obes. Metab.* **2016**, *18*, 1176–1190. [CrossRef] [PubMed]

26. Zhou, J.; Cai, X.; Huang, X.; Dai, Y.; Sun, L.; Zhang, B.; Yang, B.; Lin, H.; Huang, W.; Qian, H. A novel glucagon-like peptide-1/glucagon receptor dual agonist exhibits weight-lowering and diabetes-protective effects. *Eur. J. Med. Chem.* **2017**, *138*, 1158–1169. [CrossRef]

27. More, V.R.; Lao, J.; McLaren, D.G.; Cumiskey, A.-M.; Murphy, B.A.; Chen, Y.; Previs, S.; Stout, S.; Patel, R.; Satapati, S.; et al. Glucagon like receptor 1/ glucagon dual agonist acutely enhanced hepatic lipid clearance and suppressed de novo lipogenesis in mice. *PLoS ONE* **2017**, *12*, e0186586. [CrossRef]

28. Eslam, M.; Newsome, P.N.; Sarin, S.K.; Anstee, Q.M.; Targher, G.; Romero-Gomez, M.; Zelber-Sagi, S.; Wong, V.W.-S.; Dufour, J.-F.; Schattenberg, J.M.; et al. A new definition for metabolic dysfunction-associated fatty liver disease: An international expert consensus statement. *J. Hepatol.* **2020**, *73*, 202–209. [CrossRef]

29. Müller, W.A.; Faloona, G.R.; Aguilar-Parada, E.; Unger, R.H. Abnormal Alpha-Cell Function in Diabetes. Response to carbohydrate and protein ingestion. *N. Engl. J. Med.* **1970**, *283*, 109–115. [CrossRef]

30. Mitrakou, A.; Kelley, D.; Veneman, T.; Jenssen, T.; Pangburn, T.; Reilly, J.; Gerich, J. Contribution of Abnormal Muscle and Liver Glucose Metabolism to Postprandial Hyperglycemia in NIDDM. *Diabetes* **1990**, *39*, 1381–1390. [CrossRef]

31. Reaven, G.M.; Chen, Y.-D.I.; Golay, A.; Swislocki, A.L.M.; Jaspan, J.B. Documentation of Hyperglucagonemia Throughout the Day in Nonobese and Obese Patients with Noninsulin-Dependent Diabetes Mellitus. *J. Clin. Endocrinol. Metab.* **1987**, *64*, 106–110. [CrossRef] [PubMed]

32. Shah, P.; Vella, A.; Basu, A.; Basu, R.; Schwenk, W.F.; Rizza, R.A. Lack of Suppression of Glucagon Contributes to Postprandial Hyperglycemia in Subjects with Type 2 Diabetes Mellitus. *J. Clin. Endocrinol. Metab.* **2000**, *85*, 4053–4059. [CrossRef] [PubMed]

33. Guzman, C.B.; Zhang, X.M.; Liu, R.; Regev, A.; Shankar, S.; Garhyan, P.; Pillai, S.G.; Kazda, C.; Chalasani, N.; Hardy, T. Treatment with LY2409021, a glucagon receptor antagonist, increases liver fat in patients with type 2 diabetes. *Diabetes Obes. Metab.* **2017**, *19*, 1521–1528. [CrossRef]

34. Kazierad, D.J.; Chidsey, K.; Somayaji, V.R.; Bergman, A.J.; Calle, R.A. Efficacy and safety of the glucagon receptor antagonist PF-06291874: A 12-week, randomized, dose-response study in patients with type 2 diabetes mellitus on background metformin therapy. *Diabetes Obes. Metab.* **2018**, *20*, 2608–2616. [CrossRef] [PubMed]

35. Geary, N. Pancreatic glucagon signals postprandial satiety. *Neurosci. Biobehav. Rev.* **1990**, *14*, 323–338. [CrossRef]

36. Geary, N.; Kissileff, H.R.; Pi-Sunyer, F.X.; Hinton, V.J. Individual, but not simultaneous, glucagon and cholecystokinin infusions inhibit feeding in men. *Am. J. Physiol. Integr. Comp. Physiol.* **1992**, *262*, R975–R980. [CrossRef] [PubMed]

37. Davidson, I.W.F.; Salter, J.M.; Best, C.H. Calorigenic Action of Glucagon. *Nat. Cell Biol.* **1957**, *180*, 1124. [CrossRef]

38. Joel, C.D. Stimulation of metabolism of rat brown adipose tissue by addition of lipolytic hormones in vitro. *J. Biol. Chem.* **1966**, *241*, 814–821.

39. Doi, K.; Kuroshima, A. Modified metabolic responsiveness to glucagon in cold-acclimated and heat-acclimated rats. *Life Sci.* **1982**, *30*, 785–791. [CrossRef]

40. Nair, K.S. Hyperglucagonemia Increases Resting Metabolic Rate In Man During Insulin Deficiency. *J. Clin. Endocrinol. Metab.* **1987**, *64*, 896–901. [CrossRef]

41. Dicker, A.; Zhao, J.; Cannon, B.; Nedergaard, J. Apparent thermogenic effect of injected glucagon is not due to a direct effect on brown fat cells. *Am. J. Physiol. Content* **1998**, *275*, R1674–R1682. [CrossRef] [PubMed]

42. Beaudry, J.L.; Kaur, K.D.; Varin, E.M.; Baggio, L.L.; Cao, X.; Mulvihill, E.E.; Stern, J.H.; Campbell, J.E.; Scherer, P.E.; Drucker, D.J. The brown adipose tissue glucagon receptor is functional but not essential for control of energy homeostasis in mice. *Mol. Metab.* **2019**, *22*, 37–48. [CrossRef] [PubMed]

43. Pegorier, J.P.; Garcia-Garcia, M.V.; Prip-Buus, C.; Duee, P.H.; Kohl, C.; Girard, J. Induction of ketogenesis and fatty acid oxidation by glucagon and cyclic AMP in cultured hepatocytes from rabbit fetuses. Evidence for a decreased sensitivity of carnitine palmitoyltransferase I to malonyl-CoA inhibition after glucagon or cyclic AMP treatment. *Biochem. J.* **1989**, *264*, 93–100. [PubMed]

44. Perry, R.J.; Zhang, D.; Guerra, M.T.; Brill, A.L.; Goedeke, L.; Nasiri, A.R.; Rabin-Court, A.; Wang, Y.; Peng, L.; Dufour, S.; et al. Glucagon stimulates gluconeogenesis by INSP3R1-mediated hepatic lipolysis. *Nat. Cell Biol.* **2020**, *579*, 279–283. [CrossRef]

45. Prip-Buus, C.; Pegorier, J.P.; Duee, P.H.; Kohl, C.; Girard, J. Evidence that the sensitivity of carnitine palmitoyltransferase I to inhibition by malonyl-CoA is an important site of regulation of hepatic fatty acid oxidation in the fetal and newborn rabbit. Perinatal development and effects of pancreatic hormones in cultured rabbit hepatocytes. *Biochem. J.* **1990**, *269*, 409–415.

46. Heimberg, M.; Weinstein, I.; Kohout, M. The effects of glucagon, dibutyryl cyclic adenosine 3′,5′-monophosphate, and concentration of free fatty acid on hepatic lipid metabolism. *J. Biol. Chem.* **1969**, *244*, 5131–5139.

47. Eaton, R.P. Hypolipemic action of glucagon in experimental endogenous lipemia in the rat. *J. Lipid Res.* **1973**, *14*, 312–318.

48. Longuet, C.; Sinclair, E.M.; Maida, A.; Baggio, L.L.; Maziarz, M.; Charron, M.J.; Drucker, D.J. The Glucagon Receptor Is Required for the Adaptive Metabolic Response to Fasting. *Cell Metab.* **2008**, *8*, 359–371. [CrossRef]

49. Dresler, C.M.; Fortner, J.G.; McDermott, K.; Bajorunas, D.R. Metabolic Consequences of (Regional) Total Pancreatectomy. *Ann. Surg.* **1991**, *214*, 131–140. [CrossRef]

50. Liang, Y.; Osborne, M.C.; Monia, B.P.; Bhanot, S.; Gaarde, W.A.; Reed, C.; She, P.; Jetton, T.L.; Demarest, K.T. Reduction in glucagon receptor expression by an antisense oligonucleotide ameliorates diabetic syndrome in db/db mice. *Diabetes* **2004**, *53*, 410–417. [CrossRef]

51.    Paloyan, E.; Harper, P.V. Glucagon as a regulating factor of plasma lipids. *Metabolism* **1961**, *10*, 315–323. [PubMed]

52.    Amatuzio, D.S.; Grande, F.; Wada, S. Effect of glucagon on the serum lipids in essential hyperlipemia and in hypercholesterolemia. *Metabolism* **1962**, *11*, 1240–1249. [PubMed]

53.    Penhos, J.C.; Wu, C.H.; Daunas, J.; Reitman, M.; Levine, R.; Levune, R. Effect of Glucagon on the Metabolism of Lipids and on Urea Formation by the Perfused Rat Liver. *Diabetes* **1966**, *15*, 740–748. [CrossRef] [PubMed]

54.    Caren, R.; Corbo, L. Glucagon and cholesterol metabolism. *Metabolism* **1960**, *9*, 938–945. [PubMed]

55.    Aubry, F.; Marcel, Y.L.; Davignon, J. Effects of glucagon on plasma lipids in different types of primary hyperlipoproteinemia. *Metabolism* **1974**, *23*, 225–238. [CrossRef]

56.    Guettet, C.; Mathe, D.; Riottot, M.; Lutton, C. Effects of chronic glucagon administration on cholesterol and bile acid metabolism. *Biochim. Biophys. Acta* **1988**, *963*, 215–223. [CrossRef]

57.    Guettet, C.; Rostaqui, N.; Mathe, D.; Lécuyer, B.; Navarro, N.; Jacotot, B. Effect of chronic glucagon administration on lipoprotein composition in normally fed, fasted and cholesterol-fed rats. *Lipids* **1991**, *26*, 451–458. [CrossRef]

58.    Gu, W.; Lloyd, D.J.; Chinookswong, N.; Komorowski, R.; Sivits, G.; Graham, M.; Winters, K.A.; Yan, H.; Boros, L.G.; Lindberg, R.A.; et al. Pharmacological Targeting of Glucagon and Glucagon-Like Peptide 1 Receptors Has Different Effects on Energy State and Glucose Homeostasis in Diet-Induced Obese Mice. *J. Pharmacol. Exp. Ther.* **2011**, *338*, 70–81. [CrossRef]

59.    Sadry, S.A.; Drucker, D.J. Emerging combinatorial hormone therapies for the treatment of obesity and T2DM. *Nat. Rev. Endocrinol.* **2013**, *9*, 425–433. [CrossRef]

60.    Finan, B.; Yang, B.; Ottaway, N.; Smiley, D.L.; Ma, T.; Clemmensen, C.; Chabenne, J.; Zhang, L.; Habegger, K.M.; Fischer, K.; et al. A rationally designed monomeric peptide triagonist corrects obesity and diabetes in rodents. *Nat. Med.* **2015**, *21*, 27–36. [CrossRef]

61.    Pocai, A.; Carrington, P.E.; Adams, J.R.; Wright, M.; Eiermann, G.; Zhu, L.; Du, X.; Petrov, A.; Lassman, M.E.; Jiang, G.; et al. Glucagon-Like Peptide 1/Glucagon Receptor Dual Agonism Reverses Obesity in Mice. *Diabetes* **2009**, *58*, 2258–2266. [CrossRef] [PubMed]

62.    Day, J.W.; Ottaway, N.; Patterson, J.T.; Gelfanov, V.; Smiley, D.; Gidda, J.; Findeisen, H.; Bruemmer, D.; Drucker, D.J.; Chaudhary, N.; et al. A new glucagon and GLP-1 co-agonist eliminates obesity in rodents. *Nat. Chem. Biol.* **2009**, *5*, 749–757. [CrossRef] [PubMed]

63.    Patel, V.C.; Joharapurkar, A.; Kshirsagar, S.; Sutariya, B.; Patel, M.; Patel, H.; Pandey, D.; Patel, D.; Ranvir, R.; Kadam, S.; et al. Coagonist of GLP-1 and Glucagon Receptor Ameliorates Development of Non-Alcoholic Fatty Liver Disease. *Cardiovasc. Hematol. Agents Med. Chem.* **2018**, *16*, 35–43. [CrossRef]

64.    Younossi, Z. Non-alcoholic fatty liver disease—A global public health perspective. *J. Hepatol.* **2019**, *70*, 531–544. [CrossRef]

65.    Jung, S.; Lee, J.; Kim, J.; Lee, Y.; Kim, Y.; Kang, J.; Trautmann, M.; Hompesch, M.; Kwon, S. Potent weight loss mechanism and improvement of NASH by the long-acting GLP-1/glucagon receptor dual agonist HM12525A. In Proceedings of the European Association for the Study of Diabetes, 51st Annual Meeting, Stockholm, Sweden, 14–18 September 2015.

66.    Robertson, D.; Hansen, L.; Ambery, P.; Esterline, R.L.; Jermutus, L.; Chang, Y.-T.; Petrone, M.; Johansson, E.; Johansson, L.; Sjöberg, F.B.; et al. 354-OR: Cotadutide (medi0382), a Dual Receptor Agonist with Glucagon-Like Peptide-1 and Glucagon Activity, Modulates Hepatic Glycogen and Fat Content. *Diabetes* **2020**, *69*, 354. [CrossRef]

67.    Tan, T.; Field, B.C.; McCullough, K.A.; Troke, R.C.; Chambers, E.S.; Salem, V.; Maffe, J.G.; Baynes, K.C.; De Silva, A.; Viardot, A.; et al. Coadministration of Glucagon-Like Peptide-1 During Glucagon Infusion in Humans Results in Increased Energy Expenditure and Amelioration of Hyperglycemia. *Diabetes* **2013**, *62*, 1131–1138. [CrossRef]

68.    Cegla, J.; Troke, R.C.; Jones, B.; Tharakan, G.; Kenkre, J.; McCullough, K.A.; Lim, C.T.; Parvizi, N.; Hussein, M.; Chambers, E.S.; et al. Coinfusion of Low-Dose GLP-1 and Glucagon in Man Results in a Reduction in Food Intake. *Diabetes* **2014**, *63*, 3711–3720. [CrossRef] [PubMed]

69.    Bagger, J.I.; Holst, J.J.; Hartmann, B.; Andersen, B.; Knop, F.K.; Vilsbøll, T. Effect of Oxyntomodulin, Glucagon, GLP-1, and Combined Glucagon +GLP-1 Infusion on Food Intake, Appetite, and Resting Energy Expenditure. *J. Clin. Endocrinol. Metab.* **2015**, *100*, 4541–4552. [CrossRef] [PubMed]

70. Svendsen, B.; Larsen, O.; Gabe, M.B.N.; Christiansen, C.B.; Rosenkilde, M.M.; Drucker, D.J.; Holst, J.J. Insulin Secretion Depends on Intra-islet Glucagon Signaling. *Cell Rep.* **2018**, *25*, 1127–1134.e2. [CrossRef]

71. Moens, K.; Flamez, D.; Schravendijk, C.V.; Ling, Z.; Pipeleers, D.; Schuit, F. Dual Glucagon Recognition by Pancreatic beta-Cells via Glucagon and Glucagon-Like Peptide 1 Receptors. *Diabetes* **1998**, *47*, 66–72. [CrossRef]

72. Panjwani, N.; Mulvihill, E.E.; Longuet, C.; Yusta, B.; Campbell, J.E.; Brown, T.J.; Streutker, C.; Holland, D.; Cao, X.; Baggio, L.L.; et al. GLP-1 Receptor Activation Indirectly Reduces Hepatic Lipid Accumulation but Does Not Attenuate Development of Atherosclerosis in Diabetic Male ApoE−/− Mice. *Endocrinology* **2013**, *154*, 127–139. [CrossRef] [PubMed]

73. Younossi, Z.; Golabi, P.; De Avila, L.; Paik, J.M.; Srishord, M.; Fukui, N.; Qiu, Y.; Burns, L.; Afendy, A.; Nader, F. The global epidemiology of NAFLD and NASH in patients with type 2 diabetes: A systematic review and meta-analysis. *J. Hepatol.* **2019**, *71*, 793–801. [CrossRef] [PubMed]

74. Nair, K.S.; Halliday, D.; Matthews, D.E.; Welle, S.L. Hyperglucagonemia during insulin deficiency accelerates protein catabolism. *Am. J. Physiol.* **1987**, *253*, E208–E213. [CrossRef] [PubMed]

75. Couet, C.; Fukagawa, N.K.; Matthews, D.E.; Bier, D.M.; Young, V.R. Plasma amino acid kinetics during acute states of glucagon deficiency and excess in healthy adults. *Am. J. Physiol. Metab.* **1990**, *258*, E78–E85. [CrossRef]

76. Flakoll, P.; Borel, M.; Wentzel, L.; Williams, P.; Lacy, D.; Abumrad, N. The role of glucagon in the control of protein and amino acid metabolism in vivo. *Metabolism* **1994**, *43*, 1509–1516. [CrossRef]

77. Kraft, G.; Coate, K.C.; Winnick, J.J.; Dardevet, D.; Donahue, E.P.; Cherrington, A.D.; Williams, P.E.; Moore, M.C. Glucagon's effect on liver protein metabolism in vivo. *Am. J. Physiol. Metab.* **2017**, *313*, E263–E272. [CrossRef]

78. Boden, G.; Rezvani, I.; Owen, O.E. Effects of glucagon on plasma amino acids. *J. Clin. Investig.* **1984**, *73*, 785–793. [CrossRef]

79. Dean, E.D. A Primary Role for Alpha Cells as Amino Acid Sensors. *Diabetes* **2019**. [CrossRef]

80. Solloway, M.J.; Madjidi, A.; Gu, C.; Easthamanderson, J.; Clarke, H.J.; Kljavin, N.M.; Zavala-Solorio, J.; Kates, L.; Friedman, B.; Brauer, M.J.; et al. Glucagon Couples Hepatic Amino Acid Catabolism to mTOR-Dependent Regulation of α-Cell Mass. *Cell Rep.* **2015**, *12*, 495–510. [CrossRef]

81. Holst, J.J.; Albrechtsen, N.J.W.; Pedersen, J.; Knop, F.K. Glucagon and Amino Acids Are Linked in a Mutual Feedback Cycle: The Liver–α-Cell Axis. *Diabetes* **2017**, *66*, 235–240. [CrossRef]

82. Kim, J.; Okamoto, H.; Huang, Z.; Anguiano, G.; Chen, S.; Liu, Q.; Cavino, K.; Xin, Y.; Na, E.; Hamid, R.; et al. Amino Acid Transporter Slc38a5 Controls Glucagon Receptor Inhibition-Induced Pancreatic α Cell Hyperplasia in Mice. *Cell Metab.* **2017**, *25*, 1348–1361.e8. [CrossRef] [PubMed]

83. Dean, E.D.; Li, M.; Prasad, N.; Wisniewski, S.N.; Von Deylen, A.; Spaeth, J.; Maddison, L.; Botros, A.; Sedgeman, L.R.; Bozadjieva, N.; et al. Interrupted Glucagon Signaling Reveals Hepatic α Cell Axis and Role for L-Glutamine in α Cell Proliferation. *Cell Metab.* **2017**, *25*, 1362–1373.e5. [CrossRef] [PubMed]

84. Galsgaard, K.D.; Winther-Sørensen, M.; Ørskov, C.; Kissow, H.; Poulsen, S.S.; Vilstrup, H.; Prehn, C.; Adamski, J.; Jepsen, S.L.; Hartmann, B.; et al. Disruption of glucagon receptor signaling causes hyperaminoacidemia exposing a possible liver-alpha-cell axis. *Am. J. Physiol. Metab.* **2018**, *314*, E93–E103. [CrossRef] [PubMed]

85. Albrechtsen, N.J.W.; Færch, K.; Jensen, T.M.; Witte, D.R.; Pedersen, J.; Mahendran, Y.; Jonsson, A.E.; Galsgaard, K.D.; Winther-Sørensen, M.; Torekov, S.S.; et al. Evidence of a liver–alpha cell axis in humans: Hepatic insulin resistance attenuates relationship between fasting plasma glucagon and glucagonotropic amino acids. *Diabetologia* **2018**, *61*, 671–680. [CrossRef] [PubMed]

86. Boden, G.; Master, R.W.; Rezvani, I.; Palmer, J.P.; Lobe, T.E.; Owen, O.E. Glucagon deficiency and hyperaminoacidemia after total pancreatectomy. *J. Clin. Investig.* **1980**, *65*, 706–716. [CrossRef] [PubMed]

87. Mu, J.; Qureshi, S.A.; Brady, E.J.; Muise, E.S.; Candelore, M.R.; Jiang, G.; Li, Z.; Wu, M.S.; Yang, X.; Dallas-Yang, Q.; et al. Anti-Diabetic Efficacy and Impact on Amino Acid Metabolism of GRA1, a Novel Small-Molecule Glucagon Receptor Antagonist. *PLoS ONE* **2012**, *7*, e49572. [CrossRef] [PubMed]

88. Pedersen, J.S.; Rygg, M.O.; Kristiansen, V.B.; Olsen, B.H.; Serizawa, R.R.; Holst, J.J.; Madsbad, S.; Gluud, L.L.; Bendtsen, F.; Albrechtsen, N.J.W. Nonalcoholic Fatty Liver Disease Impairs the Liver–Alpha Cell Axis Independent of Hepatic Inflammation and Fibrosis. *Hepatol. Commun.* **2020**, *4*, 1610–1623. [CrossRef]

89.  Winther-Sørensen, M.; Galsgaard, K.D.; Santos, A.; Trammell, S.A.; Sulek, K.; Kuhre, R.E.; Pedersen, J.; Andersen, D.B.; Hassing, A.S.; Dall, M.; et al. Glucagon acutely regulates hepatic amino acid catabolism and the effect may be disturbed by steatosis. *Mol. Metab.* **2020**, 101080. [CrossRef]

90.  Gar, C.; Haschka, S.J.; Kern-Matschilles, S.; Rauch, B.; Sacco, V.; Prehn, C.; Adamski, J.; Seissler, J.; Albrechtsen, N.J.W.; Holst, J.J.; et al. The liver–alpha cell axis associates with liver fat and insulin resistance: A validation study in women with non-steatotic liver fat levels. *Diabetologia* **2020**, 1–9. [CrossRef]

91.  Felig, P. Amino Acid Metabolism in Man. *Annu. Rev. Biochem.* **1975**, *44*, 933–955. [CrossRef]

92.  Albrechtsen, N.J.W.; Junker, A.E.; Christensen, M.; Hædersdal, S.; Wibrand, F.; Lund, A.M.; Galsgaard, K.D.; Holst, J.J.; Knop, F.K.; Vilsbøll, T. Hyperglucagonemia correlates with plasma levels of non-branched-chain amino acids in patients with liver disease independent of type 2 diabetes. *Am. J. Physiol. Liver Physiol.* **2018**, *314*, G91–G96. [CrossRef] [PubMed]

93.  Eriksen, P.L.; Vilstrup, H.; Rigbolt, K.; Suppli, M.P.; Sorensen, M.; Heeboll, S.; Veidal, S.S.; Knop, F.K.; Thomsen, K.L. Non-alcoholic fatty liver disease alters expression of genes governing hepatic nitrogen conversion. *Liver Int.* **2019**. [CrossRef] [PubMed]

94.  Eriksen, P.L.; Sørensen, M.; Grønbæk, H.; Hamilton-Dutoit, S.; Vilstrup, H.; Thomsen, K.L. Non-alcoholic fatty liver disease causes dissociated changes in metabolic liver functions. *Clin. Res. Hepatol. Gastroenterol.* **2019**, *43*, 551–560. [CrossRef] [PubMed]

95.  Albrechtsen, N.J.W.; Pedersen, J.; Galsgaard, K.D.; Winther-Sorensen, M.; Suppli, M.P.; Janah, L.; Gromada, J.; Vilstrup, H.; Knop, F.K.; Holst, J.J. The liver-alpha cell axis and type 2 diabetes. *Endocr. Rev.* **2019**. [CrossRef]

96.  Suppli, M.P.; Lund, A.; Bagger, J.I.; Vilsbøll, T.; Knop, F.K. Involvement of steatosis-induced glucagon resistance in hyperglucagonaemia. *Med Hypotheses* **2016**, *86*, 100–103. [CrossRef]

97.  Suppli, M.P.; Bagger, J.I.; Lund, A.; Demant, M.; Van Hall, G.; Strandberg, C.; König, M.J.; Rigbolt, K.; Langhoff, J.L.; Albrechtsen, N.J.W.; et al. Glucagon Resistance at the Level of Amino Acid Turnover and Ureagenesis in Obese Subjects with Hepatic Steatosis. *Diabetes* **2018**, *67*, 147. [CrossRef]

98.  Schutz, Y. Protein Turnover, Ureagenesis and Gluconeogenesis. *Int. J. Vitam. Nutr. Res.* **2011**, *81*, 101–107. [CrossRef]

99.  Ramnanan, C.J.; Edgerton, D.S.; Kraft, G.; Cherrington, A.D. Physiologic action of glucagon on liver glucose metabolism. *Diabetes Obes. Metab.* **2011**, *13*, 118–125. [CrossRef]

100. Charbonneau, A.; Couturier, K.; Gauthier, M.-S.; Lavoie, J.-M. Evidence of Hepatic Glucagon Resistance Associated with Hepatic Steatosis: Reversal Effect of Training. *Int. J. Sports Med.* **2005**, *26*, 432–441. [CrossRef]

101. Charbonneau, A.; Melancon, A.; Lavoie, C.; Lavoie, J.-M. Alterations in hepatic glucagon receptor density and in Gsα and Giα2 protein content with diet-induced hepatic steatosis: Effects of acute exercise. *Am. J. Physiol. Metab.* **2005**, *289*, E8–E14. [CrossRef]

102. Charbonneau, A.; Unson, C.G.; Lavoie, J.-M. High-fat diet-induced hepatic steatosis reduces glucagon receptor content in rat hepatocytes: Potential interaction with acute exercise. *J. Physiol.* **2007**, *579*, 255–267. [CrossRef]

103. Ashford, T.P.; Porter, K.R. Cytoplasmic components in hepatic cell lysosomes. *J. Cell Biol.* **1962**, *12*, 198–202. [CrossRef]

104. Arstila, A.U.; Trump, B.F. Studies on cellular autophagocytosis. The formation of autophagic vacuoles in the liver after glucagon administration. *Am. J. Pathol.* **1968**, *53*, 687–733.

105. Deter, R.L.; Baudhuin, P.; De Duve, C. Participation of lysosomes in cellular autophagy induced in rat liver by glucagon. *J. Cell Biol.* **1967**, *35*, C11–C16. [CrossRef] [PubMed]

106. Deter, R.L. Quantitative characterization of dense body, autophagic vacuole, and acid phosphatase-bearing particle populations during the early phases of glucagon-induced autophagy in rat liver. *J. Cell Biol.* **1971**, *48*, 473–489. [CrossRef] [PubMed]

107. Guder, W.; Hepp, K.D.; Wieland, O. The catabolic action of glucagon in rat liver. The influence of age, nutritional state and adrenal function on the effect of glucagon on lysosomal N-acetyl-beta, D-glucosaminidase. *Biochim. Biophys. Acta* **1970**, *222*, 593–605. [CrossRef]

108. Becker, F.F.; Cornwall, C.C. Phlorizin induced autophagocytosis during hepatocytic glycogenolysis. *Exp. Mol. Pathol.* **1971**, *14*, 103–109. [CrossRef]

109. Amherdt, M.; Harris, V.; Renold, A.E.; Orci, L.; Unger, R.H. Hepatic Autography in Uncontrolled Experimental Diabetes and Its Relationships to Insulin and Glucagon. *J. Clin. Investig.* **1974** *54*, 188–193. [CrossRef]

110. Ruan, H.-B.; Ma, Y.; Torres, S.; Zhang, B.; Feriod, C.; Heck, R.M.; Qian, K.; Fu, M.; Li, X.; Nathanson, M.H.; et al. Calcium-dependent O-GlcNAc signaling drives liver autophagy in adaptation to starvation. *Genes Dev.* **2017**, *31*, 1655–1665. [CrossRef]

111. Ezaki, J.; Matsumoto, N.; Takeda-Ezaki, M.; Komatsu, M.; Takahashi, K.; Hiraoka, Y.; Taka, H.; Fujimura, T.; Takehana, K.; Yoshida, M.; et al. Liver autophagy contributes to the maintenance of blood glucose and amino acid levels. *Autophagy* **2011**, *7*, 727–736. [CrossRef]

112. Hansen, M.; Rubinsztein, D.C.; Walker, D.W. Autophagy as a promoter of longevity: Insights from model organisms. *Nat. Rev. Mol. Cell Biol.* **2018**, *19*, 579–593. [CrossRef] [PubMed]

113. Elmore, S.P.; Qian, T.; Grissom, S.F.; Lemasters, J.J. The mitochondrial permeability transition initiates autophagy in rat hepatocytes. *FASEB J.* **2001**, *15*, 1–17. [CrossRef] [PubMed]

114. Li, L.; Tan, J.; Miao, Y.; Lei, P.; Zhang, Q. ROS and Autophagy: Interactions and Molecular Regulatory Mechanisms. *Cell. Mol. Neurobiol.* **2015**, *35*, 615–621. [CrossRef] [PubMed]

115. Wu, W.K.K.; Zhang, L.; Chan, M.T.V. Autophagy, NAFLD and NAFLD-Related HCC. *Adv. Exp. Med. Biol.* **2018**, *1061*, 127–138. [PubMed]

116. Singh, R.; Kaushik, S.; Wang, Y.; Xiang, Y.; Novak, I.; Komatsu, M.; Tanaka, K.; Cuervo, A.M.; Czaja, M.J. Autophagy regulates lipid metabolism. *Nature* **2009**, *458*, 1131–1135. [CrossRef]

117. Lavallard, V.J.; Gual, P. Autophagy and Non-Alcoholic Fatty Liver Disease. *BioMed Res. Int.* **2014**, *2014*, 1–13. [CrossRef]

118. Zheng, L.; Zhang, W.; Zhou, Y.; Li, F.; Wei, H.; Peng, J. Recent Advances in Understanding Amino Acid Sensing Mechanisms that Regulate mTORC1. *Int. J. Mol. Sci.* **2016**, *17*, 1636. [CrossRef]

119. Hosokawa, N.; Hara, T.; Kaizuka, T.; Kishi, C.; Takamura, A.; Miura, Y.; Iemura, S.-I.; Natsume, T.; Takehana, K.; Yamada, N.; et al. Nutrient-dependent mTORC1 Association with the ULK1–Atg13–FIP200 Complex Required for Autophagy. *Mol. Biol. Cell* **2009**, *20*, 1981–1991. [CrossRef]

# Non-Alcoholic Steatohepatitis Decreases Microsomal Liver Function in the Absence of Fibrosis

**Wim Verlinden** [1,2,*], **Eugénie Van Mieghem** [1], **Laura Depauw** [1], **Thomas Vanwolleghem** [1,2], **Luisa Vonghia** [1,2], **Jonas Weyler** [1,2], **Ann Driessen** [3], **Dirk Callens** [4], **Laurence Roosens** [4], **Eveline Dirinck** [5], **An Verrijken** [5], **Luc Van Gaal** [5] **and Sven Francque** [1,2,*]

[1]   Laboratory of Experimental Medicine and Pediatrics, Division of Gastroenterology and Hepatology, University of Antwerp, 2610 Antwerp, Belgium; eugenie.vanmieghem@gmail.com (E.V.M.); laura.depauw@student.uantwerpen.be (L.D.); thomas.vanwolleghem@uza.be (T.V.); luisa.vonghia@uza.be (L.V.); jonas.weyler@uza.be (J.W.)

[2]   Department of Gastroenterology and Hepatology, Antwerp University Hospital, 2650 Antwerp, Belgium

[3]   Department of Pathology, Antwerp University Hospital, 2650 Antwerp, Belgium; ann.driessen@uza.be

[4]   Department of Clinical Biology, Antwerp University Hospital, 2650 Antwerp, Belgium; dirk.callens@uza.be (D.C.); laurence.roosens@uza.be (L.R.)

[5]   Department of Endocrinology, Diabetology and Metabolism, Antwerp University Hospital, 2650 Antwerp, Belgium; eveline.dirinck@uza.be (E.D.); an.verrijken@uza.be (A.V.); luc.vangaal@uza.be (L.V.G.)

*   Correspondence: wim.verlinden@uza.be (W.V.); sven.francque@uza.be (S.F.)

**Abstract:** The incidence of non-alcoholic fatty liver disease (NAFLD) is rising across the globe, with the presence of steatohepatitis leading to a more aggressive clinical course. Currently, the diagnosis of non-alcoholic steatohepatitis (NASH) is based on histology, though with the high prevalence of NAFLD, a non-invasive method is needed. The $^{13}$C-aminopyrine breath test (ABT) evaluates the microsomal liver function and could be a potential candidate. We aimed to evaluate a potential change in liver function in NASH patients and to evaluate the diagnostic power of ABT to detect NASH. We performed a retrospective analysis on patients suspected of NAFLD who underwent a liver biopsy and ABT. 440 patients were included. ABT did not decrease in patients with isolated liver steatosis but decreased significantly in the presence of NASH without fibrosis and decreased even further with the presence of significant fibrosis. The predictive power of ABT as a single test for NASH was low but improved in combination with ALT and ultrasonographic steatosis. We conclude that microsomal liver function of patients with NASH is significantly decreased, even in the absence of fibrosis. The ABT is thus a valuable tool in assessing the presence of NASH; and could be used as a supplementary diagnostic tool in clinical practice.

**Keywords:** NASH; steatohepatitis; aminopyrine; microsomal; liver function; breath test

## 1. Introduction

Together with the obesity epidemic, incidences of non-alcoholic fatty liver disease (NAFLD) are rising across the globe. NAFLD is defined as an accumulation of fat in >5% of hepatocytes ocurring in the absence of significant alcohol consumption or any other cause of so-called "secondary" liver steatosis or disease. NAFLD includes two pathologically distinct conditions with different prognoses: isolated steatosis or non-alcoholic fatty liver (NAFL) and non-alcoholic steatohepatitis (NASH), which implies the presence of cell damage and inflammation. The latter covers a wide spectrum of disease severity, including fibrosis, cirrhosis and hepatocellular carcinoma [1].

The [13]C-aminopyrine breath test (ABT) has been widely used to evaluate microsomal hepatocellular function. Historically, it was the first breath test proposed for the assessment of patients with liver disease and is one of the most frequently utilized and most extensively validated tests for investigating microsomal liver function. The principle of the ABT is based on the selective metabolism of [13]C-aminopyrine in the liver by the cytochrome P450 mono-oxygenase system of the microsomes [2]. In these microsomes, [13]C-aminopyrine undergoes 2-step N-demethylation and the appearance of [13]$CO_2$ in breath after administration means that the administered substance underwent microsomal liver oxidation [3,4]. Because N-demethylation of [13]C-aminopyrine has been shown to be the rate-limiting step, it has been assumed that the ABT reflects the activity of the cytochrome P450-dependent mono-oxygenase system and gives a global assessment of this system. It has been demonstrated that the N-demethylation of aminopyrine is catalyzed most efficiently by CYP2C19 and CYP2C8, followed by CYP2D6, 2C18, 1A2 and 2B6; and to a lesser extent by CYP2C9, 2A6, 1A1 and 3A4 [5,6]. Aminopyrine metabolism is mostly dependent on hepatic metabolic capacity (functional hepatic mass) rather than on portal blood flow [7]. The ABT has been shown to quantitively reflect the severity of cirrhosis, as assessed by other liver function tests [8], and the degree of fibrosis in chronic hepatitis [9–11].

Liver function assessment by breath tests based on several metabolic pathways has been studied in the context of NAFLD, mostly to non-invasively diagnose and stage the disease. These studies overall indicate a reduction of liver function in patients with NASH, though included only small groups of patients with significant fibrosis to cirrhosis in the NASH group, making it impossible to differentiate between the effect of NASH and the effect of fibrosis [4,12–15].

In this study, we aimed to evaluate a change in liver function measured by the ABT in relation to the presence of steatosis, steatohepatitis and fibrosis and the different degrees of severity hereof in a large, prospectively included cohort representing the whole spectrum of disease. Additionally, we aimed to evaluate the diagnostic power of the ABT to detect NASH and fibrosis.

## 2. Methodology

### 2.1. Study Group

We performed a single-center, retrospective study at the Antwerp University Hospital, a tertiary referral center on patient data consecutively collected between 2002 and 2018. Patients visiting the Obesity Clinic or the Hepatology Clinic due to overweight (BMI 25–29.9 kg/m$^2$), obesity (BMI $\geq$ 30 kg/m$^2$) or elevated liver enzymes with a suspicion of NAFLD (according to a pre-defined set of criteria) were included when both liver biopsy and ABT were performed. Each patient underwent a standard metabolic work-up combined with a liver-specific program (including ABT as a standard procedure), both approved by the Ethics Committee of the Antwerp University Hospital and requiring written informed consent of the patient (Reference 6/25/15, Belgian Registration Number B30020071389) [16].

### 2.2. Metabolic Work-Up

The metabolic work-up included a detailed questionnaire and a clinical examination with anthropometry. Height was measured to the nearest 0.5 cm and body weight was measured with a digital scale to the nearest 0.2 kg. BMI was calculated as weight in kilograms over height in meters squared. Waist circumference was measured at the mid-level between the lower rib margin and the iliac crest. A blood analysis included blood cell count, coagulation tests, electrolytes, kidney function tests, lipid profile (total and high density lipoprotein (HDL) cholesterols and triglycerides (TG)), liver tests (alanine aminotransferase (ALT), aspartate aminotransferase (AST), gamma glutamyl transpeptidase (GGT), alkaline phosphatase (ALP), total bilirubin and fractions), high-sensitive C-reactive protein (CRP), creatinine kinase, total protein, protein electrophoresis, glucose, insulin and thyroid function.

## 2.3. Hepatological Work-Up

The liver-specific program included additional blood analyses to exclude the classical aetiologies of liver disease (e.g., viral hepatitis and autoimmune disease): s-choline-esterase, carcino-embryonic antigen, $\alpha$-foetoprotein, anti-nuclear factor, anti-neutrophil cytoplasm antigen antibodies, anti-smooth muscle antibodies, anti-mitochondrial antibodies, anti-liver–kidney microsome antibodies, serum copper and ceruloplasmin, $\alpha$-1-antitrypsin, anti-hepatitis B core antibodies, hepatitis B surface antigen, anti-hepatitis C virus antibodies. Patients underwent a Doppler ultrasound of the abdomen with parameters of liver and spleen volume and liver vascularization and steatosis grading of the liver based on the Saverymuttu score (ultrasound steatosis, USS, scored 0–3) [17]. USS was scored as: isoechogenicity of the liver and the spleen: 0; slight increase in liver echogenicity, a slight exaggeration of liver and kidney echo discrepancy and relative preservation of echoes from the walls of the portal vein: 1; aforementioned abnormalities accompanied by loss of echoes from the walls of the portal veins, particularly from the peripheral branches, a greater posterior beam attenuation and a greater discrepancy between hepatic and renal echoes: 2; aforementioned abnormalities accompanied by a greater reduction in beam penetration, loss of echoes from most of the portal vein wall, including the main branches, and a large discrepancy between hepatic and renal echoes: 3. Patients also underwent a liver-spleen scintigraphy and an ABT.

## 2.4. Aminopyrine Breath Test

The ABT was carried out at home by the patients at rest after an overnight fasting. The $^{13}$C-labelled aminopyrine was ingested orally together with water. Aminopyrine is absorbed rapidly and almost completely and breath samples were taken at 0, 30, 60, 90 and 120 min [18]. Peak excretion (ABTpeak) was determined and cumulative excretion (ABTcum) was calculated. Values are expressed as percentage of the administered dose per hour (%dose/h) or the calculated percentage of the administered dose over two hours (%dose/120 min). The analysis of the ABT was performed in the clinical laboratory of the Antwerp University Hospital and was executed by the Automated Breath $^{13}$C Isotope Ratio Mass Spectrometer (Sercon, Crewe, UK). Normality values of the ABT are >5.4 %dose/h and >8.1 %dose/120 min for peak and cumulative excretion, respectively, based on the available literature and local experience [19].

## 2.5. Liver Biopsy

Liver biopsy was considered indicated in the presence of one or more of the following criteria: persistent abnormal liver tests (AST and/or ALT and/or GGT and/or ALP according to local lab upper limits of normal), ultrasound abnormality of the liver (enlarged liver, steatotic liver [17]), signs of liver disease on liver-spleen scintigraphy [20] and abnormal ABT [21]. A separate informed consent for liver biopsy was required. In patients who subsequently were referred to bariatric surgery, the liver biopsy was performed peri-operatively. The remaining patients were proposed for percutaneous or transjugular liver biopsy. The liver biopsy specimen was stored in formalin aldehyde. Haematoxylin–eosin stain, Sirius red (Fouchet) stain, periodic acid Schiff stain after diastase, reticulin stain (Gordon–Sweets), and Perl's iron stain were routinely performed on all biopsies and subsequently analysed by a team of experienced pathologists and hepatologists. Biopsies were re-assessed in batch by an experienced pathologist and this reading was used for further analysis. The diagnosis of NASH required the association of some degree of steatosis, some degree of ballooning, and some degree of lobular inflammation [1,22,23]. The different features were scored according to the NASH Clinical Research Network Scoring System [24]. Steatosis was graded as follows: less than 5% of liver parenchyma: 0; 5–33%: 1: 33–66%: 2; more than 66%: 3; Lobular inflammation was scored as: no foci: 0; less than two foci per x200 field: 1; 2–4 foci per x200 field: 2; more than four foci per x200 field: 3. Ballooning was scored as: none: 0; few ballooned cells: 1; many cells/prominent ballooning: 2. Fibrosis was staged: none: 0; perisinusoidal or periportal: 1; perisinusoidal and portal/periportal: 2; bridging fibrosis: 3; cirrhosis: 4. The NAFLD Activity Score (NAS) was calculated as the unweighted sum of the scores for steatosis, ballooning, and lobular inflammation [24]. The length of the biopsy and the number of portal tracts were equally so reported by the pathologist. NASH was defined as the presence of steatosis (≥1), inflammation (≥1) and ballooning (≥1). Borderline NASH was defined as the presence of NASH and a NAS of 3-4. Definite NASH was defined as the presence of NASH and a NAS ≥ 5.

## 2.6. Patient Groups

Patients were excluded from further analysis if they had significant alcohol consumption (>20 g/day for women and >30 g/day for men using self-reported alcohol consumption levels) [25], or if another liver disease was diagnosed. Based on liver biopsy, the study population was divided into different subgroups: patients without signs of steatosis (S = 0) or liver fibrosis: noNAFLD; patients without significant fibrosis (F0–F1), with signs of steatosis (S ≥ 1), and either with the absence of NASH [NAFL (non-alcoholic fatty liver)] or with the presence of NASH (activity and ballooning ≥ 1) (NASH-noF); and patients with significant fibrosis (NAFLD-F).

## 2.7. Statistical Analysis

The data analyses were performed with SPSS version 25.0 software (IBM Corporation, Armonk, NY, USA). Descriptive statistics were produced for patient characteristics. The distribution of normality was evaluated by the Kolmogorov-Smirnov test and additional visual appraisal of the W-W probability plot. Significant differences in variables between the subgroups were ascertained using independent samples $t$-test for normally distributed continuous variables, the Mann–Whitney U tests for non-normally distributed continuous variables and the Chi-square test for categorical variables. Significant correlations were determined using the Spearman's rho test. Binary logistic regression analyses were carried out for peak excretion and cumulative excretion of the 13C-ABT. Other variables that were significantly correlated with NASH were included in multivariate logistic regression analyses. A backward elimination method was used to achieve a predictive model for both peak excretion and cumulative excretion separately. Area Under the Receiver Operating Curves (AUC) were generated using the ABT and the predictive models as test variables. AUC values were interpreted as follows: fail (50–60%), poor (60–70%), fair (70–80%), good (80–90%) or excellent (90–100%) [26,27]. Single cut-off values were chosen based on the highest sum of sensitivity and specificity (Youden index). Two-cut off model values were chosen based on 90% specificity and 90% sensitivity. AUROC curves of different tests within the same population were compared according to Delong (MedCalc version 14.12.0, MedCalc Software, Ostend, Belgium) [28]. $p < 0.05$ was considered statistically significant.

## 3. Results

### 3.1. Patient Characteristics

Four hundred and forty patients with a reliable liver biopsy and ABT were included. The total population had an average age of 46.1 years (SD 13.4), median BMI of 37.6 kg/m² (IQR 33.3; 41.7) and a gender distribution of 63.6%/36.4% female to male ratio. All patients (440) were classified according to the different patient groups: noNAFLD (71; 16.1%), NAFL (72; 16.2%), NASH-noF (176; 40.0%) and NAFLD-F (121; 27.5%).

### 3.2. NoNAFLD, NAFL, NASH-noF

Characteristics of the different subgroups are represented in Table 1. There was no statistical difference of the ABTpeak and ABTcum between noNAFLD and NAFL. The ABTpeak and the ABTcum of NASH-noF were, however, significantly lower compared to both the noNAFLD and the NAFL group (Figure 1).

In the NASH-noF group, there was a trend for a decreased ABTpeak and ABTcum between patients with borderline NASH and definite NASH, though these differences did not reach statistical significance [9.20 (6.58; 11.45) vs. 7.65 (5.50; 10.48) %dose/h for ABTpeak ($p = 0.077$); and 12.90 (10.00; 16.55) vs. 10.95 (8.55; 15.13)%dose/120 min for ABTcum ($p = 0.085$), respectively].

In this population, significant positive correlations (Spearman's rho, $p < 0.05$) were found between ABTpeak and ALT (0.127), LDL cholesterol (0.124), serum albumin (0.182), and smoking (0.282) and significant negative correlations between ABTpeak and BMI (−0.199), waist (−0.157), platelet count (−0.161), steatosis grade (−0.164), lobular inflammation (−0.181), ballooning (−0.136), NAS score (−0.193) and USS (−0.136).

As for ABTcum, significant positive correlations were found with age (0.124), LDL cholesterol (0.132), albumin (0.185) and smoking (0.240) and significant negative correlations between ABTcum and BMI (−0.225), waist (−0.179), platelet count (−0.165), steatosis grade (−0.177), lobular inflammation (−0.195), ballooning (−0.158), NAS score (−0.214), fibrosis stage (−0.123) and USS (−0.145).

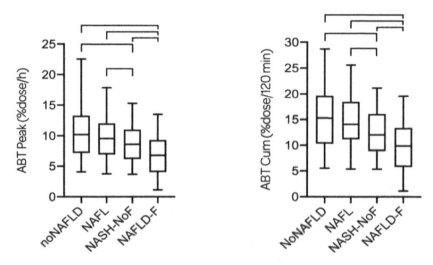

**Figure 1.** ABTpeak and ABTcum are given for the four subgroups. There was no statistical difference of the ABTpeak and ABTcum between noNAFLD [10.20 (7.20; 13.30) %dose/h and 15.30 (10.30; 19.70) %dose/120 min, respectively] and NAFL [9.55 (6.95; 12.03) %dose/h and 14.10 (11.20; 18.48) %dose/120 min, respectively]. The ABTpeak and the ABTcum of NASH-noF [8.60 (6.20; 11.00) %dose/h and 12.10 (8.90; 16.10) %dose/120 min, respectively] were significantly lower compared to both the noNAFLD and the NAFL group. The ABTpeak and the ABTcum of NAFLD-F [6.80 (4.00; 9.30) %dose/h and 9.90 (5.85; 13.45) %dose/120 min, respectively] were significantly lower compared to all three other subgroups.

The correlation between fibrosis stage and ABTcum in this group without significant fibrosis is most likely due to the confounding effect of NAS score, which was, as might be expected, lower in the NAFL and noNAFLD groups which consisted of less patients with fibrosis stage 1. When analysing this NASH-noF group, no difference of ABT could be observed between patients with fibrosis F0 or F1 [F0 8.4 (6.1–11.6) and F1 8.6 (6.3–10.2), $p = 0.423$; and F0 12.2 (8.9–16.5) and F1 12.1 (8.9–14.7), $p = 0.535$, for ABTpeak and ABTcum respectively]. In this group, there was no correlation between fibrosis stage and ABTpeak ($p = 0.803$) or ABTcum ($p = 0.833$).

*3.3. Prediction of NASH in Non-Significant Fibrosis*

In the combined groups of noNAFLD, NAFL and NASH-noF, a significant correlation ($p < 0.05$) could be found between the presence of NASH and age (0.155), waist (0.156), AST (0.227), ALT (0.268), ABTpeak (−0.174), ABTcum (−0.202) and USS (0.425). When separating ABTpeak and ABTcum, a remaining significant correlation could be found after logistic regression for ALT, USS and ABTpeak; and for ALT, USS and ABTcum. ALT and USS were significantly correlated with the NAS score ($p < 0.00001$, Spearman's rho 0.314 and 0.557, respectively). USS and ALT were significantly higher in the group of definite NASH compared to the group of borderline NASH.

**Table 1.** Patient characteristics.

| Characteristic | NoNAFLD (n = 71) | NAFL (n = 72) | NASH-noF (n = 176) | NAFLD-F (n = 121) | p noNAFLD vs. NAFL | p noNAFLD vs. NASH-noF | p NAFL vs. NASH-noF |
|---|---|---|---|---|---|---|---|
| Age (yrs) | 41.23 ± 12.19 | 45.35 ± 12.49 | 45.69 ± 12.83 | 50.03 ± 14.26 | 0.048 * | 0.013 * | 0.846 |
| Gender (female) | 60 (84.5%) | 49 (68.1%) | 111 (63.1%) | 60 (49.6%) | 0.021 * | 0.001 * | 0.456 |
| Smoking (non-smoker) | 52 (73.2%) | 55 (76.4%) | 139 (79.0%) | 89 (73.4%) | 0.659 | 0.259 | 0.554 |
| BMI (kg/m$^2$) | 36.80 (33.00; 40.30) | 37.77 (32.61; 41.40) | 37.70 (33.70; 41.80) | 38.61 (32.97; 42.85) | 0.474 | 0.187 | 0.724 |
| Waist (cm) | 111.0 ± 10.7 | 116.1 ± 15.9 | 116.9 ± 12.5 | 124.1 ± 14.6 | 0.023 * | <0.001 * | 0.682 |
| AST (U/L) | 24.0 (21.0; 29.5) | 26.0 (21.0; 29.8) | 29.0 (24.0; 37.0) | 37.0 (27.0; 52.0) | 0.268 | <0.001 * | 0.007 * |
| ALT (U/L) | 31.0 (24.0; 42.0) | 35.0 (29.3; 46.0) | 43.0 (32.0; 57.0) | 48.0 (35.0; 75.0) | 0.018 * | <0.00001 * | 0.007 * |
| GGT (U/L) | 30 (21; 49) | 32 (26; 49) | 36 (27; 49) | 50 (33; 117) | 0.13 | 0.026 * | 0.47 |
| PLT (10$^9$/L) | 282 (252; 339) | 268 (232; 323) | 290 (246; 329) | 249 (177; 302) | 0.187 | 0.92 | 0.219 |
| Tot chol (mg/dL) | 201 (170; 226) | 208 (176; 228) | 203 (177; 227) | 185 (160; 216) | 0.805 | 0.717 | 0.905 |
| HDL (mg/dL) | 50 (42; 65) | 47 (39; 56) | 46 (39; 55) | 41 (35; 51) | 0.041 * | 0.010 * | 0.993 |
| TG (mg/dL) | 118 (84; 165) | 135 (104; 204) | 147 (105; 213) | 148 (102; 208) | 0.051 | 0.002 * | 0.433 |
| LDL (mg/dL) | 118 (94; 142) | 125 (98; 151) | 120 (100; 146) | 114 (82; 139) | 0.632 | 0.672 | 0.911 |
| Tot bili (mg/dL) | 0.50 (0.40; 0.60) | 0.50 (0.40; 0.70) | 0.50 (0.40; 0.70) | 0.60 (0.41; 0.80) | 0.333 | 0.047 * | 0.473 |
| HbA1c (%) | 5.50 (5.30; 5.70) | 5.50 (5.30; 5.80) | 5.60 (5.30; 5.90) | 5.90 (5.50; 6.90) | 0.048 * | 0.011 * | 0.661 |
| Alb (g/dL) | 4.37 ± 0.37 | 4.41 ± 0.37 | 4.46 ± 0.41 | 4.21 ± 0.72 | 0.539 | 0.097 | 0.333 |
| INR | 1.00 (1.00; 1.03) | 1.01 (1.00; 1.04) | 1.02 (1.00; 1.05) | 1.04 (1.00; 1.12) | 0.537 | 0.205 | 0.56 |
| Steatosis | | | | | <0.00001 * | <0.00001 * | <0.00001 * |
| 0 | 71 (100%) | 0 | 0 | 12 (9.9%) | | | |
| 1 | 0 | 60 (83.3%) | 67 (38.1%) | 36 (29.8%) | | | |
| 2 | 0 | 11 (15.3%) | 68 (38.6%) | 37 (30.6%) | | | |
| 3 | 0 | 1 (1.4%) | 41 (23.3%) | 36 (29.8%) | | | |
| Inflammation | | | | | 0.204 | <0.00001 * | <0.00001 * |
| 0 | 59 (83.1%) | 53 (73.6%) | 0 | 24 (19.8%) | | | |
| 1 | 12 (16.9%) | 17 (23.6%) | 115 (65.3%) | 56 (46.3%) | | | |
| 2 | 0 | 2 (2.8%) | 46 (26.1%) | 26 (21.5%) | | | |
| 3 | 0 | 0 | 15 (8.5%) | 15 (12.4%) | | | |
| Ballooning | | | | | 0.003 * | <0.0001 * | <0.00001 * |
| 0 | 60 (84.5%) | 43 (59.7%) | 0 | 16 (13.2%) | | | |
| 1 | 10 (14.1%) | 22 (30.6%) | 92 (52.3%) | 48 (39.7%) | | | |
| 2 | 1 (1.4%) | 7 (9.7%) | 84 (47.7%) | 57 (47.1%) | | | |

**Table 1.** *Cont.*

| Characteristic | NoNAFLD (n = 71) | NAFL (n = 72) | NASH-noF (n = 176) | NAFLD-F (n = 121) | p noNAFLD vs. NAFL | p noNAFLD vs. NASH-noF | p NAFL vs. NASH-noF |
|---|---|---|---|---|---|---|---|
| **NAS** | | | | | | | |
| 0 | 49 (69.0%) | 0 | 0 | 6 (5.0%) | | | |
| 1 | 19 (26.8%) | 21 (29.2%) | 0 | 5 (4.1%) | | | |
| 2 | 2 (2.8%) | 36 (50.0%) | 0 | 9 (7.4%) | <0.00001 * | <0.00001 * | <0.00001 * |
| 3 | 1 (1.4%) | 13 (18.0%) | 31 (17.6%) | 18 (14.9%) | | | |
| 4 | 0 | 2 (2.8%) | 51 (29.0%) | 20 (16.5%) | | | |
| 5 | 0 | | 43 (24.4%) | 25 (20.7%) | | | |
| 6 | 0 | | 33 (18.8%) | 20 (16.5%) | | | |
| 7 | 0 | | 15 (8.5%) | 13 (10.7%) | | | |
| 8 | 0 | | 3 (1.7%) | 5 (4.1%) | | | |
| **USS** | | | | | | | |
| 0 | 25 (35.2%) | 4 (5.6%) | 6 (3.4%) | 8 (6.6%) | | | |
| 1 | 31 (43.7%) | 28 (38.9%) | 30 (17.0%) | 25 (20.7%) | <0.00001 * | <0.00001 * | 0.001 * |
| 2 | 11 (15.5%) | 20 (27.8%) | 52 (29.5%) | 26 (21.5%) | | | |
| 3 | 4 (5.6%) | 18 (25.0%) | 80 (45.5%) | 52 (43.0%) | | | |
| missing | 0 | 2 (2.8%) | 8 (4.5%) | 10 (8.3%) | | | |
| ABTpeak | 10.20 (7.20; 13.30) | 9.55 (6.95; 12.03) | 8.60 (6.20; 11.00) | 6.80 (4.00; 9.30) | 0.423 | 0.005 * | 0.031 * |
| ABTcum | 15.30 (10.30; 19.70) | 14.10 (11.20; 18.48) | 12.10 (8.90; 16.10) | 9.90 (5.85; 13.45) | 0.535 | 0.002 * | 0.007 * |

Patient characteristics of the subgroups: patients without NAFLD (noNAFLD), patients with non-alcoholic fatty liver (NAFL), patients with non-alcoholic steatohepatitis without significant fibrosis (NASH-noF) and patients with significant fibrosis (NAFLD-F). There was a significant difference between NAFLD-F and all three other subgroups for age, gender, waist circumference, AST, ALT, GGT, platelet count, total cholesterol, HDL, bilirubin, HbA1c, serum albumin, INR, steatosis, inflammation, ballooning, NAS, ABTpeak and ABTcum (full p values are given as Supplementary Table S1). LDL was significantly lower and TG higher in NAFLD-F compared to NASH-noF and noNAFLD, respectively. USS was significantly higher in NAFLD-F compared to noNAFLD and NAFL. Data are expressed as mean ± SD for normally distributed variables or as median (interquartile range) when distribution of the variable is skewed. *p*-value is calculated between different groups with * indicating statistical significance (<0.05). BMI, body mass index; AST, aspartate aminotransferase; ALT, alanine aminotransferase; GGT, gamma glutamyl transpeptidase; PLT, platelets; tot chol, total cholesterol; HDL, high density lipoprotein cholesterols; TG, triglycerides; LDL, low density lipoprotein cholesterols; tot bili, total bilirubin; HbA1c, haemoglobin A1c; Alb: albumin; INR, international normalized ratio; NAS, NAFLD activity score; USS, ultrasound steatosis score; ABTpeak, aminopyrine breath test peak value; ABTcum, aminopyrine breath test cumulative value.

Based on these data, two models were created to predict the presence of NASH:

PredABTpeak for NASH = $-1.617 + (0.025 \times ALT) + (0.909 \times USS) + (-0.094 \times ABTpeak)$

PredABTcum for NASH = $-1.457 + (0.025 \times ALT) + (0.901 \times USS) + (-0.075 \times ABTcum)$

AUROCs for the prediction of NASH and definite NASH for ABTpeak, ABTcum, ALT, USS as single tests and for the predictive models are represented in Table 2. The predictive models were significantly better ($p < 0.01$) than ABTpeak, ABTcum and ALT individually for the prediction of NASH and definite NASH, but not significantly better than USS ($p > 0.05$).

**Table 2.** AUROC to predict the presence of NASH and definite NASH.

| Test | NASH | Definite NASH |
|---|---|---|
| ABTpeak | 0.601 (0.539–0.663) | 0.612 (0.544–0.681) |
| ABTcum | 0.617 (0.555–0.679) | 0.620 (0.553–0.687) |
| ALT | 0.655 (0.595–0.715) | 0.669 (0.604–0.734) |
| USS | 0.744 (0.688–0.800) | 0.772 (0.717–0.827) |
| PredABTpeak | 0.785 (0.734–0.835) | 0.814 (0.765–0.863) |
| PredABTcum | 0.787 (0.737–0.837) | 0.819 (0.770–0.867) |

AUROC (represented with 95% confidence interval) to predict the presence of NASH and definite NASH for ABTpeak, ABTcum, ALT and US steatosis separately, and the predictive models PredABTpeak and PredABTcum combining ALT, USS and ABT.

Based on the predictive model of the ABTcum which showed a slightly higher AUROC than ABTpeak, we proposed cut-off values to determine the presence of NASH or definite NASH in Table 3. The predicted model was positively correlated to the presence of NASH. The higher the value, the higher the likelihood of NASH.

**Table 3.** Cut-off values to predict the presence of NASH and fibrosis.

| | Cut-Off Value | Sens | Spec | PPV | NPV |
|---|---|---|---|---|---|
| NASH | 0.2575 | 72.60% | 71.60% | 75.30% | 68.70% |
| Def NASH | 0.2575 | 87.60% | 61.80% | 38.10% | 92.50% |
| Sign F | 13.25 | 73.60% | 51.40% | 36.50% | 83.70% |
| Adv F | 10.1 | 63.50% | 69.90% | 30.00% | 90.50% |
| Cirrhosis | 5.05 | 51.50% | 95.30% | 52.80% | 96.00% |
| NASH | >1.1210 | | | 82.90% | |
| No NASH | <−0.6185 | | | 80.00% | |
| Def NASH | >1.1346 | | | 64.10% | |
| No def NASH | <0.0120 | | | 93.30% | |
| Sign F | <7.05 | | | 53.70% | |
| No sign F | >17.45 | | | 86.50% | |
| Adv F | <7.05 | | | 46.30% | |
| No adv F | >18.25 | | | 90.70% | |
| Cirrhosis | <6.55 | | | 30.50% | |
| No cirrhosis | >19.45 | | | 94.70% | |

Cut-off values to predict the presence of NASH in patients without significant fibrosis; and to predict fibrosis in the whole population with sensitivity, specificity, positive predictive value and negative predictive value. One and two cut-off models were created for each parameter. Using 1 cut-off, the PPV for definite NASH was low (78/162, 38.1%), but of those misclassified as definite NASH, 52% had borderline NASH. Using 2 cut-offs, the PPV for definite NASH was better (41/64, 64.1%), and with 61% of those misclassified having borderline NASH. Using two cut-off values can lead to patients with an indeterminate value. This "indeterminate" classification was present in 54%, 36%, 65%, 68% and 74% of cases for NASH, definite NASH, significant fibrosis, advanced fibrosis and cirrhosis, respectively. Def, definite NASH; Sign F, significant fibrosis; Adv F, advanced fibrosis; Sens, sensitivity; Spec, specificity; PPV, positive predictive value; NPV, negative predictive value.

## 3.4. Significant Fibrosis

This group consisted of 121 patients with 38.8% F2, 33.9% F3 and 27.3% F4 (i.e., cirrhosis); 28.1% did not have NASH, borderline NASH was present in 19.8% and definite NASH in 52.1% of these cases. In patients with significant fibrosis, ABTpeak and ABTcum are no longer significantly correlated to the presence of NASH (rho $-0.104$, $p = 0.258$ and rho $-0.072$, $p = 0.435$, respectively) nor to the NAS score (rho $-0.053$, $p = 0.566$ and $-0.020$, $p = 0.825$, respectively). In this population, fibrosis stage has a stronger (inverse) correlation with ABTpeak (rho $-0.366$, $p < 0.0001$) and ABTcum (rho $-0.347$, $p = 0.0001$). Fibrosis stage is, however, inversely correlated to the NAS score (rho $-0.203$, $p = 0.025$).

## 3.5. All Patients

In our entire population, both ABTpeak and ABTcum were independently positively correlated with smoking and serum albumin concentration and negatively correlated with BMI, the presence of NASH and fibrosis stage. Fibrosis was positively correlated with NAS (rho 0.311, $p < 0.0001$) and the presence of NASH (rho 0.222, $p < 0.0001$).

ABTpeak and ABTcum decreased significantly between each fibrosis stage; 9.1 (6.50; 11.80) and 13.40 (9.40; 17.35) for F0–1; 7.80 (6.20; 9.90) and 11.50 (8.80; 14.10) for F2; 6.70 (4.20; 9.40) and 9.50 (6.15; 13.80) for F3; and 3.50 (1.75; 6.80) and 5.00 (2.55; 10.80) for F4, respectively. Differences of ABTpeak and ABTcum for each fibrosis stage are represented in Figure 2.

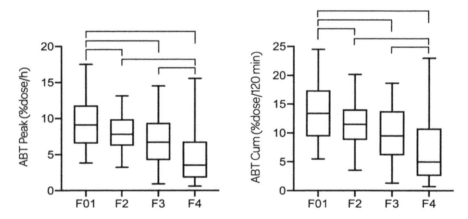

**Figure 2.** ABTpeak and ABTcum are given for every fibrosis stage in all patients. There is a significant difference of ABTpeak between F2–F4 ($p < 0.0001$) and F3–F4 ($p = 0.008$), but not between F2–F3 ($p = 0.133$). There is a significant difference of ABTcum between F2–F4 ($p < 0.0001$) and F3–F4 ($p = 0.013$), but not between F2–F3 ($p = 0.119$). The ABTpeak and ABTcum are both significantly higher for F0–1 compared to F2 ($p < 0.05$), F3 ($p < 0.001$) and F4 ($p < 0.0001$).

ABTpeak showed an AUROC of 0.612 (0.559–0.666), 0.674 (0.618–0.731), 0.718 (0.648–0.788) and 0.782 (0.682–0.882) for the prediction of NASH, significant fibrosis, advanced fibrosis and cirrhosis, respectively. ABTcum showed an AUROC of 0.616 (0.0566–0.673), 0.676 (0.619–0.732), 0.719 (0.650–0.788) and 0.769 (0.667–0.872) for the prediction of NASH, significant fibrosis, advanced fibrosis and cirrhosis, respectively.

Based on the ABTcum which showed a slightly higher AUROC than ABTpeak, we proposed cut-off values to determine the presence of significant fibrosis, advanced fibrosis or cirrhosis in Table 3.

## 4. Discussion

The $^{13}$C-aminopyrine breath test has traditionally been used to estimate functional liver reserve in advanced liver disease. In this study, we demonstrate that non-alcoholic steatohepatitis, even in the absence of significant fibrosis, is associated with a significant impairment of hepatic microsomal function as measured by the $^{13}$C-aminopyrine breath test. In the fibrotic NAFLD population, the effect of fibrosis on ABT excretion was more important than the effect of inflammation. The ABT can be used as a tool in the prediction of the presence of NASH or fibrosis in the appropriate setting.

Fibrosis has been shown to be the strongest predictor of outcome in NAFLD, which does, however, not equal that it is as such the driver of disease progression [29]. Progression of NALF to bridging fibrosis concurs with transition to NASH and several longitudinal studies have recently confirmed the direct relationship between evolution in disease activity and hepatic inflammatory changes on one hand and the evolution in fibrosis on the other hand. NASH resolution was also shown to be the strongest predictor of fibrosis regression [30,31]. Similarly, SAF activity appeared to be strongly correlated with liver fibrosis stage, further supporting the concept of disease activity as the driving force of disease progression [32,33]. These observations demonstrate that NASH and fibrosis are closely linked.

Multiple serum biomarkers have been evaluated for the prediction of the presence and/or severity of NASH, though most biomarkers failed to demonstrate accuracy. Plasma cytokeratin 18 fragment levels are a marker of hepatocyte apoptosis and represent the most extensively evaluated biomarker of steatohepatitis, although the accuracy is modest. To date, non-invasive tests cannot reliably be used solely for the diagnosis of NASH [34,35]. More extensive research has been performed on non-invasive tools to asses liver fibrosis, though most scores for fibrosis are mainly developed and validated to exclude advanced fibrosis, and do not allow the reliable categorisation of individual liver fibrosis stages [34].

The ABT has mostly been studied in the setting of cirrhosis and end stage liver disease. Smaller studies have previously shown a significant decrease of liver function in NASH patients, measured by isotope breath tests, though these studies were confounded by a limited population size and the inclusion of patients with significant fibrosis to cirrhosis in the NASH groups [4,12–15].

In this study, we included a large population of patients at risk of NAFLD, by the presence of overweight or obesity, allowing us to investigate the effect of NASH in patients without significant fibrosis and thus isolating the steatohepatitis effect. We observed a significant decrease of microsomal liver function in patients with NASH compared to patients with NAFL and overweight patients without liver steatosis. Liver function was not different between the latter two groups indicating that isolated steatosis does not significantly decrease microsomal liver function. Within the NASH population there was a trend of a decreased ABT excretion between patients with borderline NASH and definite NASH, though these differences did not reach statistical significance. Overall, this indicates that steatohepatitis as such is associated with a significant decrease in microsomal hepatocyte function, which is relevant for our understanding of the pathophysiology of NASH.

Although extraction of aminopyrine seems to be independent of portal blood flow, a role for changes in the microcirculation that have shown to occur early in the development of NASH, even in the non-fibrotic stage, might indirectly play a role [36–39]. These changes are hypothesised to cause centrolobular hypoxia by aggravating the physiological portocentral oxygen gradient [40]. Hypoxia has been shown to impact on liver microsomal function, so these mechanisms could offer an additional explanation for the presence of microsomal dysfunction early in disease development.

People with overweight or obesity and other components of the metabolic syndrome are at risk of developing fatty liver which is characterized by the presence of large vacuoles of lipids within the cytosol. In addition to macrovacuolar steatosis, NASH implies the presence of cell damage and inflammation and is histologically characterized by microvesicular steatosis, portal and lobular inflammation, and the presence of hepatocyte injury in the form of ballooning and apoptosis. All these processes ultimately stimulate fibrogenesis. At least three major events are involved in the progression of fatty liver to NASH, including overproduction of ROS (reactive oxygen species) and RNS (reactive nitrogen species), lipotoxicity and increased release of proinflammatory and profibrogenic cytokines [41]. These changes impact the microsomal activity and are probably responsible for the decreased microsomal liver function that we observed. Studies with animals and human tissue have also shown an alteration of CYP 450 enzyme activity. CYP3A, a CYP which only plays a minimal role in the ABT, is downregulated, presumably by obesity, elevated proinflammatory cytokines, noncytokine components and oxidative stress [42]. Some CYPs might not only be influenced by the presence of NASH, but could also play a causative role. It has been shown that CYP2E1 (which has no role in ABT) is overexpressed in non-alcoholic steatosis [43]. It is hypothesized that in the case of fat mobilisation as in diabetes mellitus, the hyperketonemia and other small organic molecules are both substrates and inducers of CYP2E1 that will lead to non-alcoholic fatty liver disease. This overexpressed CYP2E1 exhibits a high capacity to produce free radicals that are probably the cause of liver damage and lipid peroxidation in obese type 2 diabetes patients [44].

Since NASH seems to be the driving force for fibrosis development, its diagnosis is paramount, and the ABT could potentially help by discriminating isolated steatosis from NASH. The rising prevalence of NAFLD and the known disadvantages of liver biopsy (sampling error, cost, morbidity and mortality) illustrate the need for new non-invasive diagnostic techniques. Our current results suggest that ABT can indeed be helpful in the differentiation between patients with NASH and those with NAFL in patients without significant fibrosis. This test is non-invasive, innocuous, easy to administer and samples are transportable, which allows its use in primary and secondary care.

In our group without significant fibrosis, the ABT as a single test had rather poor predictive power, though when including ALT and USS into a predictive model, the predictive power strongly increased. A potential limitation of the use of this model in clinical practice could, however, be hampered by the absence of reliable tools to exclude significant fibrosis. Liver steatosis and ALT have both been related to the presence of NASH. Previous research has shown a correlation between the extent of steatosis (evaluated histologically or ultrasonographically) and the presence of NASH [45–47]. In line with our results, Ballestri et al. showed higher USS values in patients with NASH than in those with steatosis; and higher values in patients with definite NASH than in those with borderline NASH [48]. Although normal ALT does not exclude the presence of NASH, studies have shown that ALT levels are independently associated with NASH, even in patients with normal ALT, indicating that even a minor elevation in ALT level, albeit within normal limits, can reflect the presence of NASH-related liver damage [49].

Tribonias et al. found similar results with a substantial impairment of hepatic microsomal function as assessed by a simple non-invasive ABT in NASH patients including, however, patients with significant fibrosis in the NASH group [4]. Compared to our results, they found a higher AUROC [0.741 (0.576–0.905)] for ABTcum to diagnose the presence of NASH, though 25% of their NASH population was cirrhotic compared to 8% in our NASH population. More importantly, 31% of our patients with advanced fibrosis lost the combination of characteristics necessary for the diagnosis of NASH. This is in line with the general observation that with the progression of fibrosis, the characteristic triad of NASH and perisinusoidal fibrosis becomes less prominent or disappears [50].

In our study, we observed, apart from the effect of NASH on microsomal function, a decreasing ABT excretion with each fibrosis stage, which is in line with current literature. Previous reports support this observation and show that ABT results are associated with the severity of liver disease, and that they have a prognostic role in predicting death from liver failure in cirrhotic patients [21,51]. Moreover, we observed that from the moment significant fibrosis is present, the statistically significant influence of NASH on the ABT excretion can no longer be observed.

In our entire population, the predictive power of the cumulative ABT value was mostly higher than the peak ABT value, though not statistically significant. ABT proved to be a poor predictor of significant fibrosis as a single test with an AUROC of 0.676 for ABTcum. The power increased to a fair test to predict the presence of advanced fibrosis and cirrhosis with an AUROC of 0.719 and 0.769 for ABTcum, respectively.

Our findings clearly indicate that both steatohepatitis and fibrosis are associated with impairment of microsomal function. This implies that both these aspects should be taken into account when assessing the accuracy of the ABT as a non-invasive marker of disease. The mixing-up of both aspects may in part explain overall low accuracy and conflicting results in the literature.

ABT is not the only breath test used to investigate hepatic function. [13]C breath tests can explore either microsomal, cytosolic or mitochondrial hepatocellular subfunctions [2]. Previous research has shown that these other [13]C breath tests are also capable of distinguishing patients with various degrees of liver disease from normal subjects, as well as distinguishing patients with compensated cirrhosis from those with decompensated cirrhosis. Banasch et al. used a [13]C-methionine breath test to evaluate mitochondrial dysfunction. They showed in patients without significant fibrosis a difference of mitochondrial function between borderline and definite NASH, which was no longer present in patients with significant fibrosis [52]. In the borderline NASH group, however, 15% had significant fibrosis compared to 43% in the definite NASH group (and only 9% in the NAFL group). Correlation analyses confirmed the synergistic negative effect of NASH activity and fibrosis on individual breath test outcome. NASH activity and fibrosis were correlated as was observed in our study.

Miele et al. performed [13]C-octanoate breath tests (OBT) in patients with NAFLD and demonstrated the relationship between the presence of fibrosis and the impairment of liver function, expressed by lower OBT results than those of controls [53]. Park et al. showed that the [13]C-caffeine breath test, another test for microsomal function, reflected the extent of hepatic fibrosis in NALFD and was an independent predictor of significant fibrosis in these patients. They showed impaired liver function in NASH patients, but induced by the presence of significant fibrosis, as they found no correlation with steatosis or inflammation [14].

In our study, ABT results were found to have an inverse correlation with BMI, which is consistent with previous findings as increasing BMI has been repeatedly shown to be associated with worse liver histologic lesions in the NAFLD patients [4,54].

A weakness of our study is the fact that the majority of patients were obese, but the sample included relatively few diabetic patients. The generalizability of the findings to NAFLD patients with a different metabolic profile hence needs to be studied. Furthermore, there is the confounding effect of patient characteristics on the ABT and the cross-sectional nature of the study. Enzymatic functions explored by the ABT may be influenced by hormones, malnutrition, heart or renal failure, sex or xenobiotics such as medication or smoking [2]. No data concerning menstrual cycle or exogenous female sex hormones were obtained during our diagnostic work-up. Smoking induces CYP450 enzymes (primarily CYP1A2); hence a higher peak and cumulative excretion can be expected in smokers [55]. In our non-fibrotic population, smoking was independently correlated with ABT values, though smoking habits did not differ between our subpopulations. In the literature, older age and female gender are correlated with lower ABT values, which could not be observed in our population [56]. Genetic polymorphisms in CYPs are a major cause of the inter individual variation in drug metabolism. Several of the CYPs important for the aminopyrine metabolisation (such as CYP2C19, 2D6, 1A2, 2C9, 2A6) are known to be functionally polymorphic [44]. Rapid metabolisers will have higher ABT results compared to slow metabolisers. In this study, determination of CYP polymorphisms was not performed. Most likely it will not have influenced our findings due to the large subgroups. The strength of our study is first of all the large patient population, which allows us to compare groups independent from the impact of significant fibrosis and which decreases the confounding effect of ABT influencers in individual patients. Furthermore, a large proportion of the patients came in for a problem of overweight or obesity and underwent a liver assessment without a priori suspicion of liver disease. This implies that all patients underwent ABT, and not only those selected because of elevated liver tests or other indicators of liver disease, avoiding a lot of potential bias of which many biopsy-proven NAFLD cohort studies suffer. This methodological approach more closely resembles the context of use in which biomarkers for NAFLD will be used in the future and reinforces the validity of these results and their relevance for routine clinical practice.

To confirm our results, more studies should be performed in large patient groups without the confounding factor of significant or advanced fibrosis. Other compounds than aminopyrine can be used to assess the decreased microsomal function in NASH patients, such as caffeine, phenacetin or methacetin.

The observations in this study open new possibilities for the use of the ABT in NAFLD. The ABT can be incorporated in the diagnostic toolset for NASH (in our model, together with ALT and USS) or fibrosis assessment. A decreased microsomal liver function in patients with NASH might indicate a decreased metabolism of xenobiotics, which has a major impact considering the high global prevalence of NASH. Future studies of NASH medication should take this into account. The ABT could be used to monitor disease progression of inflammation in the absence of fibrosis. Furthermore, the ABT could be an additional tool the evaluate the potential improvement upon (new) therapeutic interventions.

## 5. Conclusions

The present study shows a decreased microsomal function in NASH patients without significant fibrosis compared to patients with simple steatosis, as assessed by ABT. Fibrosis, when present, has a stronger impact on ABT excretion compared to inflammation and decreases ABT excretion with each fibrosis stage. ABT might be a useful tool for the decision to conduct a liver biopsy in the NAFLD patients and potentially also for the prospective monitoring of disease progression or of the potential benefits after therapeutic interventions.

**Author Contributions:** Conceptualization, W.V., S.F., L.V.G.; methodology, W.V. and S.F.; validation, E.V.M., L.D., W.V. and S.F.; formal analysis, E.V.M., L.D., W.V.; investigation, E.V.M., L.D., T.V., L.V., A.D., D.C., L.R., E.D., A.V., J.W., W.V.; data curation, A.V.; writing—original draft preparation, W.V.; writing—review and editing, S.F.; visualization, W.V.; supervision, S.F. and L.V.G.; project administration, S.F. All authors have read and agreed to the published version of the manuscript.

## References

1.   Marchesini, G.; Day, C.P.; Dufour, J.F.; Canbay, A.; Nobili, V.; Ratziu, V.; Tilg, H.; Roden, M.; Gastaldelli, A.; Yki-Jarvinen, H.; et al. EASL-EASD-EASO Clinical Practice Guidelines for the management of non-alcoholic fatty liver disease. *J. Hepatol.* **2016**, *64*, 1388–1402. [CrossRef] [PubMed]

2.   Armuzzi, A.; Candelli, M.; Zocco, M.A.; Andreoli, A.; De Lorenzo, A.; Nista, E.C.; Miele, L.; Cremonini, F.; Cazzato, I.A.; Grieco, A.; et al. Review article: Breath testing for human liver function assessment. *Aliment. Pharmacol. Ther.* **2002**, *16*, 1977–1996. [CrossRef] [PubMed]

3.   Afolabi, P.; Wright, M.; Wootton, S.A.; Jackson, A.A. Clinical utility of 13C-liver-function breath tests for assessment of hepatic function. *Dig. Dis. Sci.* **2013**, *58*, 33–41. [CrossRef] [PubMed]

4.   Tribonias, G.; Margariti, E.; Tiniakos, D.; Pectasides, D.; Papatheodoridis, G.V. Liver function breath tests for differentiation of steatohepatitis from simple fatty liver in patients with nonalcoholic fatty liver disease. *J. Clin. Gastroenterol.* **2014**, *48*, 59–65. [CrossRef] [PubMed]

5.   Niwa, T.; Sato, R.; Yabusaki, Y.; Ishibashi, F. Contribution of human hepatic cytochrome P450s and steroidogenic CYP17 to the N-demethylation of aminopyrine. *Xenobiotica* **1999**, *29*, 187–193. [CrossRef] [PubMed]

6.   Niwa, T.; Imagawa, Y. Substrate specificity of human cytochrome P450 (CYP) 2C subfamily and effect of azole antifungal agents on CYP2C8. *J. Pharm. Pharm. Sci.* **2016**, *19*, 423–429. [CrossRef] [PubMed]

7.   Brockmöller, J.; Ivar, R. Assessment of Liver Metabolic Function: Clinical Implications. *Clin. Pharmacokinet.* **1994**, *27*, 216–248. [CrossRef]

8.   Bircher, J.; Küpfer, A.; Gikalov, I.; Preisig, R. Aminopyrine demethylation measured by breath analysis in cirrhosis. *Clin. Pharmacol. Ther.* **1976**, *20*, 484–492. [CrossRef]

9.   Monroe, P.; Baker, A.; Schneider, J.; Krager, P.; Klein, P.; Schoeller, D. The aminopyrine breath test and serum bile acids reflect histologic severity in chronic hepatitis. *Hepatology* **1982**, *2*, 317–322. [CrossRef]

10.  Giannini, E.; Fasoli, A.; Chiarbonello, B.; Malfatti, F.; Romagnoli, P.; Botta, F.; Testa, E.; Polegato, S.; Fumagalli, A.; Testa, R. 13C-aminopyrine breath test to evaluate severity of disease in patients with chronic hepatitis C virus infection. *Aliment. Pharmacol. Ther.* **2002**, *16*, 717–725. [CrossRef]

11.  Herold, C.; Heinz, R.; Niedobitek, G.; Schneider, T.; Hahn, E.G.; Schuppan, D. Quantitative testing of liver function in relation to fibrosis in patients with chronic hepatitis B and C. *Liver* **2001**, *21*, 260–265. [CrossRef] [PubMed]

12. Fierbinteanu-Braticevici, C.; Plesca, D.A.; Tribus, L.; Panaitescu, E.; Braticevici, B. The role of 13C-methacetin breath test for the non-invasive evaluation of nonalcoholic fatty liver disease. *J. Gastrointest. Liver Dis.* **2013**, *22*, 149–156.

13. Portincasa, P.; Grattagliano, I.; Lauterburg, B.H.; Palmieri, V.O.; Palasciano, G.; Stellaard, F. Liver breath tests non-invasively predict higher stages of non-alcoholic steatohepatitis. *Clin. Sci.* **2006**, *111*, 135–143. [CrossRef] [PubMed]

14. Park, G.; Wiseman, E.; George, J.; Katelaris, P.; Seow, F.; Fung, C.; Ngu, M. Non-invasive estimation of liver fibrosis in non-alcoholic fatty liver disease using the 13 C-caffeine breath test. *J. Gastroenterol. Hepatol.* **2011**, *26*, 1411–1416. [PubMed]

15. Schmilovitz-Weiss, H.; Niv, Y.; Pappo, O.; Halpern, M.; Sulkes, J.; Braun, M.; Barak, N.; Rotman, Y.; Cohen, M.; Waked, A.; et al. The 13C-Caffeine Breath Test Detects Significant Fibrosis in Patients With Nonalcoholic Steatohepatitis. *J. Clin. Gastroenterol.* **2008**, *42*, 408–412. [CrossRef] [PubMed]

16. Francque, S.; Verrijken, A.; Caron, S.; Prawitt, J.; Paumelle, R.; Derudas, B.; Lefebvre, P.; Taskinen, M.; Van Hul, W.; Mertens, I.; et al. PPARα gene expression correlates with severity and histological treatment response in patients with non-alcoholic steatohepatitis. *J. Hepatol.* **2015**, *63*, 164–173. [CrossRef] [PubMed]

17. Saverymuttu, S.H.; Joseph, A.E.A.; Maxwell, J.D. Ultrasound scanning in the detection of hepatic fibrosis and steatosis. *Br. Med. J. (Clin. Res. Ed).* **1986**, *292*, 13–15. [CrossRef]

18. Volz, M.; Kellner, H. Kinetics and metabolism of pyrazolones (propyphenazone, aminopyrine and dipyrone). *Br. J. Clin. Pharmacol.* **1980**, *10*, 299S–308S. [CrossRef]

19. Giannini, E.G.; Fasoli, A.; Borro, P.; Botta, F.; Malfatti, F.; Fumagalli, A.; Testa, E.; Polegato, S.; Cotellessa, T.; Milazzo, S.; et al. 13C-galactose breath test and 13C-aminopyrine breath test for the study of liver function in chronic liver disease. *Clin. Gastroenterol. Hepatol.* **2005**, *3*, 279–285. [CrossRef]

20. Taylor, K.J.W.; Sullivan, D.; Simeone, J.; Rosenfield, A.T. Scintigraphy, ultrasound and CT scanning of the liver. *Yale J. Biol. Med.* **1977**, *50*, 437–455. [CrossRef]

21. Merkel, C.; Bolognesi, M.; Bellon, S.; Bianco, S.; Honisch, B.; Lampe, H.; Angeli, P.; Gatta, A. Aminopyrine breath test in the prognostic evaluation of patients with cirrhosis. *Gut* **1992**, *33*, 836–842. [CrossRef] [PubMed]

22. Brunt, E.M.; Kleiner, D.E.; Wilson, L.A.; Belt, P.; Neuschwander-Tetri, B.A. NASH Clinical Research Network The NAS and the histopathologic diagnosis in NAFLD: Distinct clinicopathologic meanings. *Hepatology* **2011**, *53*, 810–820. [CrossRef] [PubMed]

23. Chalasani, N.; Younossi, Z.; Lavine, J.E.; Charlton, M.; Cusi, K.; Rinella, M.; Harrison, S.A.; Brunt, E.M.; Sanyal, A.J. The diagnosis and management of nonalcoholic fatty liver disease: Practice guidance from the American Association for the Study of Liver Diseases. *Hepatology* **2018**, *67*, 328–357. [CrossRef] [PubMed]

24. Kleiner, D.E.; Brunt, E.M.; Van Natta, M.; Behling, C.; Contos, M.J.; Cummings, O.W.; Ferrell, L.D.; Liu, Y.C.; Torbenson, M.S.; Unalp-Arida, A.; et al. Design and validation of a histological scoring system for nonalcoholic fatty liver disease. *Hepatology* **2005**, *41*, 1313–1321. [CrossRef] [PubMed]

25. Ratziu, V.; Bellentani, S.; Cortez-Pinto, H.; Day, C.; Marchesini, G. A position statement on NAFLD/NASH based on the EASL 2009 special conference. *J. Hepatol.* **2010**, *53*, 372–384. [CrossRef] [PubMed]

26. Tape, T.G. Interpreting Diagnostic Tests: The Area under an ROC Curve. University of Nebraska Medical Center. Available online: http://gim.unmc.edu/dxtests/ROC3.htm (accessed on 18 November 2020).

27. Mandrekar, J.N. Receiver operating characteristic curve in diagnostic test assessment. *J. Thorac. Oncol.* **2010**, *5*, 1315–1316. [CrossRef] [PubMed]

28. DeLong, E.; DM, D.; Clarke-Pearson, D. Comparing the areas under two or more correlated receiver operating characteristic curves: A nonparametric approach. *Biometrics* **1988**, *44*, 837–845. [CrossRef]

29. Dulai, P.S.; Singh, S.; Patel, J.; Soni, M.; Prokop, L.; Younossi, Z.; Sebastiani, G.; Ekstedt, M.; Hagstrom, H.; Nasr, P.; et al. Increased risk of mortality by fibrosis stage in non-alcoholic fatty liver disease: Systematic review and meta-analysis. *Hepatology* **2017**, *65*, 1557–1565. [CrossRef]

30. Kleiner, D.E.; Brunt, E.M.; Wilson, L.A.; Behling, C.; Guy, C.; Contos, M.; Cummings, O.; Yeh, M.; Gill, R.; Chalasani, N.; et al. Association of histologic disease activity with progression of nonalcoholic fatty liver disease. *JAMA Netw. Open* **2019**, *2*, e1912565. [CrossRef]

31. Bunney, P.E.; Zink, A.N.; Holm, A.A.; Billington, C.J.; Kotz, C.M. Orexin activation counteracts decreases in nonexercise activity thermogenesis (NEAT) caused by high-fat diet. *Physiol. Behav.* **2017**, *176*, 139–148. [CrossRef]

32. Nascimbeni, F.; Bedossa, P.; Fedchuk, L.; Pais, R.; Charlotte, F.; Lebray, P.; Poynard, T.; Ratziu, V.; LIDO (Liver Injury in Diabetes and Obesity) Study Group. Clinical validation of the FLIP algorithm and the SAF score in patients with non-alcoholic fatty liver disease. *J. Hepatol.* **2020**, *72*, 828–838. [CrossRef] [PubMed]

33. Bedossa, P. Utility and appropriateness of the fatty liver inhibition of progression (FLIP) algorithm and steatosis, activity, and fibrosis (SAF) score in the evaluation of biopsies of nonalcoholic fatty liver disease. *Hepatology* **2014**, *60*, 565–575. [CrossRef] [PubMed]

34. Francque, S.; Lanthier, N.; Verbeke, L.; Reynaert, H.; van Steenkiste, C.; Vonghia, L.; Kwanten, W.; Weyler, J.; Trépo, E.; Cassiman, D.; et al. The Belgian Association for Study of the Liver guidance document on the management of adult and paediatric non-alcoholic fatty liver disease. *Acta Gastroenterol. Belgica* **2018**, *81*, 55–81.

35. Wai-Sun Wong, V.; Adams, L.; de Lédinghen, V.; Lai-Hung Wong, G.; Sookoian, S. Noninvasive biomarkers in NAFLD and NASH—Current progress and future promise. *Nat. Rev. Gastroenterol. Hepatol.* **2018**, *15*, 461–478. [CrossRef]

36. Hori, Y.; Shimizu, Y.; Aiba, T. Altered hepatic drug-metabolizing activity in rats suffering from hypoxemia with experimentally induced acute lung impairment. *Xenobiotica* **2018**, *48*, 576–583. [CrossRef]

37. Francque, S.; Laleman, W.; Verbeke, L.; Van Steenkiste, C.; Casteleyn, C.; Kwanten, W.; Van Dyck, C.; D'Hondt, M.; Ramon, A.; Vermeulen, W.; et al. Increased intrahepatic resistance in severe steatosis: Endothelial dysfunction, vasoconstrictor overproduction and altered microvascular architecture. *Lab. Investig.* **2012**, *92*, 1428–1439. [CrossRef]

38. Francque, S.; Verrijken, A.; Mertens, I.; Hubens, G.; Van Marck, E.; Pelckmans, P.; Van Gaal, L.; Michielsen, P. Noncirrhotic human nonalcoholic fatty liver disease induces portal hypertension in relation to the histological degree of steatosis. *Eur. J. Gastroenterol. Hepatol.* **2010**, *22*, 1449–1457. [CrossRef]

39. van der Graaff, D.; Kwanten, W.J.; Couturier, F.J.; Govaerts, J.S.; Verlinden, W.; Brosius, I.; D'Hondt, M.; Driessen, A.; De Winter, B.Y.; De Man, J.G.; et al. Severe steatosis induces portal hypertension by systemic arterial hyporeactivity and hepatic vasoconstrictor hyperreactivity in rats. *Lab. Investig.* **2018**, *98*, 1263–1275. [CrossRef]

40. van der Graaff, D.; Kwanten, W.J.; Francque, S.M. The potential role of vascular alterations and subsequent impaired liver blood flow and hepatic hypoxia in the pathophysiology of non-alcoholic steatohepatitis. *Med. Hypotheses* **2019**, *122*, 188–197. [CrossRef]

41. Begriche, K.; Massart, J.; Robin, M.A.; Bonnet, F.; Fromenty, B. Mitochondrial adaptations and dysfunctions in nonalcoholic fatty liver disease. *Hepatology* **2013**, *58*, 1497–1507. [CrossRef]

42. Cobbina, E.; Akhlaghi, F. Non-alcoholic fatty liver disease (NAFLD)–pathogenesis, classification, and effect on drug metabolizing enzymes and transporters. *Drug Metab. Rev.* **2017**, *49*, 197–211. [CrossRef] [PubMed]

43. Niemelä, O.; Parkkila, S.; Juvonen, R.O.; Viitala, K.; Gelboin, H.V.; Pasanen, M. Cytochromes P450 2A6, 2E1, and 3A and production of protein-aldehyde adducts in the liver of patients with alcoholic and non-alcoholic liver diseases. *J. Hepatol.* **2000**, *33*, 893–901. [CrossRef]

44. Elfaki, I.; Mir, R.; Almutairi, F.M.; Abu Duhier, F.M. Cytochrome P450: Polymorphisms and roles in cancer, diabetes and atherosclerosis. *Asian Pac. J. Cancer Prev.* **2018**, *19*, 2057–2070. [CrossRef] [PubMed]

45. Zardi, E.M.; De Sio, I.; Ghittoni, G.; Sadun, B.; Palmentieri, B.; Roselli, P.; Persico, M.; Caturelli, E. Which clinical and sonographic parameters may be useful to discriminate NASH from steatosis? *J. Clin. Gastroenterol.* **2011**, *45*, 59–63. [CrossRef]

46. Chalasani, N.; Wilson, L.; Kleiner, D.E.; Cummings, O.W.; Brunt, E.M.; Ünalp, A. Relationship of steatosis grade and zonal location to histological features of steatohepatitis in adult patients with non-alcoholic fatty liver disease. *J. Hepatol.* **2008**, *48*, 829–834. [CrossRef]

47. Liang, R.J.; Wang, H.H.; Lee, W.J.; Liew, P.L.; Lin, J.T.; Wu, M.S. Diagnostic value of ultrasonographic examination for nonalcoholic steatohepatitis in morbidly obese patients undergoing laparoscopic bariatric surgery. *Obes. Surg.* **2007**, *17*, 45–56. [CrossRef]

48. Ballestri, S.; Lonardo, A.; Romagnoli, D.; Carulli, L.; Losi, L.; Day, C.P.; Loria, P. Ultrasonographic fatty liver indicator, a novel score which rules out NASH and is correlated with metabolic parameters in NAFLD. *Liver Int.* **2012**, *32*, 1242–1252. [CrossRef]

49. Fracanzani, A.L.; Valenti, L.; Bugianesi, E.; Andreoletti, M.; Colli, A.; Vanni, E.; Bertelli, C.; Fatta, E.; Bignamini, D.; Marchesini, G.; et al. Risk of severe liver disease in nonalcoholic fatty liver disease with normal aminotransferase levels: A role for insulin resistance and diabetes. *Hepatology* **2008**, *48*, 792–798. [CrossRef]

50. Ahmed, M. Non-alcoholic fatty liver disease in 2015. *World J. Hepatol.* **2015**, *7*, 1450–1459. [CrossRef]

51. Herold, C.; Ganslmayer, M.; Ocker, M.; Zopf, S.; Gailer, B.; Hahn, E.; Schuppan, D. Inducibility of microsomal liver function may differentiate cirrhotic patients with maintained compared with severely compromised liver reserve. *J. Gastroenterol. Hepatol.* **2003**, *18*, 445_449. [CrossRef]

52. Banasch, M.; Ellrichmann, M.; Tannapfel, A.; Schmidt, W.E.; Goetze, O. The non-invasive 13C-methionine breath test detects hepatic mitochondrial dysfunction as a marker of disease activity in non-alcoholic steatohepatitis. *Eur. J. Med. Res.* **2011**, *16*, 258–264. [CrossRef] [PubMed]

53. Miele, L.; Greco, A.; Armuzzi, A.; Candelli, M.; Forgione, A.; Gasbarrini, A.; Gasbarrini, G. Hepatic mitochondrial beta-oxidation in patients with nonalcoholic steatohepatitis assessed bij 13C-octanoate breath test. *Am. J. Gastroenterol.* **2003**, *98*, 2335–2336. [CrossRef] [PubMed]

54. Dixon, J.B.; Bhathal, P.S.; O'Brien, P.E. Nonalcoholic fatty liver disease: Predictors of nonalcoholic steatohepatitis and liver fibrosis in the severely obese. *Gastroenterology* **2001**, *121*, 91–100. [CrossRef] [PubMed]

55. Hukkanen, J.; Jacob, P.; Peng, M.; Dempsey, D.; Benowitz, N.L. Effect of nicotine on cytochrome P450 1A2 activity. *Br. J. Clin. Pharmacol.* **2011**, *72*, 836–838. [CrossRef]

56. Caubet, M.S.; Laplante, A.; Caillé, J.; L, B.J. 13C aminopyrine and 13C caffeine breath test: Influence of gender, cigarette smoking and oral contraceptives intake. *Isot. Environ. Health Stud.* **2002**, *38*, 71–77. [CrossRef]

# Non-Alcoholic Steatohepatitis (NASH): Risk Factors in Morbidly Obese Patients

Alexandre Losekann [1], Antonio C. Weston [2], Angelo A. de Mattos [1], Cristiane V. Tovo [1], Luis A. de Carli [2], Marilia B. Espindola [2], Sergio R. Pioner [2] and Gabriela P. Coral [1,*]

[1]  Post-Graduation Program, Hepatology at Universidade Federal de Ciências da Saúde de Porto Alegre (UFCSPA), Porto Alegre 90.050-170, Brasil; alosekann@gmail.com (A.L.); angeloamattos@gmail.com (A.A.M.); cris.tovo@terra.com.br (C.V.T.)

[2]  Centro de Tratamento da Obesidade (CTO), Hospital Santa Casa de Misericórdia de Porto Alegre, Porto Alegre 92.010-300, Brasil; drweston@terra.com.br (A.C.W.); luizdecarli@plugin.com.br (L.A.C.); mariliae@brturbo.com.br (M.B.E.); srpioner@terra.com.br (S.R.P.)

*  Author to whom correspondence should be addressed; g.coral@terra.com.br

Academic Editors: Amedeo Lonardo and Giovanni Targher

**Abstract:** The aim was to investigate the prevalence of non-alcoholic steatohepatitis (NASH) and risk factors for hepatic fibrosis in morbidly obese patients submitted to bariatric surgery. This retrospective study recruited all patients submitted to bariatric surgery from January 2007 to December 2012 at a reference attendance center of Southern Brazil. Clinical and biochemical data were studied as a function of the histological findings of liver biopsies done during the surgery. Steatosis was present in 226 (90.4%) and NASH in 176 (70.4%) cases. The diagnosis of cirrhosis was established in four cases (1.6%) and fibrosis in 108 (43.2%). Risk factors associated with NASH at multivariate analysis were alanine aminotransferase (ALT) >1.5 times the upper limit of normal (ULN); glucose $\geq$ 126 mg/dL and triglycerides $\geq$ 150 mg/dL. All patients with ALT $\geq$1.5 times the ULN had NASH. When the presence of fibrosis was analyzed, ALT > 1.5 times the ULN and triglycerides $\geq$ 150 mg/dL were risk factors, furthermore, there was an increase of 1% in the prevalence of fibrosis for each year of age increase. Not only steatosis, but NASH is a frequent finding in MO patients. In the present study, ALT $\geq$ 1.5 times the ULN identifies all patients with NASH, this finding needs to be further validated in other studies. Moreover, the presence of fibrosis was associated with ALT, triglycerides and age, identifying a subset of patients with more severe disease.

**Keywords:** NAFLD; NASH; morbidly obese; liver fibrosis

## 1. Introduction

Nonalcoholic fatty liver disease (NAFLD) embraces a wide range of manifestations that includes simple steatosis (SS), non-alcoholic steatohepatitis (NASH), cirrhosis and hepatocellular carcinoma [1,2]. The real prevalence of NASH is not known, as the disease is usually asymptomatic and that the definitive diagnosis is possible only by the histopathological assessment [3,4]. In a study conducted in a tertiary public hospital in south Brazil, the prevalence of NASH was 3.18% in obese patients without diabetes mellitus (DM) [5].

Morbidly obese (MO) patients, defined as body mass index (BMI) $\geq$35 and experiencing obesity-related health conditions or $\geq$40 kg/m$^2$, are a subgroup with higher risk of NAFLD. In these patients, the prevalence of NAFLD is estimated from 84% to 96% and of NASH from 25% to 55%. In those with NASH, there is bridging fibrosis or cirrhosis at a rate of 12% and 2% respectively [4,6].

This study aimed to estimate the prevalence of NASH and the risk factors for fibrosis in MO patients submitted to bariatric surgery (BS).

## 2. Results

A total of 250 patients were evaluated; 200 (80%) were women, with an average age of 36.8 ± 10.2 years. The average BMI was 43.6 ± 5.2 kg/m$^2$. Type 2 diabetes was identified in 12.8% and arterial hypertension in 41.3%.

Simple steatosis was present in 226 (90.4%) patients and were classified as mild in 76 (30.4%); moderate in 71 (28.4%) and severe in 79 (31.6%). NASH was diagnosed in 176 (70.4%) cases, being mild degree in 120 (48.4%) cases; moderate in 50 (20%) cases, and severe in 6 (2.4%) cases. Fibrosis was reported in 108 (43.2%) biopsies, 95 (38%) of them were mild; 2 (0.8%) moderate; and 7 severe (2.8%). Cirrhosis was diagnosed in 4 (1.6%) cases.

The risk factors related to NASH in bivariate analysis (Table 1) were: Mean value of AST, mean value of ALT, ALT ≥ 1.5 times the ULN, mean value of TG, TG ≥ 150 mg/dL and mean value of glucose. All patients with ALT ≥1.5 times the ULN had NASH. After the adjustment by the multivariate model, the following variables remain associated with NASH (Table 2): ALT > 1.5 times the ULN; glucose ≥ 126 mg/dL and TG ≥ 150 mg/dL.

Some risk factors associated to fibrosis by bivariate analysis (Table 3) were the same as those associated with NASH: Mean value of AST, mean value of ALT, ALT > 1.5 times the ULN, mean value of TG, TG ≥ 150 mg/dL and mean value of glucose. In addition, glucose ≥ 126 mg/dL and age were also associated with fibrosis. The mean age of patients with fibrosis was 40.0 ± 11.4 and without fibrosis, 34.8 ± 9.3 ($p$ = 0.001). After the adjustment by the multivariate model (Table 2), the following variables remain associated with fibrosis: ALT > 1.5 times the ULN, TG ≥ 150 mg/dL and age: For a year of age increase, there is an increase of 1% in the prevalence of fibrosis (PR = 1.01; 95% CI = 1.00–1.02; $p$ = 0.006).

**Table 1.** Bivariate analysis according to the presence of non-alcoholic steatohepatitis (NASH).

| Variable * | Total Sample | With NASH | Without NASH | $p$ |
|---|---|---|---|---|
| Age (years) | 37.2 ± 10.6 ($n$ = 183) | 37.6 ± 11.0 ($n$ = 141) | 35.5 ± 9.0 ($n$ = 42) | 0.208 |
| Female | 153 (80.1) ($n$ = 191) | 113 (79) ($n$ = 143) | 40 (83.3) ($n$ = 48) | 0.661 |
| BMI (kg/m$^2$) | 43.7 ± 5.2 ($n$ = 191) | 43.5 ± 5.0 ($n$ = 143) | 44.1 ± 5.7 ($n$ = 48) | 0.535 |
| Ferritin (μ/L) | 119 (67–208) ($n$ = 169) | 123 (75–239) ($n$ = 128) | 97 (58.5–173) ($n$ = 41) | 0.120 |
| Iron (μ/L) | 76.4 ± 25.2 ($n$ = 163) | 75.8 ± 24.1 ($n$ = 125) | 78.4 ± 29.1 ($n$ = 38) | 0.587 |
| ** AST (U/L) | 24 (19–31) ($n$ = 183) | 25 (20–34) ($n$ = 139) | 21.5 (16.3–26.8) ($n$ = 44) | 0.007 |
| ** ALT (U/L) | 29 (21–47.8) ($n$ = 183) | 32 (23–51) ($n$ = 139) | 25 (17–29.5) ($n$ = 44) | <0.001 |
| ALT > 1.5 × U/L | 28 (15.2) ($n$ = 183) | 28 (20.1) ($n$ = 139) | 0 (0.0) ($n$ = 44) | 0.002 |
| Glucose (mg/dL) | 103.7 ± 34.3 ($n$ = 188) | 106.7 ± 37.7 ($n$ = 142) | 94.5 ± 17.9 ($n$ = 46) | 0.036 |
| Glucose ≥ 126 mg/dL | 24 (12.8) ($n$ = 188) | 22 (15.5) ($n$ = 142) | 2 (4.3) ($n$ = 46) | 0.086 |
| Platelets (10$^3$/mm$^3$) | 278.5 ± 68.6 ($n$ = 172) | 283.3 ± 64.8 ($n$ = 131) | 269 ± 68.8 ($n$ = 41) | 0.233 |
| Total cholesterol (mg/dL) | 193 ± 42 ($n$ = 186) | 196.6 ± 42.8 ($n$ = 138) | 182.9 ± 38.3 ($n$ = 48) | 0.052 |
| LDL-C (mg/dL) | 116 ± 41 ($n$ = 186) | 117.4 ± 41.1 ($n$ = 138) | 112 ± 41.1 ($n$ = 48) | 0.438 |
| HDL-C (mg/dL) | 48.9 ± 13.7 ($n$ = 186) | 48.4 ± 13.5 ($n$ = 138) | 50.2 ± 14.3 ($n$ = 48) | 0.427 |
| TG (mg/dL) | 122 (91–193) ($n$ = 186) | 134 (96–198) ($n$ = 138) | 105 (72–135) ($n$ = 48) | 0.004 |
| TG ≥ 150 mg/dL | 68 (36.3) ($n$ = 186) | 58 (42.0) ($n$ = 138) | 9 (18.8) ($n$ = 48) | 0.007 |

* Variables described by mean ± standard deviation, median (percentiles 25–75) or $n$ (%); ** Normal values for ALT: 14–42 U/L and for AST: 10–42 U/L; $n$ = number of cases; NASH = nonalcoholic steatohepatitis; BMI = body mass index; AST = aspartate aminotransferase; ALT = alanine aminotransferase; LDL-C = low density lipoprotein; HDL-C = high density lipoprotein.

**Table 2.** Multivariate analysis according to the presence of NASH and fibrosis.

| Variables | NASH | | Fb | |
|---|---|---|---|---|
| | PR (95% CI) | $p$ | PR (95% CI) | $p$ |
| ALT > 1.5 ULN | 1.31 (1.22–1.41) | <0.001 | 1.22 (1.00–1.48) | 0.048 |
| Glucose $\geq$ 126 mg/dL | 1.16 (1.02–1.32) | 0.022 | 1.22 (0.99–1.50) | 0.058 |
| TGs $\geq$ 150 mg/dL | 1.15 (1.01–1.30) | 0.035 | 1.24 (1.07–1.45) | 0.005 |
| Age | * | * | 1.01 (1.00–1.02) | 0.006 |

* did not present a $p$ value <0.20 in the bivariate analysis.

**Table 3.** Bivariate analysis according to the presence of fibrosis.

| Variable * | With Fb | Without Fb | $p$ |
|---|---|---|---|
| Age (years) | 40.0 ± 11.4 ($n$ = 83) | 34.8 ± 9.3 ($n$ = 100) | 0.001 |
| Female | 67 (79.8) ($n$ = 84) | 86 (80.4) ($n$ = 107) | 1.000 |
| BMI (kg/m$^2$) | 43.4 ± 5.4 ($n$ = 84) | 43.9 ± 5.0 ($n$ = 107) | 0.479 |
| Ferritin ($\mu$/L) | 127 (81–293) ($n$ = 73) | 109 (56–97) ($n$ = 96) | 0.080 |
| Iron ($\mu$/L) | 75.8 ± 22.5 ($n$ = 73) | 76.9 ± 27.4 ($n$ = 90) | 0.790 |
| ** AST (U/L) | 25 (19–43) ($n$ = 83) | 24 (18–28) ($n$ = 100) | 0.040 |
| ** ALT (U/L) | 30 (24–54) ($n$ = 83) | 26 (19–39) ($n$ = 100) | 0.008 |
| ** ALT > 1.5 × U/L | 19 (22.9) ($n$ = 83) | 9 (8.9) ($n$ = 100) | 0.015 |
| Glycemia (mg/dL) | 110.9 ± 40 ($n$ = 83) | 98.0 ± 27.9 ($n$ = 105) | 0.014 |
| Glycemia $\geq$ 126 mg/dL | 17 (20.5) ($n$ = 83) | 7 (6.7) ($n$ = 105) | 0.009 |
| Platelets ($10^3$/mm$^3$) | 273.6 ± 59.3 ($n$ = 77) | 285 ± 70.6 ($n$ = 95) | 0.261 |
| Total cholesterol (mg/dL) | 198.9 ± 42.3 ($n$ = 80) | 188.7 ± 41.4 ($n$ = 106) | 0.102 |
| LDL-C (mg/dL) | 116.3 ± 38.4 ($n$ = 80) | 115.8 ± 43.1 ($n$ = 106) | 0.934 |
| HDL-C (mg/dL) | 49.2 ± 14.2 ($n$ = 80) | 48.6 ± 13.3 ($n$ = 106) | 0.776 |
| TG (mg/dL) | 148.5 (100–199) ($n$ = 80) | 112.5 (83.8–158) ($n$ = 106) | 0.005 |
| TG $\geq$ 150 mg/dL | 40 (50) ($n$ = 80) | 27 (25.5) ($n$ = 106) | 0.001 |

* Variables described by mean ± standard deviation, median (percentiles 25–75) or n (%); ** Normal values for ALT: 14–42 U/L and for AST: 10–42 U/L; $n$ = number of cases; Fb = fibrosis; BMI = body mass index; AST = aspartate aminotransferase; ALT = alanine aminotransferase; LDL-C = low density lipoprotein; HDL-C = high density lipoprotein; TG = triglycerides.

## 3. Discussion

More recently, BS has become an accepted therapeutic option for MO patients and has been associated with histological improvement of NAFLD [7–10]. When liver biopsies performed before and after the weight loss caused by the surgery were compared, it was shown that this treatment determines an improvement or stabilization of SS, NASH and fibrosis [9,10]. However, in cirrhosis, the likelihood of regression is reduced and there is an increase in morbidity and mortality after BS [8–12].

In the present study, NAFLD was present in 90.4% of the MO patients submitted to BS. This result is consistent with the literature that reports a prevalence varying between 84% and 96% of NAFLD [4,13]. In the same way, the degree of steatosis was uniformly distributed in 30.4%, 28.4% and 31.6%, as mild, moderate and severe degree respectively, and NASH was found in approximately 70%, with a moderate correlation with the degree of steatosis. Other authors found a prevalence of NASH between 55% and 60%, but in these cases, the histopathological diagnostic criteria were not homogeneous, which makes the actual prevalence of NASH difficult to be established [3,11].

Bedossa *et al.* [14] proposed recently a score and algorithm for the histopathological definition of NASH in patients with MO. Patients should be classified as having NASH only if they have unequivocal hepatocyte ballooning. According to these criteria, a prevalence of NASH in 34% in patients with MO was found, which is lower than the observed in other studies [3,11], including ours. A possible explanation for this finding is that Bedossa *et al.* used more specific criteria for the diagnosis of NASH. In the present study, fibrosis was present in 48.3% of patients; out of these, 38% were mild and only 4.4% were considered severe. Although cirrhosis is not a contraindication for BS, there is a risk of hepatic decompensation with rapid weight loss [15].

New noninvasive clinical and biochemical markers of fibrosis in NASH have been evaluated [3]. Age, obesity, hypertension, DM, the levels of bilirubin and the ALT/AST ratio greater than 1 has been associated with the presence of NASH or fibrosis [3,13,16–18]. Contrary to other studies [19,20], the present results did not show a positive correlation of BMI with the degree of steatosis, NASH and fibrosis. BMI does not always properly reflect the degree of visceral adiposity, significantly more involved in the physiopathology of NAFLD. It is possible that there is a closer correlation between the liver damage and the measure of abdominal circumference; however, this data was not evaluated in the present study.

The results of the present study demonstrated that all patients whose ALT values were greater than 1.5 times the ULN (15% of the sample) presented NASH, and ALT was also strongly associated with fibrosis. This data can represent a cutoff and has not yet been reported in the literature for this subgroup of patients.

This study showed an association among serum levels of TG and glucose with NASH. These findings were already described in former studies concerning the risk factors of NASH [13,18,21]. In addition to high levels of TG, we found that the presence of fibrosis was also correlated with age; this association has been described before [20,22]. Furthermore, an increase in age raises the prevalence of fibrosis linearly.

Although several non-invasive markers for prediction of advanced fibrosis are available (aspartate aminotransferase-to-platelet ratio index - APRI; NAFLD fibrosis score; body mass index, ASL/ALT ratio and diabetes mellitus - BARD; FIB-4) [16,23–25], the present study suggests that patients with MO and more advanced age, high levels of ALT and TG should best be submitted to a full diagnostic evaluation such as liver biopsy to better assessment of hepatic damage.

In conclusion, this study showed a high prevalence of NASH in patients with MO and identifies a subset of patients with a higher risk of more advanced disease.

## 4. Experimental Section

This is a retrospective cohort study, where MO patients were submitted to BS from 2007 to 2012 at the Obesity Treatment Center of a tertiary reference center (Santa Casa de Porto Alegre, SCPA) in southern Brazil. Age, gender, the presence of comorbidities (diabetes, arterial hypertension) and body mass index (BMI) were evaluated. The dosage of ferritin, aspartate (AST) and alanine (ALT) aminotransferases, fasting glucose, platelets, total cholesterol, triglycerides (TG), high (HDL-C) and low (LDL-C) density lipoproteins was done up to 90 days before procedure. These variables were compared with the histological results of liver biopsies obtained in the trans-operative period.

Patients aged less than 18 years, those who presented serological markers for viral hepatitis, as well as patients with other causes of chronic liver disease and history of alcohol intake >20 g/day were excluded.

Liver biopsies were routinely stained with Hematoxylin-Eosin, Perls and Masson's trichrome and evaluated by the same liver pathologist who was blinded to the clinical data.

Simple steatosis (SS) was considered to be present over 5% of the sample and scored as suggested by Brunt: Mild steatosis was defined when present in 5% to 33%; moderate steatosis when present in 33% to 66%, and severe steatosis when greater than 66% [26]. To diagnose NASH, steatosis associated with hepatocyte ballooning and/or inflammatory infiltrate were the main findings, and was classified using NAFLD Activity Score (NAS) as mild (A1), moderate (A2) and severe (A3), according to classification described by the Pathology Committee of the NASH Clinical Research Network. The degree of fibrosis (Fb) was classified as stage A1, when sinusoidal/discrete cellular Fb was present; degree 1B, when sinusoidal/dense and diffuse Fb was identified; and 1c for portal Fb. Stage 2 was considered when there was pericellular/perisinusoidal associated with periportal Fb, and stage 3 in the presence of the anterior changes associated to bridging Fb. Finally, stage 4 corresponds to cirrhosis [27]. In the statistical analysis, the degree of Fb was classified as mild (stages 1A, 1B, 1C); moderate (stage 2); severe (stage 3) or cirrhosis (stage 4).

The data were analyzed using the SPSS (Statistical Package for the Social Sciences) Inc., Chicago, IL, USA, version 18.0. The sample size supports a minimum difference between groups of 20%, power of 85% and a significance level of 5%. To control confounding factors and analyze the variables independently associated with NASH and fibrosis, the Poisson regression analysis was applied. To evaluate the association, the prevalence ratio (PR) was used, with the 95% confidence interval (CI) to estimate the risk in the population. To control the multicollinearity, two regression models were made, one of them inserting the glycemia and the other the TG. The criteria for entering the variable in the multivariate model was that it should have a value of $p < 0.20$ in the bivariate analysis. To evaluate the association between the categorical variables, the Pearson chi-square test was applied, and for the continuous or ordinal variables, the Spearman ($r_s$) correlation test was used. $p$ values of <0.05 were considered significant. This study was approved by the Institutional review board of SCPA. For this type of study formal consent was not required.

**Author Contributions:** Alexandre Losekann and Gabriela P. Coral conceptualized and designed this manuscript; Alexandre Losekann, Antonio C. Weston, Luiz A. de Carli, Marilia B. Espindola and Sergio R. Pioner collected and analyzed the data; Alexandre Losekann, Angelo A. de Mattos, Cristiane V. Tovo and Gabriela P. Coral reviewed the literature and wrote the paper; all authors approved the final version of the manuscript.

## Abbreviations

ALT: alanine aminotransferase; AST: aspartate aminotransferase; APRI: aspartate aminotransferase-to-platelet ratio index; BARD: body mass index, ASL/ALT ratio and diabetes mellitus; BMI: body mass index; BS: bariatric surgery CI: confidence interval; DM: diabetes mellitus; Fb: fibrosis; HDL-C: high density lipoproteins; LDL-C: low density lipoproteins; MO: morbidly obese; NAFLD: Nonalcoholic fatty liver disease; NAS: NAFLD Activity Score; NASH: non-alcoholic steatohepatitis; PR: prevalence ratio; $r_s$:Spearman correlation test; SCPA: Santa Casa de Porto Alegre; SPSS: Statistical Package for the Social Sciences; SS: simple steatosis; TG: triglycerides; ULN: upper limit of normal.

## References

1.  Brunt, E.M. Nonalcoholic steatohepatitis. *Semin. Liver Dis.* **2004**, *24*, 3–20.

2.  White, D.L.; Kanwal, F.; El-Serag, H.B. Associations between nonalcoholic fatty liver disease and risk for hepatocellular cancer based on systematic review. *Clin. Gastroenterol. Hepatol.* **2012**, *10*, 1342–1359.

3.  Musso, G.; Gambino, R.; Cassader, M.; Pagano, G. Meta-analysis: natural history of non-alcoholic fatty liver disease (NAFLD) and diagnostic accuracy of non-invasive tests for liver disease severity. *Ann. Med.* **2011**, *43*, 617–649. [CrossRef] [PubMed]

4.  Clark, J.M. The epidemiology of nonalcoholic fatty liver disease in adults. *J. Clin. Gastroenterol.* **2006**, *40*, 5–10.

5.  Zamin, I., Jr.; de Mattos, A.A.; Zettler, C.G. Nonalcoholic steatohepatitis in nondiabetic obese patients. *Can. J. Gastroenterol.* **2002**, *16*, 303–307. [PubMed]

6.  Ratziu, V.; Giral, P.; Charlotte, F.; Bruckert, E.; Thibault, V. Liver fibrosis in overweight patients. *Gastroenterology* **2000**, *118*, 1117–1123. [CrossRef]

7.  Chalasani, N.; Younossi, Z.; Lavine, J.E.; Diehl, A.M.; Brunt, E.M.; Cusi, K.; Charlton, M.; Sanyal, A.J. The diagnosis and management of non-alcoholic fatty liver disease: Practice Guideline by the American Association for the Study of Liver Diseases, American College of Gastroenterology, and the American Gastroenterological Association. *Hepatology* **2012**, *55*, 2005–2023. [CrossRef] [PubMed]

8.  De Andrade, A.R.; Cotrim, H.P.; Alves, E.; Soares, D.; Rocha, R. Nonalcoholic fatty liver disease in severely obese individuals: The influence of bariatric surgery. *Ann. Hepatol.* **2008**, *7*, 364–368. [PubMed]

9.  Mathurin, P.; Hollebecque, A.; Arnalsteen, L.; Buob, D.; Leteurtre, E.; Caiazzo, R.; Pigeyre, M.; Verkindt, H.; Dharancy, S.; Louvet, A.; *et al.* Prospective study of the long-term effects of bariatric surgery on liver injury in patients without advanced disease. *Gastroenterology* **2009**, *137*, 532–540. [CrossRef] [PubMed]

10. Moretto, M.; Kupski, C.; da Silva, V.D.; Padoin, A.V.; Mottin, C.C. Effect of bariatric surgery on liver fibrosis. *Obes. Surg.* **2012**, *22*, 1044–1049. [PubMed]

11. Mummadi, R.R.; Kasturi, K.S.; Chennareddygari, S.; Sood, G.K. Effect of bariatric surgery on nonalcoholic fatty liver disease: systematic review and meta-analysis. *Clin. Gastroenterol. Hepatol.* **2008**, *6*, 1396–1402. [CrossRef] [PubMed]

12. Mosko, J.D.; Nguyen, G.C. Increased perioperative mortality following bariatric surgery among patients with cirrhosis. *Clin. Gastroenterol. Hepatol.* **2011**, *9*, 897–901. [CrossRef] [PubMed]

13. Ong, J.P.; Elariny, H.; Collantes, R.; Younoszai, A.; Chandhoke, V.; Reines, H.D.; Goodman, Z.; Younossi, Z.M. Predictors of nonalcoholic steatohepatitis and advanced fibrosis in morbidly obese patients. *Obes. Surg.* **2005**, *15*, 310–315. [CrossRef] [PubMed]

14. Bedossa, P.; Poitou, C.; Veyrie, N.; Bouillot, J.L.; Basdevant, A.; Paradis, V.; Tordjman, J.; Clement, K. Histopathological algorithm and scoring system for evaluation of liver lesions in morbidly obese patients. *Hepatology* **2012**, *56*, 1751–1759. [CrossRef] [PubMed]

15. D'Albuquerque, L.A.C.; Gonzalez, A.M.; Whale, R.C.; de Oliveira Souza, E.; Mancero, J.M.; de Oliveira e Silva, A. Liver transplantation for subacute hepatocellular failure due to massive steatohepatitis after bariatric surgery. *Liver Transpl.* **2008**, *14*, 881–885. [CrossRef] [PubMed]

16. Angulo, P. Long-term mortality in nonalcoholic fatty liver disease: Is liver histology of any prognostic significance? *Hepatology* **2010**, *51*, 373–375. [CrossRef] [PubMed]

17. Chisholm, J.; Seki, Y.; Toouli, J.; Stahl, J.; Collins, J.; Kow, L. Serologic predictors of nonalcoholic steatohepatitis in a population undergoing bariatric surgery. *Surg. Obes. Relat. Dis.* **2012**, *8*, 416–422. [CrossRef] [PubMed]

18. Praveenraj, P.; Gomes, R.M.; Kumar, S.; Karthikeyan, P.; Shankar, A.; Parthasarathi, R.; Senthilnathan, P.; Rajapandian, S.; Palanivelu, C. Prevalence and predictors of non-alcoholic fatty liver disease in morbidly obese south indian patients undergoing bariatric surgery. *Obes. Surg.* **2015**, *25*, 2078–2087. [PubMed]

19. Pagano, G.; Pacini, G.; Musso, G.; Gambino, R.; Mecca, F.; Depetris, N.; Cassader, M.; David, E.; Cavallo-Perin, P.; Rizzetto, M. Nonalcoholic steatohepatitis, insulin resistance, and metabolic syndrome: further evidence for an etiologic association. *Hepatology* **2002**, *35*, 367–372. [CrossRef] [PubMed]

20. Rocha, R.; Cotrim, H.P.; Carvalho, F.M.; Siqueira, A.C.; Braga, H.; Freitas, L.A. Body mass index and waist circumference in non-alcoholic fatty liver disease. *J. Hum. Nutr. Diet.* **2005**, *18*, 365–370. [CrossRef] [PubMed]

21. Chitturi, S.; Abeygunasekera, S.; Farrell, G.C.; Holmes-Walker, J.; Hui, J.M.; Fung, C. NASH and insulin resistance: Insulin hypersecretion and specific association with the insulin resistance syndrome. *Hepatology* **2002**, *35*, 373–379. [CrossRef] [PubMed]

22. Guidorizzi de Siqueira, A.C.; Cotrim, H.P.; Rocha, R.; Carvalho, F.M.; de Freitas, L.A.; Barreto, D.; Gouveia, L.; Landeiro, L. Non-alcoholic fatty liver disease and insulin resistance: Importance of risk factors and histological spectrum. *Eur. J. Gastroenterol. Hepatol.* **2005**, *17*, 837–841. [CrossRef] [PubMed]

23. Kruger, F.C.; Daniels, C.R.; Kidd, M.; Swart, G.; Brundyn, K.; van Rensburg, C.; Kotze, M. APRI: A simple bedside marker for advanced fibrosis that can avoid liver biopsy in patients with NAFLD/NASH. *South Afr. Med. J.* **2011**, *101*, 477–480.

24. Harrison, S.A.; Oliver, D.; Arnold, H.L.; Gogia, S.; Neuschwander-Tetri, B.A. Development and validation of a simple NAFLD clinical scoring system for identifying patients without advanced disease. *Gut* **2008**, *57*, 1441–1447. [CrossRef] [PubMed]

25. Shah, A.G.; Lydecker, A.; Murray, K.; Tetri, B.N.; Contos, M.J.; Sanyal, A.J.; Nash Clinical Research Network. Use of the FIB4 index for non-invasive evaluation of fibrosis in nonalcoholic fatty liver disease. *Clin. Gastroenterol. Hepatol.* **2009**, *7*, 1104–1112. [CrossRef] [PubMed]

26. Brunt, E.M.; Janney, C.G.; Di Bisceglie, A.M.; Neuschwander-Tetri, B.A.; Bacon, B.R. Nonalcoholic steatohepatitis: A proposal for grading and staging the histological lesions. *Am. J. Gastroenterol.* **1999**, *94*, 2467–2474. [CrossRef] [PubMed]

27. Kleiner, D.E.; Brunt, E.M.; van Natta, M.; Behling, C.; Contos, M.J.; Cummings, O.W.; Ferrell, L.D.; Liu, Y.C.; Torbenson, M.S.; Unalp-Arida, A.; *et al.* Design and validation of a histological scoring system for nonalcoholic fatty liver disease. *Hepatology* **2005**, *41*, 1313–1321. [CrossRef] [PubMed]

# 4

# Low Serum Lysosomal Acid Lipase Activity Correlates with Advanced Liver Disease

**Eyal Shteyer** [1,2,*,†], **Rivka Villenchik** [1,†], **Mahmud Mahamid** [3,4], **Nidaa Nator** [1] and **Rifaat Safadi** [1,4]

[1]   The Liver Unit, Gastroenterology Institute, Hadassah Medical Center, Hadassah Medical School, The Hebrew University, Jerusalem 9112001, Israel; eshteyer@hotmail.com (R.V.); nidaa@hadassah.org.il (N.N.); safadi@hadassah.org.il (R.S.)
[2]   Pediatric Gastroenterology Institute, Shaare Zedek Medical Center, Hadassah Medical School, The Hebrew University, Jerusalem 9103102, Israel
[3]   Liver Unit, Gastroenterology Institute, Shaare Zedek Medical Center, Hadassah Medical School, The Hebrew University, Jerusalem 9112001, Israel; mmahamid@szmc.org.il
[4]   Liver Unit, Holy Family Hospital; Safed Medical School, Bar Ilan University, Nazareth 1641110, Israel
*   Correspondence: eyals@szmc.org.il
†   These authors contributed equally to this work.

Academic Editors: Amedeo Lonardo and Giovanni Targher

**Abstract:** Fatty liver has become the most common liver disorder and is recognized as a major health burden in the Western world. The causes for disease progression are not fully elucidated but lysosomal impairment is suggested. Here we evaluate a possible role for lysosomal acid lipase (LAL) activity in liver disease. To study LAL levels in patients with microvesicular, idiopathic cirrhosis and nonalcoholic fatty liver disease (NAFLD). Medical records of patients with microvesicular steatosis, cryptogenic cirrhosis and NAFLD, diagnosed on the basis of liver biopsies, were included in the study. Measured serum LAL activity was correlated to clinical, laboratory, imaging and pathological data. No patient exhibited LAL activity compatible with genetic LAL deficiency. However, serum LAL activity inversely predicted liver disease severity. A LAL level of 0.5 was the most sensitive for detecting both histologic and noninvasive markers for disease severity, including lower white blood cell count and calcium, and elevated γ-glutamyltransferase, creatinine, glucose, glycated hemoglobin, uric acid and coagulation function. Serum LAL activity <0.5 indicates severe liver injury in patients with fatty liver and cirrhosis. Further studies should define the direct role of LAL in liver disease severity and consider the possibility of replacement therapy.

**Keywords:** lysosomal acid lipase; cholesteryl ester storage disease; non-alcoholic liver disease; non-alcoholic steatohepatitis; cirrhosis

## 1. Introduction

Fatty liver has become the most common liver disorder [1] and is recognized as a major health burden in the Western world. The spectrum of histological abnormalities includes simple steatosis (steatosis without other liver injuries) and nonalcoholic steatohepatitis in its more extreme forms [2]. Over 30% of adults in developed countries suffer from hepatic fat accumulation [3]. Among these patients, 60% are diabetic, obese or morbidly obese [3–5].

The earliest stage of nonalcoholic fatty liver disease (NAFLD) consists of hepatic steatosis or lipid deposition in the cytoplasm of hepatocytes [6,7]. Hepatic steatosis may progress to the more aggressive necro-inflammatory form of NAFLD, nonalcoholic steatohepatitis (NASH) [2]. NASH patients, as compared to those with steatosis, have a much greater risk for developing liver cirrhosis, a significant risk factor for development of hepatocellular carcinoma [7–9]. It is still unclear what leads to the progression from simple steatosis to advanced liver disease. In some cases hepatic steatosis is merely a marker for other diseases, such as microvesicular steatosis in metabolic diseases [10] and in viral hepatitis [11].

An emerging cause for fatty liver and hepatic dysfunction is lysosomal acid lipase deficiency (LAL-d). Pronounced LAL-d is a rare autosomal recessive storage disorder, leading to lysosomal accumulation of lipids, predominately cholesteryl esters and triglycerides in various tissues and cell types. In LAL-deficient hepatocytes increased levels of cholesterol lead to substantial increases in very low-density lipoprotein (VLDL)-cholesterol production and secretion, the normal way of exporting cholesterol from the liver. This in turn leads to enhanced low-density lipoprotein (LDL)-cholesterol secretion and thus may be an important enhancer of hypercholesterolemia in LAL-d [12]. LAL-d is classified as either Wolman disease (WD) or cholesteryl ester storage disease (CESD), both characterized by very low LAL activity [13–15]. CESD usually has a later onset than WD, and primarily affects the liver, with a wide spectrum of involvement ranging from early onset disease with severe cirrhosis to later onset of slowly progressive hepatic disease with survival into adulthood. Subsequently, complications of fatty liver disease with mixed hyperlipidemia lead to accelerated atherosclerosis, which dominates the clinical picture. Moreover, CESD patients exhibit many abnormalities that overlap with those in more common liver disorders such as nonalcoholic fatty liver disease (NAFLD), making the diagnosis of CESD much more challenging. Therefore, the importance of LAL-d in dyslipidemia and liver dysfunction was recently suggested for the NAFLD spectrum [9]. Furthermore, low LAL activity has been reported only in patients with NAFLD, underscoring the potential role of LAL in NAFLD [16].

The aim of the current study was to further evaluate LAL activity in patients with liver diseases that may be attributed to LAL-d: fatty liver with microvesicular steatosis, cryptogenic cirrhosis and NAFLD.

## 2. Results

### 2.1. Basic Characterization of the Study Population

Seventy-four patients diagnosed with cirrhosis according to the International Classification of Diseases 9 (ICD9) classification, and having an available liver biopsy were identified. Sixty-three were excluded due to clear etiology for their liver disease, thus not meeting the diagnostic criteria for cryptogenic cirrhosis. Two of the remaining patients underwent liver transplantation and five others declined to participate in the study. From the 15 patients with histology of microvesicular steatosis, two were excluded due to other overt etiology and four patients refused to participate in the trial. Nine NAFLD-patients with macrovesicular steatosis were also included. Altogether, the 22 patients in the study were analyzed as one group and as two groups, designated as higher-risk for LAL-d (13 patients, nine with microvesicular steatosis and four with cryptogenic cirrhosis) and lower-risk for LAL-d (nine patients with metabolic syndrome and NAFLD).

The mean age of all 22 patients participating in the study was $32.4 \pm 23.3$ (range 3.0–71.8) years, with similar distribution of males and females (Table 1). The ethnic origin of most participants was Arab and the rest were defined as Ashkenazi or Sephardi Jews. The age of the high-risk group was significantly lower ($p = 0.001$), while the rate of consanguinity and family history of fatty liver or cirrhosis were higher in this group ($p > 0.05$). As expected, systemic blood pressure, body mass index (BMI), and waist circumference were significantly higher in the low-risk group ($p = 0.023$–$0.028$, $p = 0.006$ and $p = 0.006$, respectively).

**Table 1.** Baseline characteristics of participants.

| Parmeters | Discriptors | High Risk $n$ = 13 | Low Risk $n$ = 9 | Total $n$ = 22 | $p$ |
|---|---|---|---|---|---|
| Age, years | Mean ± SD | 17.2 ± 12.3 | 54.3 ± 17.1 | 32.4 ± 23.3 | 0.0001 |
| | Median | 14.2 | 59.2 | 24.9 | - |
| | Range | 3.0–39.9 | 21.7–71.8 | 3.0–71.8 | - |
| Gender, Male, % | - | 61.5 | 44.4 | 54.5 | 0.666 |
| Origin, % | Ashkenazi Jew | 15.4 | 22.2 | 18.2 | 1.000 |
| | Sephardi Jew | 7.7 | 11.1 | 9.1 | - |
| | Arab | 76.9 | 66.7 | 72.7 | - |
| Consanguinity, % | - | 58.3 | 22.2 | 42.9 | 0.184 |
| Familial Fatty liver, % | - | 58.3 | 12.5 | 40 | 0.070 |
| Familial Cirrhosis, % | - | 33.3 | 0 | 21.1 | 0.245 |
| Smoking, % | - | 15.4 | 33.3 | 22.7 | 0.609 |
| SBP, mmHg | Mean ± SD | 116.9 ± 10.3 | 128.2 ± 10.3 | 121.8 ± 11.6 | 0.028 |
| | Median | 117.0 | 131.0 | 125.0 | - |
| DBP, mmHg | Mean ± SD | 66.1 ± 14.8 | 77.9 ± 6.1 | 71.1 ± 13.1 | 0.023 |
| | Median | 69.5 | 79.0 | 74.0 | - |
| BMI, kg/m² | Mean ± SD | 22.1 ± 6.8 | 33.4 ± 8.5 | 28.0 ± 89.5 | 0.006 |
| | Median | 19.95 | 30.1 | 26.2 | - |
| Waist C., m | Mean ± SD | 0.79 ± 0.11 | 1.07 ± 0.16 | 0.98 ± 0.2 | 0.006 |
| | Median | 0.80 | 1.01 | 0.95 | - |

SBP = Systolic blood pressure; DBP = Diastolic blood pressure; BMI = Body mass index; Waist C. = Waist circumference; SD = Standard deviation; m = meters; $n$ = number of patients. $p$ Value calculated by: Fisher's Exact Test, Exact Significance (2-sided); Mann-Whitney Test, Exact Significance (2*(1-tailed Sig.)).

Differences between groups were found for several laboratory tests. Alkaline phosphatase serum levels were significantly higher in the high-risk group (198.5 ± 76 $vs.$ 94 ± 33. $p < 0.001$); this may be attributed to the younger age of the patients in this group. In contrast, the low-risk group had significantly higher levels of urea (8.3 ± 2 $vs.$ 11.9 ± 2.9 $p < 0.006$), uric acid (234.8 ± 50 $vs.$ 347 ± 66, $p < 0.006$) and hematocrit (36.3 ± 5 $vs.$ 41 ± 4, $p < 0.03$). A significant difference was also noted in white blood cell count (WBC), glycated hemoglobin (HbA1c) and thyroid-stimulating hormone (TSH). Abdominal imaging and liver histologic assessments showed higher fibrosis scorings in the high-risk group ($p = 0.01$). However, imaging signs of portal hypertension and NAS biopsy scores were similar (Table 2).

**Table 2.** Imaging and histologic characterization of participants.

| Total ($n$ = 22) | High Risk Study Group ($n$ = 13) | Low Risk Control Group ($n$ = 9) | Total ($n$ = 22) | $p$ Value |
|---|---|---|---|---|
| Fatty liver, Imaging test, $n$ | 4 (31%) | 9 (100%) | 13 (59%) | 0.002 |
| Hepatomegaly, Imaging test, $n$ | 6 (46%) | 2 (22%) | 8 (36%) | 0.380 |
| Splenomegaly, Imaging test, $n$ | 6 (46%) | 3 (33%) | 9 (41%) | 0.674 |
| Hepatic Fibrosis, Imaging test, $n$ | 3 (23%) | 1 (11%) | 4 (18%) | 0.616 |
| Portal Hypertension, Imaging test, $n$ | 3 (23%) | 1 (11%) | 4 (18%) | 0.616 |
| Macrovesicular steatosis, Liver pathology, $n$ | 7 (54%) | 2 (22%) | 9 (41%) | 0.620 |
| Microvesicular steatosis, Liver pathology, $n$ | 7 (54%) | 0 | 7 (32%) | 0.044 |
| Liver fibrosis score, mean ± SD | 2.4 ± 1.1 | 1 ± 1.3 | 1.9 ± 1.3 | 0.01 |
| NAS scoring, Liver pathology | 2.8 ± 2 | 2.2 ± 2.2 | 2.6 ± 2 | 1.000 |

Imaging test = Ultrasound (US), Computed tomography (CT) or Magnetic resonance imaging (MRI); $p$ value calculated by Fisher's Exact Test, Exact Significance (2-sided).

## 2.2. Lysosomal Acid Lipase (LAL) Activity

Mean LAL activity was 0.74 (median 0.8, ±0.28) nmol/punch/h, and was similar in both risk groups. Subsequently, the entire cohort was analyzed according to two LAL cutoffs: 0.5 and

0.6 nmol/punch/h. Characterization of the cohort according to the cutoffs revealed similar composition with respect to age, gender, origin, weight, MBI, waist circumference, smoking rate, consanguinity, family history (of fatty liver or cirrhosis) and blood pressure (Table 3).

**Table 3.** Baseline characteristics of participants according to LAL cutoffs.

| Parmeters | Discriptors | LAL 0.5 Cutoff | | | LAL 0.6 Cutoff | | |
|---|---|---|---|---|---|---|---|
| | | <0.5 (n = 6) | ≥0.5 (n = 16) | p | <0.6 (n = 7) | ≥0.6 (n = 15) | p |
| Age, years | Mean ± SD | 46.3 ± 18.4 | 27.2 ± 23.3 | 0.08 | 40.7 ± 22.4 | 28.5 ± 23.5 | 0.26 |
| | Median | 52.5 | 18.6 | | 47.4 | 21.7 | |
| Males, n | | 2 | 10 | 0.34 | 3 | 9 | 0.65 |
| Jew, n | Ashkenazi | 2 | 2 | | 2 | 2 | |
| Jew, n | Sephardi | 0 | 2 | 0.57 | 0 | 2 | 0.60 |
| Arab, n | Palestinian | 4 | 12 | | 5 | 11 | |
| Consanguinity , n | | 2 | 7 | 1.00 | 3 | 6 | 1.00 |
| Familial Fatty liver, n | | 2 | 6 | 1.00 | 2 | 6 | 1.00 |
| Familial Cirrhosis, n | | 0 | 4 | 1.00 | 0 | 4 | 0.53 |
| Smoking, n | | 1 | 4 | 1.00 | 1 | 4 | 1.00 |
| SBP, mmHg | Mean ± SD | 122.17 ± 9.95 | 121.60 ± 12.52 | 0.97 | 121.14 ± 9.48 | 122.07 ± 12.85 | 0.69 |
| | Median | 122.50 | 126.00 | | 120.00 | 126.00 | |
| DBP, mmHg | Mean ± SD | 79.17 ± 8.59 | 67.93 ± 13.39 | 0.09 | 75.86 ± 11.75 | 68.79 ± 13.47 | 0.29 |
| | Median | 77.50 | 70.00 | | 74.00 | 71.50 | |
| BMI, kg/m² | Mean ± SD | 33.89 ± 12.77 | 25.66 ± 7.07 | 0.19 | 33.89 ± 12.77 | 25.66 ± 7.07 | 0.19 |
| | Median | 36.33 | 24.96 | | 36.33 | 24.96 | |
| Waist C., m | Mean ± SD | 1.16 ± 0.21 | 0.90 ± 0.13 | 0.08 | 1.16 ± 0.21 | 0.90 ± 0.13 | 0.08 |
| | Median | 1.19 | 0.94 | | 1.19 | 0.94 | |

SBP = Systolic blood pressure; DBP = Diastolic blood pressure; BMI = Body mass index; SD = Standard deviation; m = meters; n = number of patients; Waist C. = Waist Circumference. p Value calculated by: Fisher's Exact Test, Exact Significance (2-sided); Mann-Whitney Test, Exact Significance (2*(1-tailed Sig.)).

Table 4 shows selected parameters that differed significantly when analyzed according to LAL cutoffs. Significant differences were found for WBC, platelets (PLT), International Normalized Ratio (INR), $\gamma$-glutamyltransferase ($\gamma$GT), total protein, albumin, calcium, uric acid, creatinine, glucose and HbA1c. Other parameters that were analyzed but were not significantly different included hematological (hemoglobin, hematocrit (HCT)), biochemical (sodium, alanine aminotransferase (ALT), aspartate aminotransferase (AST), alkaline phosphatase (ALP), total bilirubin, direct bilirubin, phosphorous, urea, triglycerides, low-density lipoproteins (LDL), high-density lipoproteins (HDL) and total cholesterol), metabolic and inflammatory markers (TSH, vitamin D 25, ammonia, ferritin, C-reactive protein (CRP)), as well as $\alpha$-fetoprotein ($\alpha$FP). A threshold of LAL <0.5 was found to characterize six patients. All had marked macrosteatosis and hepatomegaly. LAL <0.5 identified eight severity markers of liver disease, including low calcium levels, a low WBC, high creatinine levels, high uric acid, high glucose and HbA1c, and high $\gamma$GT and prolonged INR. The seven patients with a LAL threshold <0.6 were the six mentioned above (for the LAL <0.5 threshold) and a child from the high-risk group with severe microvesicular steatosis and liver fibrosis complicated by portal hypertension. LAL <0.6 identified seven additional markers, including lower serum calcium, total protein and platelets, and increased glucose, HbA1c, uric acid and INR.

**Table 4.** Laboratory results of participants, according to LAL cutoffs.

| Parmeters | LAL Cutoff 0.5 | | | | | | | | | | LAL Cutoff 0.6 | | | | | | | | | |
| | LAL < 0.5 n = 6 | | | LAL ≥ 0.5 n = 16 | | | p | LAL < 0.6 n = 7 | | | LAL ≥ 0.6 n = 15 | | | p |
| | Mean | Median | SD | Mean | Median | SD | | Mean | Median | SD | Mean | Median | SD | |
|---|---|---|---|---|---|---|---|---|---|---|---|---|---|---|
| WBC | 6.64 | 7.01 | 1.36 | 9.33 | 8.76 | 3.31 | **0.029** | 6.95 | 7.11 | 1.49 | 9.37 | 8.59 | 3.43 | 0.079 |
| PLT(x1000) | 193 | 207 | 96 | 292 | 273 | 110 | 0.095 | 194 | 200 | 87 | 298 | 284 | 111 | **0.046** |
| INR | 1.25 | 1.17 | 0.28 | 1.06 | 1.02 | 0.11 | **0.046** | 1.23 | 1.09 | 0.26 | 1.05 | 1.02 | 0.12 | **0.022** |
| γGT | 147.02 | 135.50 | 104.84 | 61.70 | 35.00 | 59.41 | **0.036** | 129.44 | 108.00 | 106.41 | 64.84 | 37.50 | 60.91 | 0.100 |
| Total protein | 66.80 | 67.00 | 10.83 | 75.86 | 76.00 | 6.14 | 0.070 | 66.67 | 67.00 | 9.69 | 76.62 | 76.00 | 5.66 | **0.012** |
| Albumin | 38.17 | 43.00 | 10.94 | 43.80 | 44.00 | 5.68 | 0.178 | 37.86 | 43.00 | 10.02 | 44.36 | 44.50 | 5.46 | **0.056** |
| Calcium | 2.34 | 2.38 | 0.19 | 2.53 | 2.46 | 0.12 | **0.012** | 2.34 | 2.38 | 0.19 | 2.53 | 2.46 | 0.12 | **0.012** |
| Uric acid | 382.25 | 380.26 | 64.44 | 269.43 | 280.00 | 64.18 | **0.020** | 382.25 | 380.26 | 64.44 | 269.43 | 280.00 | 64.18 | **0.020** |
| Creatinine | 64.14 | 62.03 | 20.71 | 44.78 | 45.00 | 17.75 | **0.049** | 60.12 | 60.00 | 21.69 | 45.37 | 45.76 | 18.22 | 0.142 |
| Glucose | 6.60 | 6.46 | 0.80 | 5.18 | 5.01 | 0.91 | **0.005** | 6.70 | 6.72 | 0.78 | 5.04 | 4.90 | 0.74 | **<0.001** |
| HbA1c | 6.12 | 6.10 | 0.55 | 5.51 | 5.50 | 0.18 | **0.048** | 6.12 | 6.10 | 0.55 | 5.51 | 5.50 | 0.18 | **0.048** |

$p = p$ value, calculated by Mann-Whitney Test, Exact Significance [2*(1-tailed Sig)]. Significant values are in bold.

Abdominal imaging and liver histologi c characterization were also analyzed according to the LAL cutoffs (Table 5). There were no significant differences between LAL-groups. However, in the $\geqslant 0.5$ group the NAS score was significantly higher and the fibrosis score was marginally higher compared to the <0.5 group ($p = 0.06$) (Table 5). In conclusion, the LAL 0.5 threshold was the most sensitive for detecting both histologic and noninvasive markers for disease severity.

**Table 5.** Imaging and histologic characterization of participants according to LAL cutoffs.

| LAL Cutoff | LAL 0.5 | | | LAL 0.6 | | |
|---|---|---|---|---|---|---|
| | <0.5 (*n* = 6) | $\geqslant$0.5 (*n* = 16) | *p* | <0.6 (*n* = 7) | $\geqslant$0.6 (*n* = 15) | *p* |
| Fatty liver, Image, *n* | 4 | 9 | 1.0 | 4 | 9 | 1.0 |
| Hepatomegaly, Image, *n* | 2 | 6 | 1.0 | 3 | 5 | 1.0 |
| Splenomegaly, Image, *n* | 4 | 5 | 0.18 | 5 | 4 | 0.07 |
| Cirrhosis Liver, Image, *n* | 1 | 3 | 1.0 | 1 | 3 | 1.0 |
| PTH, Image, *n* | 2 | 2 | 0.29 | 3 | 1 | 0.08 |
| NAS score | 2.1 | 3.7 | 0.03 | 3.3 | 2 | 0.1 |
| Fibrosis score | 1.75 | 3 | 0.06 | 1.8 | 2.75 | 0.1 |

*p* = *p*-value, calculated by Fisher's Exact Test, Exact Significance (2-sided); NAS: Nonalcoholic steatohepatitis score, PTH = Portal Hypertension.

## 3. Discussion

Fatty liver disease is emerging as the leading liver disease with no current effective treatment. Although in most cases a metabolic syndrome is the cause of hepatic steatosis, other causes of fatty liver should also be considered. One of those diagnoses is lysosomal acid lipase deficiency (LAL-d), which is hopefully soon to be treatable with encouraging results from enzyme replacement therapy (Sebelipase Alfa, Kanuma®, New Haven, CT, USA). This was indeed our initial motivation for the current study. We aimed to assess LAL activity in patients with liver disease in order to provide suitable therapy. Thus, we measured levels of LAL in patients with cryptogenic cirrhosis, microvesicular steatosis and nonalcoholic fatty liver disease (NAFLD) related to a metabolic syndrome. Although no LAL-d was found, and no patient was eligible for enzyme replacement therapy, we did find that low LAL activity was associated with liver disease severity.

Our initial aim in the study was to compare patients with higher likelihood of genetically-low LAL activity (cryptogenic cirrhosis and microvesicular steatosis) to patients with NAFLD who we thought would be less likely to have low LAL activity. However, Baratta *et al.* [16] reported recently that patients with NAFLD have low LAL activity. As we could not find any statistical difference in LAL levels when we compared the two groups, we concluded that our study supports the study by Baratta *et al.* [16]. Subsequently, we analyzed our data according to two LAL levels. The analysis revealed significant differences that could be attributed to liver disease severity. A LAL threshold of 0.5 identified six patients with significantly higher histologic scorings and eight noninvasive markers (including low calcium levels and white blood cell count, and high creatinine, uric acid, glucose and HbA1c, and γGT levels and prolonged INR). A LAL threshold of 0.6 detected seven patients with seven markers (including low PLT count, calcium levels and total protein; prolonged INR; and high uric acid, glucose and HbA1c), but could not differentiate on the basis of histologic severity.

The blood work that was found to be different in patients with low LAL activity levels signifies indirect measures for liver disease severity. Low platelets and white blood counts serve as indirect markers for cirrhosis because of portal hypertension and hypersplenism. An elevated creatinine level, which is a marker of advanced liver disease and a strong predictor of survival in cirrhosis and [17] hepatorenal syndrome patients [18–20], was also observed in the lower-risk LAL group. With respect to insulin resistance, higher glucose and HbA1c levels were also observed for patients in the low LAL group and may signify more advanced fatty liver disease [21]. Interestingly, higher γGT levels were observed in the lower risk LAL group. This observation corresponds with the other disease severity markers, as γGT is regarded to be an independent predictive marker of morbidity and mortality in cardiovascular-related disorders, including coronary arterial disease, and congestive heart failure [17,22–25]. Higher uric acid levels may be a result of hypovolemia but also of advanced liver injury, accompanied by malnutrition and protein breakup, or a secondary renal injury [21]. Furthermore, when assessing the NAS score we found higher scores for NASH and fibrosis at low LAL levels. Taken together, all measures that were found to be different in the low LAL group signify hepatic and overall disease severity.

The association between low LAL activity and severity of liver injury merits further discussion. It may be considered that low LAL activity in patients with severe liver disease is merely a consequence of an overall decrease in viable hepatocytes that leads to lower protein production. On the other hand, various studies in animal models suggest that lower LAL activity may be part of the pathogenesis of fatty liver disease. The mechanism of lipid accumulation in hepatocytes is not completely elucidated but the role of lipases, including LAL is significant [26]. Autophagy is the key process in hepatic lipid metabolism and steatosis [27], and is the common pathway for the other liver diseases included in our study. Thus, other enzymes may be affected in our cohort. Nevertheless, the importance of measuring LAL activity lies in the potential for treatment with enzyme replacement therapy. Furthermore, the lysosomal-associated NK cells are crucial to prevent fibrosis progression in liver diseases [28,29] and LAL decrease uncovers an additional possible mechanism.

The major limitation of the study is the number of patients and the age range. Despite these limitations we still observed significant differences between the groups of patients with lower and higher LAL activity. It is hard to draw clear conclusions from these observation but they may set a basis for further studies to elucidate the role of LAL in each group of patients within a larger cohort.

## 4. Materials and Methods

### 4.1. Study Design

This study was conducted in the Liver Unit, Hadassah Medical Center, Jerusalem, Israel. The local ethics committee of Hadassah Medical Center approved the study (application 920120061, 24/05/2012) and written informed consent was obtained from all the participants or legal guardians in cases of minors. Patients aged 1–75 years who underwent liver biopsy during the years 2006–2012 were screened for the diagnosis of cryptogenic cirrhosis (according to ICD9 registration), microvesicular steatosis (according to liver pathology reports) and NAFLD with macrovesicular steatosis.

Exclusion criteria included daily alcohol intake >10 g/day, exposure to any other hepatotoxic agents, or evidence of other liver disease. Therefore, patients were excluded with the presence of serum hepatitis B surface antigen (HBsAg), hepatitis C viral (HCV) antibodies, HCV RNA, positive autoimmune serology, evidence for hemochromatosis, Wilson's disease (low ceruloplasmin serum levels and high liver tissue copper content) or α-1-antitrypsin disease (low α-1-antitrypsin levels with suggestive biopsy). Abdominal ultrasound was performed to exclude masses, obstruction of bile or blood vessels, but also provided features of liver steatosis and cirrhosis.

### 4.2. Study Groups

The cohort of patients was analyzed both as a whole group and as two groups: one consisting of patients with cryptogenic cirrhosis or microvesicular steatosis, and a second consisting of patients with NAFLD and macrovesicular steatosis.

### 4.3. Clinical Characterizations

Body mass index (BMI), blood pressure, waist circumference, concomitant diseases and medications were recorded at the time of LAL evaluation. Any results of abdominal imaging (Abdominal Ultrasound, Computerized Tomography and Magnetic Resonance) were documented, focusing on fatty liver appearance, hepatomegaly and splenomegaly and hepatic fibrosis (irregular hepatic appearance).

## 4.4. NAFLD Activity Score (NAS)

This score represented the sum of scores for steatosis, lobular inflammation, and ballooning, ranging from 0 to 8 according to Kleiner *et al.* [30]. Subjects with a NAS activity score of 0–2 were considered as having NAFLD. Biopsies with an activity score of 3 or more were considered as NASH. Fibrosis was ranked as follows: 0-none, 1-perisinusoidal or periportal, 2-perisinusoidal and periportal, 3-bridging fibrosis, 4-cirrhosis.

## 4.5. LAL Activity in Dried Blood Spots (DBS)

The test was performed as described previously by Hamilton *et al.* [31]. DBS values of 0.37–2.30 nmol/punch/h were interpreted as normal, 0.15–0.40 nmol/punch/h as carriers and <0.03 nmol/punch/h as CESD patients.

## 4.6. Statistical Analysis

All clinical, laboratory, imaging and pathological parameters were compared between the two groups using the $t$-test and the nonparametric Mann-Whitney $U$ test. Categorical parameters were compared using Fisher's exact test. All statistical tests were bilateral and a $p$-value of 5% or less was considered statistically significant.

## 5. Conclusions

In the current study we found that LAL activity correlates with hepatic steatosis and dysfunction. Our findings suggest a possible role for LAL in the pathogenesis of liver dysfunction and future studies may assist in finding subseta of patients who will benefit from enzyme replacement therapy. As our cohort is small, further larger groups should be studied in order to substantiate our findings.

**Acknowledgments:** This study was supported by grants from the Israel Scientific Foundation (ISF), the Chief Scientist of the Israeli Ministry of Health, and the Israel-American Bi-national Scientific Foundation (BSF) awards.

**Author Contributions:** Eyal Shteyer and Rifaat Safadi conceived and designed the experiments; Rivka Villenchik, Mahmud Mahamid and Nidaa Nator recruited the patients; Eyal Shteyer, Rivka Villenchik and Rifaat Safadi analyzed the data; Eyal Shteyer, Rivka Villenchik and Rifaat Safadi wrote the paper.

## References

1. Bellentani, S.; Marino, M. Epidemiology and natural history of non-alcoholic fatty liver disease (NAFLD). *Ann. Hepatol.* **2009**, *8*, S4–S8. [PubMed]
2. Sun, B.; Karin, M. Obesity, inflammation, and liver cancer. *J. Hepatol.* **2012**, *56*, 704–713. [CrossRef] [PubMed]
3. Machado, M.V.; Cortez-Pinto, H. Non-alcoholic fatty liver disease: What the clinician needs to know. *World J. Gastroenterol.* **2014**, *20*, 12956–12980. [CrossRef] [PubMed]
4. Gupte, P.; Amarapurkar, D.; Agal, S.; Baijal, R.; Kulshrestha, P.; Pramanik, S.; Patel, N.; Madan, A.; Amarapurkar, A. Non-alcoholic steatohepatitis in type 2 diabetes mellitus. *J. Gastroenterol. Hepatol.* **2004**, *19*, 854–858. [CrossRef] [PubMed]
5. Del Gaudio, A.; Boschi, L.; del Gaudio, G.A.; Mastrangelo, L.; Munari, D. Liver damage in obese patients. *Obes. Surg.* **2002**, *12*, 802–804. [CrossRef] [PubMed]
6. Baffy, G.; Brunt, E.M.; Caldwell, S.H. Hepatocellular carcinoma in non-alcoholic fatty liver disease: An emerging menace. *J. Hepatol.* **2012**, *56*, 1384–1391. [CrossRef] [PubMed]
7. Cohen, J.C.; Horton, J.D.; Hobbs, H.H. Human fatty liver disease: Old questions and new insights. *Science* **2011**, *332*, 1519–1523. [CrossRef] [PubMed]
8. Michelotti, G.A.; Machado, M.V.; Diehl, A.M. NAFLD, NASH and liver cancer. *Nat. Rev. Gastroenterol. Hepatol.* **2013**, *10*, 656–665. [CrossRef] [PubMed]

9. Reiner, Z.; Guardamagna, O.; Nair, D.; Soran, H.; Hovingh, K.; Bertolini, S.; Jones, S.; Ćorić, M.; Calandra, S.; Hamilton, J.; *et al.* Lysosomal acid lipase deficiency—An under-recognized cause of dyslipidaemia and liver dysfunction. *Atherosclerosis* **2014**, *235*, 21–30. [CrossRef] [PubMed]

10. Bernstein, D.L.; Hulkova, H.; Bialer, M.G.; Desnick, R.J. Cholesteryl ester storage disease: Review of the findings in 135 reported patients with an underdiagnosed disease. *J. Hepatol.* **2013**, *58*, 1230–1243. [CrossRef] [PubMed]

11. Haga, Y.; Kanda, T.; Sasaki, R.; Nakamura, M.; Nakamoto, S.; Yokosuka, O. Nonalcoholic fatty liver disease and hepatic cirrhosis: Comparison with viral hepatitis-associated steatosis. *World J. Gastroenterol.* **2015**, *21*, 12989–12995. [CrossRef] [PubMed]

12. Ginsberg, H.N.; Le, N.A.; Short, M.P.; Ramakrishnan, R.; Desnick, R.J. Suppression of apolipoprotein B production during treatment of cholesteryl ester storage disease with lovastatin. Implications for regulation of apolipoprotein B synthesis. *J. Clin. Investig.* **1987**, *80*, 1692–1697. [CrossRef] [PubMed]

13. Aslanidis, C.; Ries, S.; Fehringer, P.; Buchler, C.; Klima, H.; Schmitz, G. Genetic and biochemical evidence that CESD and Wolman disease are distinguished by residual lysosomal acid lipase activity. *Genomics* **1996**, *33*, 85–93. [CrossRef] [PubMed]

14. Saito, S.; Ohno, K.; Suzuki, T.; Sakuraba, H. Structural bases of Wolman disease and cholesteryl ester storage disease. *Mol. Genet. Metab.* **2012**, *105*, 244–248. [CrossRef] [PubMed]

15. Pagani, F.; Pariyarath, R.; Garcia, R.; Stuani, C.; Burlina, AB.; Ruotolo, G.; Rabusin, M.; Baralle, F.E. New lysosomal acid lipase gene mutants explain the phenotype of Wolman disease and cholesteryl ester storage disease. *J. Lipid Res.* **1998**, *39*, 1382–1388. [PubMed]

16. Baratta, F.; Pastori, D.; del Ben, M.; Polimeni, L.; Labbadia, G.; di Santo, S.; Piemonte, F.; Tozzi, G.; Violi, F.; Angelico, F. Reduced lysosomal acid lipase activity in adult patients with non-alcoholic fatty liver disease. *EBioMedicine* **2015**, *2*, 750–754. [CrossRef] [PubMed]

17. Jiang, S.; Jiang, D.; Tao, Y. Role of γ-glutamyltransferase in cardiovascular diseases. *Exp. Clin. Cardiol.* **2013**, *18*, 53–56. [PubMed]

18. Li, G.; Shi, W.; Hug, H.; Chen, Y.; Liu, L.; Yin, D. Nonalcoholic fatty liver disease associated with impairment of kidney function in nondiabetes population. *Biochem. Med.* **2012**, *22*, 92–99. [CrossRef]

19. Lau, T.; Ahmad, J. Clinical applications of the model for end-stage liver disease (MELD) in hepatic medicine. *Hepat. Med.* **2013**, *5*, 1–10. [PubMed]

20. Hartleb, M.; Gutkowski, K. Kidneys in chronic liver diseases. *World J. Gastroenterol.* **2012**, *18*, 3035–3049. [CrossRef] [PubMed]

21. Miyake, T.; Kumagi, T.; Furukawa, S.; Tokumoto, Y.; Hirooka, M.; Abe, M.; Hiasa, Y.; Matsuura, B.; Onji, M. Non-alcoholic fatty liver disease: Factors associated with its presence and onset. *J. Gastroenterol. Hepatol.* **2013**, *28*, 71–78. [CrossRef] [PubMed]

22. Lee, D.S.; Evans, J.C.; Robins, S.J.; Wilson, P.W.; Albano, I.; Fox, C.S.; Wang, T.J.; Benjamin, E.J.; D'Agostino, R.B.; Vasan, R.S. γ Glutamyl transferase and metabolic syndrome, cardiovascular disease, and mortality risk: The framingham heart study. *Arterioscler Thromb. Vasc. Biol.* **2007**, *27*, 127–133. [CrossRef] [PubMed]

23. Onat, A.; Can, G.; Ornek, E.; Cicek, G.; Ayhan, E.; Dogan, Y. Serum γ-glutamyltransferase: Independent predictor of risk of diabetes, hypertension, metabolic syndrome, and coronary disease. *Obesity* **2012**, *20*, 842–848. [CrossRef] [PubMed]

24. Liu, C.F.; Zhou, W.N.; Fang, N.Y. γ-Glutamyltransferase levels and risk of metabolic syndrome: A meta-analysis of prospective cohort studies. *Int. J. Clin. Pract.* **2012**, *66*, 692–698. [CrossRef] [PubMed]

25. Nakchbandi, I.A. Osteoporosis and fractures in liver disease: Relevance, pathogenesis and therapeutic implications. *World J. Gastroenterol.* **2014**, *20*, 9427–9438. [PubMed]

26. Czaja, M.J. Autophagy in health and disease. 2. Regulation of lipid metabolism and storage by autophagy: Pathophysiological implications. *Am. J. Physiol. Cell Physiol.* **2010**, *298*, C973–C978. [CrossRef] [PubMed]

27. Singh, R.; Kaushik, S.; Wang, Y.; Xiang, Y.; Novak, I.; Komatsu, M.; Keiji, T.; Cuervo, A.M.; Czaja, M.J. Autophagy regulates lipid metabolism. *Nature* **2009**, *458*, 1131–1135. [CrossRef] [PubMed]

28. Melhem, A.; Muhanna, N.; Bishara, A.; Alvarez, C.E.; Ilan, Y.; Bishara, T.; Horani, A.; Nassar, M.; Friedman, S.L.; Safadi, R. Anti-fibrotic activity of NK cells in experimental liver injury through killing of activated HSC. *J. Hepatol.* **2006**, *45*, 60–71. [CrossRef] [PubMed]

29. Gur, C.; Doron, S.; Kfir-Erenfeld, S.; Horwitz, E.; Abu-Tair, L.; Safadi, R.; Mandelboim, O. NKp46-mediated killing of human and mouse hepatic stellate cells attenuates liver fibrosis. *Gut* **2012**, *61*, 885–893. [CrossRef] [PubMed]
30. Kleiner, D.E.; Brunt, E.M.; van Natta, M.; Polimeni, L.; Labbadia, G.; di Santo, S.; Piemonte, F.; Tozzi, G.; Violi, F.; Angelico, F. Design and validation of a histological scoring system for nonalcoholic fatty liver disease. *Hepatology* **2005**, *41*, 1313–1321. [CrossRef] [PubMed]
31. Hamilton, J.; Jones, I.; Srivastava, R.; Galloway, P. A new method for the measurement of lysosomal acid lipase in dried blood spots using the inhibitor Lalistat 2. *Clin. Chim. Acta* **2012**, *413*, 1207–1210. [CrossRef] [PubMed]

# 5

# Extracellular Vesicles: A New Frontier in Biomarker Discovery for Non-Alcoholic Fatty Liver Disease

**Linda A. Ban [1], Nicholas A. Shackel [2] and Susan V. McLennan [1,\*]**

[1]   Greg Brown Diabetes and Endocrine Laboratory, Charles Perkins Centre, University of Sydney, NSW 2006, Australia; linda.ban@sydney.edu.au

[2]   Liver Cell Biology Laboratory, Centenary Institute of Cancer Medicine and Cell Biology, Camperdown, NSW 2006, Australia; n.shackel@centenary.usyd.edu.au

\*   Correspondence: sue.mclennan@sydney.edu.au

Academic Editors: Amedeo Lonardo and Giovanni Targher

**Abstract:** In recent years, the global burden of obesity and diabetes has seen a parallel rise in other metabolic complications, such as non-alcoholic fatty liver disease (NAFLD). This condition, once thought to be a benign accumulation of hepatic fat, is now recognized as a serious and prevalent disorder that is conducive to inflammation and fibrosis. Despite the rising incidence of NAFLD, there is currently no reliable method for its diagnosis or staging besides the highly invasive tissue biopsy. This limitation has resulted in the study of novel circulating markers as potential candidates, one of the most popular being extracellular vesicles (EVs). These submicron membrane-bound structures are secreted from stressed and activated cells, or are formed during apoptosis, and are known to be involved in intercellular communication. The cargo of EVs depends upon the parent cell and has been shown to be changed in disease, as is their abundance in the circulation. The role of EVs in immunity and epigenetic regulation is widely attested, and studies showing a correlation with disease severity have made these structures a favorable target for diagnostic as well as therapeutic purposes. This review will highlight the research that is available on EVs in the context of NAFLD, the current limitations, and projections for their future utility in a clinical setting.

**Keywords:** biomarkers; diagnosis; exosomes; extracellular vesicles; microvesicles; NAFLD; non-alcoholic steatohepatitis (NASH); steatosis; steatohepatitis

## 1. Introduction

Obesity is rapidly evolving into a global pandemic, and poses a significant healthcare and socioeconomic burden. Its increased prevalence in both developed and developing nations has seen a rise in other serious metabolic complications, such as cardiovascular disease, type 2 diabetes mellitus and non-alcoholic fatty liver disease (NAFLD). Although diabetes is a common risk factor for NAFLD progression and *vice versa* [1–4], lean or non-diabetic patients also develop NAFLD [5–7], and so biochemical rather than anthropometric parameters would likely be of greater utility in diagnosis or prognosis of the disease.

To address this issue, the World Gastroenterology Organisation (WGO) recently published a set of comprehensive guidelines on the assessment and management of NAFLD [8], with emphasis on the distinction between simple steatosis and non-alcoholic steatohepatitis (NASH). The latter represents the advanced manifestation of the NAFLD spectrum whereby inflammation and fibrosis are also present, and is a condition which is much easier to identify than simple steatosis. However, limitations with current diagnostic methods, such as unreliable imaging techniques and serum markers, have meant that tissue biopsy remains the gold standard for NASH diagnosis [9–14]. Irrespective of this, biopsy is a highly invasive procedure and subject to variability through sampling error [15–17].

Moreover, it cannot predict disease progression, and, for this reason, there is increasing emphasis on the identification of stable non-invasive markers specific for liver disease progression.

At this stage, effective early detection is poor as patients usually do not report symptoms until they have progressed to NASH or cirrhosis. Serum biochemistry that reveals elevated liver transaminases in the absence of excessive alcohol consumption or other liver disease is the most typical indicator of NAFLD, while anthropometric data such as a high body mass index (considered obese if above 35 kg/m$^2$) may warrant further screening for visceral fat accumulation in the liver [8]. It must nonetheless be stressed that despite the increased likelihood, not all obese individuals will develop NAFLD/NASH, and so probing for markers of steatosis in global metabolic disorders should therefore address what is known about the mechanisms of disease within the target organ. Ideal marker candidates should reflect not only the presence of NAFLD, but also the severity of disease, which is vital for early diagnosis as well grading progression [13].

This review aims to introduce the concept of using circulating cell-derived vesicles as novel markers of NAFLD, with an emphasis on their role in diagnosis and the assessment of disease pathology. Drawing on recent evidence from the literature, the paradigm of "marker *versus* mediator" will be discussed, as well as insight into their potential as therapeutic targets.

## 2. Novel Biomarkers in Liver Disease

In the latter half of the last century, shedding of vesicles from the cell membrane was identified as an inconsequential by-product of cell degradation [18,19]. However, clinical studies supported by research findings have recently pointed to the regulated secretion of these extracellular vesicles and their role in intercellular communication. Moreover, the abundance as well as the phenotype of circulating vesicles is reported to change in many disease states, including liver diseases [20–23] and metabolic disorders such as diabetes and obesity [24–27]. As such, much interest has been invested in characterising these structures for their potential utility in diagnostics, especially for conditions where this is otherwise notoriously difficult, such as NAFLD.

### 2.1. Extracellular Vesicles: What Are They?

Extracellular vesicles (EVs) are collectively represented by three subclasses of membrane-bound structures that are distinguished based on their size, typical markers, and biogenesis [28–30] (see Figure 1). Exosomes are the smallest vesicles, usually below 100 nm in diameter, and are formed within multivesicular bodies (MVB) that release their contents into the interstitium upon fusion with the cell membrane. These exocytosed EVs are characterised by their expression of membrane tetraspanins, most notably CD63, as well as the endosomal sorting complex required for transport (ESCRT)-associated protein Alix, both of which reflect the MVB origin of exosomes [29,31,32].

In contrast, microvesicles (MVs) are shed directly from the cell membrane by a "budding" process and typically range in size from around 100 to 1000 nm, although these values are somewhat arbitrary and subclass overlap may exist [29]. MVs are identified by the expression of phosphatidylserine (PS) on their surface, which is indicative of their release from activated or apoptotic cells. In these cells PS is externalized, whereas in quiescent cells the membrane PS has a cytosolic orientation [33,34]. Most studies utilise the fact that Annexin V—a soluble protein used in the detection of apoptotic cells—binds with high affinity to PS and is therefore a useful marker of the MV subclass. Meanwhile, some groups have argued that a majority of circulating MVs are in fact PS-negative, whilst others have proposed that measurement of lactadherin may be a more sensitive alternative to Annexin V [35–37]. Despite ongoing controversies in their characterisation, both EV populations have ultimately been shown to impart functional properties of their parent cells through the transfer of proteins, mRNAs, and particularly microRNAs (or miRNAs) that are subsequently involved in epigenetic regulation [38,39].

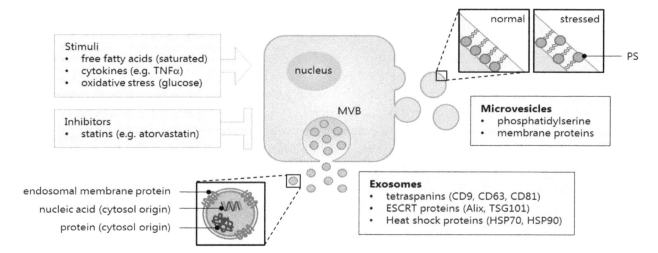

**Figure 1.** Extracellular vesicle characterisation. Cells respond to a variety of stimuli that cause inflammation and metabolic stress, which result in their activation, impaired functioning, or apoptosis. This mechanism drives the release of extracellular vesicles (EVs), which signal to paracrine or distal effectors the condition of the cell microenvironment. Effector cells may, in turn, respond by selectively imparting regulatory molecules—small nucleic acids (mRNA and miRNA), lipids, and proteins—contained within EVs, that are taken up by the recipient cell. The EV subclasses are identified by membrane markers that denote the site of their biogenesis. Exosomes typically express endosomal membrane proteins, such as tetraspanins, while microvesicles are understood to contain phosphatidylserine. These lipoproteins are normally oriented towards the cytosol to maintain the cell membrane asymmetry, but during conditions that stimulate EV release, the molecules become everted. Abbreviations: ESCRT = endosomal sorting complex required for transport; MVB = multivesicular body; PS = phosphatidylserine.

Finally, apoptotic bodies represent the largest EV subclass in terms of their size, ranging from one to four microns. Since this is comparable with platelets, studies that use size exclusion techniques to isolate circulating EVs, such as ultracentrifugation or filtration, will usually lose this population of vesicles with larger contaminants [40]. Furthermore, as apoptotic bodies are formed during the compartmentalization of apoptotic cells, they are generally assumed to be inert particles destined for phagocytosis, although their horizontal gene-transfer capacity has been documented [41,42].

*2.2. Role of Extracellular Vesicles in Liver Disease*

Almost all cell types ubiquitously release low levels of extracellular vesicles. In normal physiology, most circulating EVs are derived from platelets and endothelial cells, and have been shown to be important in common haemostatic events such as coagulation [43]. While vesicles of the same origin have been implicated in disease complications of a pro-coagulative nature [44,45], there is still a paucity of knowledge regarding the dynamics of EV secretion by different cell types and in particular how the secreted EVs interact to advance the pathogenesis of a given disease. Controlled *in vitro* experiments have provided the most direct lines of evidence for EV regulation, including how the stimulus for release may affect their phenotype [46]. There is a wealth of research using liver injury models to explore EV-mediated fibrosis [47–49], transcriptomic signalling [50–54], and targeted immunotherapy [55–57] in artificial cell culture systems. However, *in vivo* studies present an added degree of complexity due to the difficulty of identifying liver specific EVs within the circulating pool. For this reason, most studies have opted to focus on circulating vesicle characterisation and their temporal changes in relation to liver disease development [58–63], while others have pointed to roles in extrahepatic cancer metastasis to the liver [64–66], although functional relationships have yet to be explored.

Some groups have approached the study of EVs from a more organ-targeted perspective, assessing their role as paracrine mediators. Most of these studies evaluate the effect of EVs in fibrogenesis, for example, the shuttling of pro-fibrogenic connective tissue growth factor (CTGF) between hepatic stellate cells on the one hand [47], or the CTGF inhibiting miRNA-214 between stellate cells and hepatocytes or adjacent stellate cells on the other hand [48]. Immune-mediated modulation has also been suggested; one study had demonstrated a role for T cell-derived EVs in the induction of stellate cell fibrolytic activity, as defined by an increase in the gene expression of matrix metalloproteinases (MMPs) [49]. The findings concluded that this response from the stellate cells was likely mediated by the homodimeric interaction of CD147 at the EV-cell interface. A pro-inflammatory glycoprotein, CD147 had previously been implicated in liver disease pathogenesis by our group [67,68] as well as having a well document role in tumour metastasis, which more recently had been attributed to EV-mediated translocation [69–71]. Secreted vesicles have also been linked to paracrine signalling in the tumour microenvironment, whereby miRNAs shuttled from hepatoma cells were able to modulate protein expression in adjacent hepatocytes and to increase their proliferative potential [50,51]. Silencing of these miRNAs, in turn, had abrogated the pro-tumorigenic effects, while another study had suggested a role for liver stem cell-derived EVs in miRNA-mediated tumour suppression [52].

### 2.3. Markers or Mediators of Liver Disease?

Taken together, this body of evidence highlights the growing expanse of EV research pertaining to liver disease, and on the contrary, a relative paucity of data regarding the involvement of EVs in NAFLD progression to NASH. Additionally, it introduces the "marker *versus* mediator" paradigm when addressing the functionality of EVs. This plays an important role in EV analysis; for instance, in the context of NAFLD, global changes in the circulating pool (marker) may not reflect the local interactions within specific tissues, such as the liver, that drive pathogenesis at these sites (mediator). However, a circulating profile that is unique to a given disease etiology would still substantiate the use of EVs as non-invasive diagnostic markers, a concept that is discussed further in the section below.

## 3. Studies in Non-Alcoholic Fatty Liver Disease

Liver research involving EVs as disease mediators faces a number of inherent challenges. The most important of these is finding a link between the circulating EV populations and a specific contribution from the liver. From a biomarker perspective, it could be argued that a quantitative or phenotypic change in circulating EVs with disease may validate their diagnostic utility, especially if these changes are intensified with NAFLD progression (see Table 1). Unfortunately, given the complex biological determinants of EV secretion, rather than a linear relationship we are more likely to see dynamic responses from different tissues during the course of pathogenesis (see Figure 2). For a start, NAFLD is not an isolated condition and, generally speaking, occurs as a complication of other metabolic disorders where global insulin resistance is also present. Therefore, multiple tissues may be affected by the resulting oxidative stress and fatty acid flux, which in turn promotes the activation of immune cells and their migration to these sites. Consequently, the extrahepatic release of EVs may in fact mask the pathogenesis of NAFLD. For this reason, and the lack of a specifically hepatic molecular marker, ideal studies should examine the circulating EVs against their liver-derived counterparts, where possible.

**Table 1.** Extracellular vesicle markers in non-alcoholic fatty liver disease (NAFLD) studies.

| Vesicle Source | | Marker(s) | Key Study Findings | Citation |
|---|---|---|---|---|
| Circulating | Lymphoid cells | CD4<br>CD8<br>Va24/Vb11 | Enriched in NAFLD, positively correlated with serum ALT and liver biopsy | [72] |
| | Myeloid cells | CD14<br>CD15 | Variable; CD14$^+$ (monocyte origin) enriched in NAFLD, positively correlated with serum ALT; CD15$^+$ (neutrophil origin) opposite trend | [72] |
| | Erythrocytes | TER119 | Comprise the majority of circulating EVs during Western diet | [73] |
| | Platelets | CD41<br>CD62P | Conflicting data for abundance in NAFLD; reduced with statin intervention | [72,74] |
| | Liver | ASGPR1<br>CES1<br>miR-122<br>miR-192 | Enriched in NAFLD; miR-122 and miR-192 correlated with decreased liver expression | [75–77] |
| | Endothelial | CD144 | Enriched in NAFLD; reduced with statin intervention | [74] |
| Tissue derived | Adipose | adiponectin<br>IL-6<br>MCP-1<br>MIF | Enriched in adipose origin; with the exception of adiponectin, enriched in visceral *versus* subcutaneous adipose | [78] |
| | Hepatocytes | Vanin-1 | Enriched in steatotic hepatocytes (HepG2 cells treated with palmitate) | [76] |

Abbreviations: ALT = alanine transaminase; ASGPR1 = asialoglycoprotein receptor 1; CES1 = (liver) carboxylesterase 1; IL-6 = interleukin 6; iNKT = invariant natural killer T [cell]; MCP-1 = monocyte chemotactic protein 1; MIF = (macrophage) migration inhibitory factor; NAFLD = non-alcoholic fatty liver disease; Va24/Vb11 = T cell receptor covariants a24/b11.

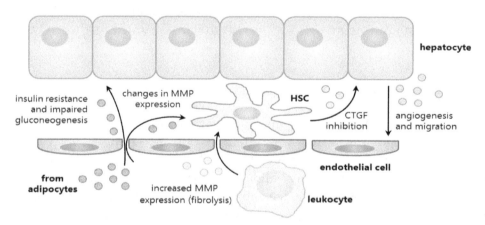

**Figure 2.** Extracellular vesicle roles in non-alcoholic fatty liver disease (NAFLD). EVs are involved in intercellular communication within the liver tissue, between hepatic cells as well as other tissues involved in mediating NAFLD pathogenesis, such as adipose and circulating (liver-homing) leukocytes. Collectively, these EVs are involved in a dynamic response that may exacerbate tissue injury, as well as promoting repair and matrix remodelling. Abbreviations: CTGF = connective tissue growth factor; HSC = hepatic stellate cell; MMP = matrix metalloproteinase.

## 3.1. Animal Studies

The fact that such issues remain to be addressed can be explained by the relative infancy of this field of research. To date, there are fewer than a dozen studies to have documented a role for EV signalling in a model of NAFLD, the earliest reported as late as 2009 in mice [79]. To better define a role for EVs in the development of hepatic steatosis, researchers have sought to replicate the clinical observations in rodent models of NAFLD, simulated by administering a choline-deficient diet (CDD) or high-fat diet (HFD) *ad libitum* for several weeks, the latter of which more accurately reflects the development of human metabolic syndrome. It should also be noted, that while CDD animals have comparable liver triglycerides to HFD animals, and a much more rapid progression to hepatic fibrosis, other typical changes such as increased body weight and fat depots, insulin resistance, and elevated fasting glucose and fatty acids are not observed [80]. This is due to the fact that, while HFD feeding increases lipid production, choline deficiency results in mitochondrial dysfunction and hence prevents the normal breakdown of lipids [81]. In saying that, contrary to what would be expected, EV studies in rodent models of NAFLD showed similar trends for both diets (see Table 2).

**Table 2.** Important findings for extracellular vesicles in the context of NAFLD.

| | Key Study Findings | Disease Model | Vesicle Source | Methods | Citation |
|---|---|---|---|---|---|
| Rodent | NAFLD-inducing diet increases circulating EV abundance | HFD CDD | plasma | FC | [74–76] |
| | Circulating EV abundance correlates with NAFLD progression | CDD | plasma | FC | [75,76] |
| | NAFLD-inducing diet increases circulating liver-derived EVs | HFD CDD | plasma serum | RT-qPCR | [75–77] |
| | NAFLD-inducing diet changes circulating EV contents | CDD | plasma | LCMS WB | [75,76] |
| | NAFLD-inducing diet changes circulating EV interactions with cells | HFD | plasma | FC | [79] |
| Human | Circulating EV abundance correlates with NAFLD progression | NASH | plasma | FC | [72] |
| | Circulating EV contents can distinguish NAFLD from other liver diseases | NASH | plasma serum | FC microarray | [72,82] |

Abbreviations: CDD = choline deficient diet, EV = extracellular vesicle, FC = flow cytometry, HFD = high-fat diet, LCMS = liquid chromatography with mass spectrometry, NAFLD = non-alcoholic fatty liver disease, NASH = non-alcoholic steatohepatitis, RT-qPCR = real-time quantitative polymerase chain reaction, WB = western blot.

In the original study, Deng and colleagues described a phenomenon in their chronic HFD model whereby circulating EVs that were adoptively transferred to healthy animals were engulfed by myeloid cells that subsequently accumulated in the liver [79]. This phenotype was not observed when EVs were transferred from animals on a normal chow diet, which may suggest a selective, EV-driven mechanism for hepatic inflammation as a concomitant to steatosis. While these findings are yet to be reproduced, other groups have instead begun to more comprehensively examine the profile of circulating EVs to better understand their temporal regulation, contents, and possible intervention strategies. Indeed it was shown that vesicles tend to increase on a background of NAFLD, and do so in a time-dependent manner, according to data obtained from flow cytometry experiments [74–76].

To evaluate how the liver contributes to this population, EVs were assessed for their expression of miRNA-122, a molecule that is enriched in mammalian livers and is shown to be involved in early NAFLD progression [83–85]. Consistent with previous findings, rodent studies confirmed an increase in circulating EV-associated miRNA-122 accompanied by a decrease in the liver expression of this molecule [75–77]. Furthermore, one study demonstrated that when miRNA-122 was trafficked in EVs, it was not associated with its protein binding partner Argonaute 2, a phenomenon that is otherwise typically observed in non-disease conditions [75]. While other miRNAs and proteins were not correlated against disease severity, Povero and colleagues had employed mass spectrometry to identify an EV-specific proteome in NAFLD that was distinct from healthy controls [75]. These findings complement a previous study done by the group, in which they confirm a role for EV-bound Vanin-1 in hepatocyte vesicle uptake by an endothelial cell line, with subsequent angiogenic behaviour that is only observed when EVs are derived from hepatocytes subjected to lipotoxic stress [76].

Taken together, these studies establish a solid foundation for understanding the role of EVs in NAFLD, however, some notable limitations exist. Firstly, changes in EV phenotype were not correlated against histological severity of liver disease, which would otherwise give some insight into their prognostic value. Furthermore, perhaps an emphasis on distinguishing NAFLD from other underlying liver pathologies would give EVs a stronger diagnostic utility, as had been addressed in the clinical studies below.

### 3.2. Human Studies

The pioneering study to involve human subjects was published three years later by Kornek and colleagues, who for the first time had suggested a correlation between the circulating abundance of leukocyte-derived EVs and disease severity, as determined by liver transaminase levels, biopsy grade, and NAFLD activity score (NAS) [72]. These findings still provide the most compelling evidence in clinical samples for the prognostic value of EVs in NASH development, and have been extensively cited. The authors have additionally noted a distinction between the circulating NAFLD EV profile and that seen in hepatitis C patients. This is further supported by another study where transcriptomic analysis revealed that serum exosome-derived miRNAs are capable of differentiating multiple aetiologies of liver disease, as well as disease from normal liver controls [82]. Similar to the first study, it was shown that the expression level of some miRNAs was regulated either positively or negatively with histological features of disease, such as inflammation and fibrosis. However, these results were limited to the cohort with chronic hepatitis and no such data was available for NAFLD progression to NASH.

More recent studies have described the modulation of hepatocyte and stellate cell activity by EVs isolated from visceral (peritoneal) adipose tissue. While the subjects did not necessarily present with NAFLD, the *ex vivo* experimental designs instead aimed to establish a role for EVs in potentially mediating this disease. As such, Kranendonk and colleagues showed that adipocyte EVs from non-obese patients were capable of interfering with insulin signalling and gluconeogenesis when directly exposed to a hepatocyte cell line [78]. Furthermore, the concentration of EVs correlated positively with expression of liver transaminases, which supports the evidence for their role in hepatocyte dysfunction. In another study, albeit on a smaller scale, adipose tissue isolated from obese patients released EVs in culture that subsequently altered the gene expression of an MMP inhibitor, TIMP-1, in both hepatocytes and stellate cells [86]. Collectively, these findings suggest a novel mechanism of NAFLD pathogenesis by EVs through adipocyte-mediated hepatic cell stress and tissue remodelling.

## 4. Understanding the Role of Secreted Vesicles

With the urgency to develop a non-invasive biomarker for the diagnosis and staging of NAFLD, research into the biology of extracellular vesicles has provided an opportunity to explore a novel mechanism of disease pathogenesis that can also be harnessed as a clinical tool. However, there is still a long way to go before EV-related assays will have translational utility. Besides the obvious question of disease and tissue specificity, current techniques used in the isolation and characterisation of EVs remain laborious, and suffer from a lack of standardization, as well as high variability. It will undoubtedly take a few years before the processing of EVs from blood and other bodily fluids as "liquid biopsies" becomes economically viable, reproducible and validated. Until then we are unlikely to see their use in routine clinical practice.

While much can be learned from the studies described in this review, the concept of analysing EVs in the context of NAFLD is still very much a small niche in the literature. One reason could be the limitations mentioned above, or a focus on more accessible biochemistries such as liver transaminases and soluble miRNA-122. But then why look at circulating EVs? Perhaps the answer lies in their active role in disease; they may not only confirm the presence of NAFLD, but also give an insight into which tissues are interacting and how this is driving pathogenesis. It has been shown that adipose tissue EVs taken from obese individuals are capable of signalling to hepatic cells to remodel their extracellular milieu, while these cells in turn may communicate via EVs with the sinusoid to promote angiogenesis [76,86]. Circulating vesicles have also been implicated in the innate immune response that accompanies steatosis, pointing to a role in the progression from early NAFLD to NASH [72,79]. From a physiological perspective, it makes sense to encapsulate certain molecules that are otherwise prone to enzymatic degradation, especially in a complex or unpredictable disease environment. However, if preservation of these molecules within EVs leads to a heightened stimulation of inflammatory cells, as previously suggested, this mechanism may in turn be responsible for the exacerbation of tissue injury.

Whether EVs can be considered as friend or foe in metabolic diseases is still a grey area, and likely depends on the tissue of origin. Their use as a biomarker is further complicated by the possibility of temporal fluctuation or waning, as is seen with liver enzymes in models of NAFLD [87,88], which limits their predictive value. Furthermore, high-powered micrographs of liver sections have shown that hepatic EVs are predominantly located in the perisinusoidal region [75,76], which may indicate their entrapment in the liver, contrary to previous findings described in this review and also within the same studies. This idea is supported by the fact that the sinusoidal endothelium undergoes defenestration with progressive fibrosis, as well as aging [89], which may restrict the normal flux of vesicles and macromolecules within the liver. Alternatively, the accumulation of fibrous tissue in the perisinusoid may also limit the passage of EVs, or provide selective permeability to smaller vesicles. However, whether this is a protective mechanism or passive consequence of disease is yet to be elucidated.

*What Does the Future Hold?*

The multifaceted nature of EVs suggests that these structures may have potential value beyond their use as circulating biomarkers in NAFLD. For instance, cancer studies have explored the transfer of oncogenes and an oncogenic phenotype through EV uptake in cell culture models [41,90,91], which may provide a target for therapeutic intervention. Indeed, it was shown that incubating hepatoma cells with various anti-cancer drugs promoted the secretion of immunogenic EVs that were capable of enhancing natural killer (NK) cell responses [55,56]. Conversely, exposing macrophages to such drugs may induce the release of EV-derived miRNAs, which suppress cancer growth by epigenetic regulation [57]. This concept has been extended to NAFLD models, where it was found that administering cholesterol-lowering drugs to high-fat fed rodents can attenuate the release of EVs, however the exact implication of this was not discussed, except for a potential reduction in liver cell death [73,74].

Another approach is to use the vesicles themselves as a mode or target of therapy, not simply a marker of injury. This idea has been investigated since the late 1980s, whereby synthetic EVs were used as a vehicle for drug delivery in both *in vitro* and *in vivo* models of liver injury [92,93]. It is also possible that in the future, endogenous EVs may be harvested for similar purposes, providing an efficient technique for tissue-specific delivery of molecules. The advantage of this autologous transfer system is that the vesicles are less likely to be rejected by the patient, however still sufficiently immunogenic to elicit a response [79].

## 5. Conclusions

With the rapid advancement of technology, it can be expected that once EVs become a routine parameter for assessment of disease status—of especial value in conditions that are difficult to diagnose, such as NAFLD—their utility may be further projected to the treatment of disease in its early stages, and potentially the reversal of chronic disorders like NASH. While there is still a long way to go, for the time being it is important to focus on controlling the underlying metabolic disorders through traditional intervention methods and lifestyle changes, which would also slow the progression of its comorbidities. However, detection of NAFLD and its staging continues to be a problem with invasive techniques such as biopsy being the gold standard. For this reason, EV analysis has promise as a non-invasive diagnostic tool.

**Acknowledgments:** Linda A. Ban is supported by a grant from the Greg Brown Diabetes and Endocrine Trust Fund.

**Author Contributions:** Linda A. Ban and Susan V. McLennan conceived the study; Linda A. Ban and Nicholas A. Shackel designed the figures; Susan V. McLennan and Nicholas A. Shackel reviewed/edited the manuscript; Linda A. Ban researched the data and wrote the manuscript.

## Abbreviations

The following abbreviations are used in this manuscript:

| | |
|---|---|
| ALT | alanine transaminase |
| ASGPR1 | asialoglycoprotein receptor 1 |
| CDD | choline-deficient diet |
| CES1 | carboxylesterase 1 |
| CTGF | connective tissue growth factor |
| ESCRT | endosomal sorting complex required for transport |
| EV | extracellular vesicle |
| FC | flow cytometry |
| HFD | high-fat diet |
| HSC | hepatic stellate cell |
| IL-6 | interleukin 6 |
| iNKT cell | invariant natural killer T cell |
| LC-MS/MS | liquid chromatography with tandem mass spectrometry |
| MCP-1 | monocyte chemotactic protein 1 |
| MIF | [macrophage] migration inhibitory factor |
| miRNA | microRNA |
| MMP | matrix metalloproteinase |
| MV | microvesicle |
| MVB | multivesicular body |
| NAFLD | non-alcoholic fatty liver disease |
| NAS | NAFLD activity score |
| NASH | non-alcoholic steatohepatitis |
| NK cell | natural killer cell |
| PS | phosphatidylserine |
| RT-qPCR | real-time quantitative polymerase chain reaction |
| TEM | transmission electron microscopy |
| TIMP-1 | tissue inhibitor of metalloproteinase 1 |
| WB | western blot |
| WGO | World Gastroenterology Organisation |

## References

1. Hui, E.; Xu, A.; Bo Yang, H.; Lam, K.S. Obesity as the common soil of non-alcoholic fatty liver disease and diabetes: Role of adipokines. *J. Diabetes Investig.* **2013**, *4*, 413–425. [CrossRef] [PubMed]
2. Bugianesi, E.; Vanni, E.; Marchesini, G. NASH and the risk of cirrhosis and hepatocellular carcinoma in type 2 diabetes. *Curr. Diabetes Rep.* **2007**, *7*, 175–180. [CrossRef]

3.  Williams, K.H.; Shackel, N.A.; Gorrell, M.D.; McLennan, S.V.; Twigg, S.M. Diabetes and nonalcoholic fatty liver disease: A pathogenic duo. *Endocr. Rev.* **2013**, *34*, 84–129. [CrossRef] [PubMed]

4.  Adams, L.A.; Harmsen, S.; St Sauver, J.L.; Charatcharoenwitthaya, P.; Enders, F.B.; Therneau, T.; Angulo, P. Nonalcoholic fatty liver disease increases risk of death among patients with diabetes: A community-based cohort study. *Am. J. Gastroenterol.* **2010**, *105*, 1567–1573. [CrossRef] [PubMed]

5.  Feng, R.N.; Du, S.S.; Wang, C.; Li, Y.C.; Liu, L.Y.; Guo, F.C.; Sun, C.H. Lean-non-alcoholic fatty liver disease increases risk for metabolic disorders in a normal weight chinese population. *World J. Gastroenterol.* **2014**, *20*, 17932–17940. [PubMed]

6.  Kumar, R.; Rastogi, A.; Sharma, M.K.; Bhatia, V.; Garg, H.; Bihari, C.; Sarin, S.K. Clinicopathological characteristics and metabolic profiles of non-alcoholic fatty liver disease in indian patients with normal body mass index: Do they differ from obese or overweight non-alcoholic fatty liver disease? *Indian J. Endocrinol. Metab.* **2013**, *17*, 665–671. [CrossRef] [PubMed]

7.  Younossi, Z.M.; Stepanova, M.; Negro, F.; Hallaji, S.; Younossi, Y.; Lam, B.; Srishord, M. Nonalcoholic fatty liver disease in lean individuals in the united states. *Medicine* **2012**, *91*, 319–327. [CrossRef] [PubMed]

8.  LaBrecque, D.R.; Abbas, Z.; Anania, F.; Ferenci, P.; Khan, A.G.; Goh, K.L.; Hamid, S.S.; Isakov, V.; Lizarzabal, M.; Penaranda, M.M.; *et al.* World gastroenterology organisation global guidelines: Nonalcoholic fatty liver disease and nonalcoholic steatohepatitis. *J. Clin. Gastroenterol.* **2014**, *48*, 467–473. [CrossRef] [PubMed]

9.  Deffieux, T.; Gennisson, J.L.; Bousquet, L.; Corouge, M.; Cosconea, S.; Amroun, D.; Tripon, S.; Terris, B.; Mallet, V.; Sogni, P.; *et al.* Investigating liver stiffness and viscosity for fibrosis, steatosis and activity staging using shear wave elastography. *J. Hepatol.* **2015**, *62*, 317–324. [CrossRef] [PubMed]

10. Khov, N.; Sharma, A.; Riley, T.R. Bedside ultrasound in the diagnosis of nonalcoholic fatty liver disease. *World J. Gastroenterol.* **2014**, *20*, 6821–6825. [CrossRef] [PubMed]

11. Myers, R.P.; Pomier-Layrargues, G.; Kirsch, R.; Pollett, A.; Beaton, M.; Levstik, M.; Duarte-Rojo, A.; Wong, D.; Crotty, P.; Elkashab, M. Discordance in fibrosis staging between liver biopsy and transient elastography using the FibroScan XL probe. *J. Hepatol.* **2012**, *56*, 564–570. [CrossRef] [PubMed]

12. Myers, R.P.; Pomier-Layrargues, G.; Kirsch, R.; Pollett, A.; Duarte-Rojo, A.; Wong, D.; Beaton, M.; Levstik, M.; Crotty, P.; Elkashab, M. Feasibility and diagnostic performance of the FibroScan XL probe for liver stiffness measurement in overweight and obese patients. *Hepatology* **2012**, *55*, 199–208. [CrossRef] [PubMed]

13. Pais, R.; Charlotte, F.; Fedchuk, L.; Bedossa, P.; Lebray, P.; Poynard, T.; Ratziu, V.; Group, L.S. A systematic review of follow-up biopsies reveals disease progression in patients with non-alcoholic fatty liver. *J. Hepatol.* **2013**, *59*, 550–556. [CrossRef] [PubMed]

14. Zelber-Sagi, S.; Yeshua, H.; Shlomai, A.; Blendis, L.; Leshno, M.; Levit, S.; Halpern, Z.; Oren, R. Sampling variability of transient elastography according to probe location. *Eur. J. Gastroenterol. Hepatol.* **2011**, *23*, 507–514. [CrossRef] [PubMed]

15. Athyros, V.G.; Katsiki, N.; Karagiannis, A.; Mikhailidis, D.P. Statins and nonalcoholic fatty liver disease: A bright future? *Expert Opin. Investig. Drugs* **2013**, *22*, 1089–1093. [CrossRef] [PubMed]

16. Angulo, P. Long-term mortality in nonalcoholic fatty liver disease: Is liver histology of any prognostic significance? *Hepatology* **2010**, *51*, 373–375. [CrossRef] [PubMed]

17. Arun, J.; Jhala, N.; Lazenby, A.J.; Clements, R.; Abrams, G.A. Influence of liver biopsy heterogeneity and diagnosis of nonalcoholic steatohepatitis in subjects undergoing gastric bypass. *Obes. Surg.* **2007**, *17*, 155–161. [CrossRef] [PubMed]

18. Wolf, P. The nature and significance of platelet products in human plasma. *Br. J. Haematol.* **1967**, *13*, 269–288. [CrossRef] [PubMed]

19. Dalton, A.J. Microvesicles and vesicles of multivesicular bodies *versus* "virus-like" particles. *J. Natl. Cancer Inst.* **1975**, *54*, 1137–1148.

20. Bala, S.; Petrasek, J.; Mundkur, S.; Catalano, D.; Levin, I.; Ward, J.; Alao, H.; Kodys, K.; Szabo, G. Circulating microRNAs in exosomes indicate hepatocyte injury and inflammation in alcoholic, drug-induced, and inflammatory liver diseases. *Hepatology* **2012**, *56*, 1946–1957. [CrossRef] [PubMed]

21. Kornek, M.; Schuppan, D. Microparticles: Modulators and biomarkers of liver disease. *J. Hepatol.* **2012**, *57*, 1144–1146. [CrossRef] [PubMed]

22. Lemoinne, S.; Thabut, D.; Housset, C.; Moreau, R.; Valla, D.; Boulanger, C.M.; Rautou, P.E. The emerging roles of microvesicles in liver diseases. *Nat. Rev. Gastroenterol. Hepatol.* **2014**, *11*, 350–361. [CrossRef] [PubMed]

23. Royo, F.; Falcon-Perez, J.M. Liver extracellular vesicles in health and disease. *J. Extracell. Vesicles* **2012**, *1*. [CrossRef] [PubMed]

24. Ferrante, S.C.; Nadler, E.P.; Pillai, D.K.; Hubal, M.J.; Wang, Z.; Wang, J.M.; Gordish-Dressman, H.; Koeck, E.; Sevilla, S.; Wiles, A.A.; *et al.* Adipocyte-derived exosomal miRNAs: A novel mechanism for obesity-related disease. *Pediatr. Res.* **2015**, *77*, 447–454. [CrossRef] [PubMed]

25. Goichot, B.; Grunebaum, L.; Desprez, D.; Vinzio, S.; Meyer, L.; Schlienger, J.L.; Lessard, M.; Simon, C. Circulating procoagulant microparticles in obesity. *Diabetes Metab.* **2006**, *32*, 82–85. [CrossRef]

26. Nomura, S.; Inami, N.; Shouzu, A.; Urase, F.; Maeda, Y. Correlation and association between plasma platelet-, monocyte- and endothelial cell-derived microparticles in hypertensive patients with type 2 diabetes mellitus. *Platelets* **2009**, *20*, 406–414. [CrossRef] [PubMed]

27. Wang, Y.; Chen, L.M.; Liu, M.L. Microvesicles and diabetic complications—Novel mediators, potential biomarkers and therapeutic targets. *Acta Pharmacol. Sin.* **2014**, *35*, 433–443. [CrossRef] [PubMed]

28. Akers, J.C.; Gonda, D.; Kim, R.; Carter, B.S.; Chen, C.C. Biogenesis of extracellular vesicles (EV): Exosomes, microvesicles, retrovirus-like vesicles, and apoptotic bodies. *J. Neuro-Oncol.* **2013**, *113*, 1–11. [CrossRef] [PubMed]

29. Cocucci, E.; Meldolesi, J. Ectosomes and exosomes: Shedding the confusion between extracellular vesicles. *Trends Cell Biol.* **2015**, *25*, 364–372. [CrossRef] [PubMed]

30. Kreimer, S.; Belov, A.M.; Ghiran, I.; Murthy, S.K.; Frank, D.A.; Ivanov, A.R. Mass-spectrometry-based molecular characterization of extracellular vesicles: Lipidomics and proteomics. *J. Proteome Res.* **2015**, *14*, 2367–2384. [CrossRef] [PubMed]

31. Hurley, J.H.; Odorizzi, G. Get on the exosome bus with ALIX. *Nat. Cell Biol.* **2012**, *14*, 654–655. [CrossRef] [PubMed]

32. Pols, M.S.; Klumperman, J. Trafficking and function of the tetraspanin CD63. *Exp. Cell Res.* **2009**, *315*, 1584–1592. [CrossRef] [PubMed]

33. Schutters, K.; Reutelingsperger, C. Phosphatidylserine targeting for diagnosis and treatment of human diseases. *Apoptosis Int. J. Program. Cell Death* **2010**, *15*, 1072–1082. [CrossRef] [PubMed]

34. Spronk, H.M.; ten Cate, H.; van der Meijden, P.E. Differential roles of tissue factor and phosphatidylserine in activation of coagulation. *Thromb. Res.* **2014**, *133*, S54–S56. [CrossRef] [PubMed]

35. Albanyan, A.M.; Murphy, M.F.; Rasmussen, J.T.; Heegaard, C.W.; Harrison, P. Measurement of phosphatidylserine exposure during storage of platelet concentrates using the novel probe lactadherin: A comparison study with annexin V. *Transfusion* **2009**, *49*, 99–107. [CrossRef] [PubMed]

36. Connor, D.E.; Exner, T.; Ma, D.D.; Joseph, J.E. The majority of circulating platelet-derived microparticles fail to bind annexin V, lack phospholipid-dependent procoagulant activity and demonstrate greater expression of glycoprotein Ib. *Thromb. Haemost.* **2010**, *103*, 1044–1052. [CrossRef] [PubMed]

37. Dasgupta, S.K.; Guchhait, P.; Thiagarajan, P. Lactadherin binding and phosphatidylserine expression on cell surface-comparison with annexin A5. *Transl. Res. J. Lab. Clin. Med.* **2006**, *148*, 19–25. [CrossRef] [PubMed]

38. Quesenberry, P.J.; Goldberg, L.R.; Aliotta, J.M.; Dooner, M.S.; Pereira, M.G.; Wen, S.; Camussi, G. Cellular phenotype and extracellular vesicles: Basic and clinical considerations. *Stem Cells Dev.* **2014**, *23*, 1429–1436. [CrossRef] [PubMed]

39. Xiong, W.; Sun, L.P.; Chen, X.M.; Li, H.Y.; Huang, S.A.; Jie, S.H. Comparison of microRNA expression profiles in HCC-derived microvesicles and the parental cells and evaluation of their roles in HCC. *J. Huazhong Univ. Sci. Technol. Med. Sci.* **2013**, *33*, 346–352. [CrossRef] [PubMed]

40. Witwer, K.W.; Buzas, E.I.; Bemis, L.T.; Bora, A.; Lasser, C.; Lotvall, J.; Nolte-'t Hoen, E.N.; Piper, M.G.; Sivaraman, S.; Skog, J.; *et al.* Standardization of sample collection, isolation and analysis methods in extracellular vesicle research. *J. Extracell. Vesicles* **2013**, *2*. [CrossRef] [PubMed]

41. Bergsmedh, A.; Szeles, A.; Henriksson, M.; Bratt, A.; Folkman, M.J.; Spetz, A.L.; Holmgren, L. Horizontal transfer of oncogenes by uptake of apoptotic bodies. *Proc. Natl. Acad. Sci. USA* **2001**, *98*, 6407–6411. [CrossRef] [PubMed]

42. Elmore, S. Apoptosis: A review of programmed cell death. *Toxicol. Pathol.* **2007**, *35*, 495–516. [CrossRef] [PubMed]

43. Lynch, S.F.; Ludlam, C.A. Plasma microparticles and vascular disorders. *Br. J. Haematol.* **2007**, *137*, 36–48. [CrossRef] [PubMed]

44. Ogasawara, F.; Fusegawa, H.; Haruki, Y.; Shiraishi, K.; Watanabe, N.; Matsuzaki, S. Platelet activation in patients with alcoholic liver disease. *Tokai J. Exp. Clin. Med.* **2005**, *30*, 41–48. [PubMed]

45. Stravitz, R.T.; Bowling, R.; Bradford, R.L.; Key, N.S.; Glover, S.; Thacker, L.R.; Gabriel, D.A. Role of procoagulant microparticles in mediating complications and outcome of acute liver injury/acute liver failure. *Hepatology* **2013**, *58*, 304–313. [CrossRef] [PubMed]

46. Bernimoulin, M.; Waters, E.K.; Foy, M.; Steele, B.M.; Sullivan, M.; Falet, H.; Walsh, M.T.; Barteneva, N.; Geng, J.G.; Hartwig, J.H.; *et al.* Differential stimulation of monocytic cells results in distinct populations of microparticles. *J. Thromb. Haemost.* **2009**, *7*, 1019–1028. [CrossRef] [PubMed]

47. Charrier, A.; Chen, R.; Chen, L.; Kemper, S.; Hattori, T.; Takigawa, M.; Brigstock, D.R. Exosomes mediate intercellular transfer of pro-fibrogenic connective tissue growth factor (CCN2) between hepatic stellate cells, the principal fibrotic cells in the liver. *Surgery* **2014**, *156*, 548–555. [CrossRef] [PubMed]

48. Chen, L.; Charrier, A.; Zhou, Y.; Chen, R.; Yu, B.; Agarwal, K.; Tsukamoto, H.; Lee, L.J.; Paulaitis, M.E.; Brigstock, D.R. Epigenetic regulation of connective tissue growth factor by microRNA-214 delivery in exosomes from mouse or human hepatic stellate cells. *Hepatology* **2014**, *59*, 1118–1129. [CrossRef] [PubMed]

49. Kornek, M.; Popov, Y.; Libermann, T.A.; Afdhal, N.H.; Schuppan, D. Human t cell microparticles circulate in blood of hepatitis patients and induce fibrolytic activation of hepatic stellate cells. *Hepatology* **2011**, *53*, 230–242. [CrossRef] [PubMed]

50. Kogure, T.; Lin, W.L.; Yan, I.K.; Braconi, C.; Patel, T. Intercellular nanovesicle-mediated microRNA transfer: A mechanism of environmental modulation of hepatocellular cancer cell growth. *Hepatology* **2011**, *54*, 1237–1248. [CrossRef] [PubMed]

51. Kogure, T.; Yan, I.K.; Lin, W.L.; Patel, T. Extracellular vesicle-mediated transfer of a novel long noncoding RNA TUC339: A mechanism of intercellular signaling in human hepatocellular cancer. *Genes Cancer* **2013**, *4*, 261–272. [CrossRef] [PubMed]

52. Fonsato, V.; Collino, F.; Herrera, M.B.; Cavallari, C.; Deregibus, M.C.; Cisterna, B.; Bruno, S.; Romagnoli, R.; Salizzoni, M.; Tetta, C.; *et al.* Human liver stem cell-derived microvesicles inhibit hepatoma growth in scid mice by delivering antitumor microRNAs. *Stem Cells* **2012**, *30*, 1985–1998. [CrossRef] [PubMed]

53. Momen-Heravi, F.; Bala, S.; Kodys, K.; Szabo, G. Exosomes derived from alcohol-treated hepatocytes horizontally transfer liver specific miRNA-122 and sensitize monocytes to LPS. *Sci. Rep.* **2015**, *5*, 9991. [CrossRef] [PubMed]

54. Takahashi, K.; Yan, I.K.; Kogure, T.; Haga, H.; Patel, T. Extracellular vesicle-mediated transfer of long non-coding RNA ror modulates chemosensitivity in human hepatocellular cancer. *FEBS Open Bio* **2014**, *4*, 458–467. [CrossRef] [PubMed]

55. Lv, L.H.; Wan, Y.L.; Lin, Y.; Zhang, W.; Yang, M.; Li, G.L.; Lin, H.M.; Shang, C.Z.; Chen, Y.J.; Min, J. Anticancer drugs cause release of exosomes with heat shock proteins from human hepatocellular carcinoma cells that elicit effective natural killer cell antitumor responses *in vitro*. *J. Biol. Chem.* **2012**, *287*, 15874–15885. [CrossRef] [PubMed]

56. Xiao, W.; Dong, W.; Zhang, C.; Saren, G.; Geng, P.; Zhao, H.; Li, Q.; Zhu, J.; Li, G.; Zhang, S.; *et al.* Effects of the epigenetic drug MS-275 on the release and function of exosome-related immune molecules in hepatocellular carcinoma cells. *Eur. J. Med. Res.* **2013**, *18*, 61. [CrossRef] [PubMed]

57. Zhang, J.; Shan, W.F.; Jin, T.T.; Wu, G.Q.; Xiong, X.X.; Jin, H.Y.; Zhu, S.M. Propofol exerts anti-hepatocellular carcinoma by microvesicle-mediated transfer of miR-142–3p from macrophage to cancer cells. *J. Transl. Med.* **2014**, *12*, 279. [CrossRef] [PubMed]

58. Li, Y.; Zhang, L.; Liu, F.; Xiang, G.; Jiang, D.; Pu, X. Identification of endogenous controls for analyzing serum exosomal miRNA in patients with hepatitis B or hepatocellular carcinoma. *Dis. Markers* **2015**, *2015*, 893594. [CrossRef] [PubMed]

59. Sugimachi, K.; Matsumura, T.; Hirata, H.; Uchi, R.; Ueda, M.; Ueo, H.; Shinden, Y.; Iguchi, T.; Eguchi, H.; Shirabe, K.; *et al.* Identification of a bona fide microRNA biomarker in serum exosomes that predicts hepatocellular carcinoma recurrence after liver transplantation. *Br. J. Cancer* **2015**, *112*, 532–538. [CrossRef] [PubMed]

60. Sun, L.; Hu, J.; Xiong, W.; Chen, X.; Li, H.; Jie, S. MicroRNA expression profiles of circulating microvesicles in hepatocellular carcinoma. *Acta Gastro-Enterol. Belg.* **2013**, *76*, 386–392.

61.  Wang, H.; Hou, L.; Li, A.; Duan, Y.; Gao, H.; Song, X. Expression of serum exosomal microRNA-21 in human hepatocellular carcinoma. *BioMed Res. Int.* **2014**, *2014*, 864894. [CrossRef] [PubMed]

62.  Brodsky, S.V.; Facciuto, M.E.; Heydt, D.; Chen, J.; Islam, H.K.; Kajstura, M.; Ramaswamy, G.; Aguero-Rosenfeld, M. Dynamics of circulating microparticles in liver transplant patients. *J. Gastrointest. Liver Dis.* **2008**, *17*, 261–268.

63.  Freeman, C.M.; Quillin, R.C., 3rd; Wilson, G.C.; Nojima, H.; Johnson, B.L., 3rd; Sutton, J.M.; Schuster, R.M.; Blanchard, J.; Edwards, M.J.; Caldwell, C.C.; *et al.* Characterization of microparticles after hepatic ischemia-reperfusion injury. *PLoS ONE* **2014**, *9*, e97945. [CrossRef] [PubMed]

64.  Costa-Silva, B.; Aiello, N.M.; Ocean, A.J.; Singh, S.; Zhang, H.; Thakur, B.K.; Becker, A.; Hoshino, A.; Mark, M.T.; Molina, H.; *et al.* Pancreatic cancer exosomes initiate pre-metastatic niche formation in the liver. *Nat. Cell Biol.* **2015**, *17*, 816–826. [CrossRef] [PubMed]

65.  Eldh, M.; Olofsson Bagge, R.; Lasser, C.; Svanvik, J.; Sjostrand, M.; Mattsson, J.; Lindner, P.; Choi, D.S.; Gho, Y.S.; Lotvall, J. MicroRNA in exosomes isolated directly from the liver circulation in patients with metastatic uveal melanoma. *BMC Cancer* **2014**, *14*, 962. [CrossRef] [PubMed]

66.  Wang, X.; Ding, X.; Nan, L.; Wang, Y.; Wang, J.; Yan, Z.; Zhang, W.; Sun, J.; Zhu, W.; Ni, B.; *et al.* Investigation of the roles of exosomes in colorectal cancer liver metastasis. *Oncol. Rep.* **2015**, *33*, 2445–2453. [CrossRef] [PubMed]

67.  Calabro, S.R.; Maczurek, A.E.; Morgan, A.J.; Tu, T.; Wen, V.W.; Yee, C.; Mridha, A.; Lee, M.; d'Avigdor, W.; Locarnini, S.A.; *et al.* Hepatocyte produced matrix metalloproteinases are regulated by CD147 in liver fibrogenesis. *PLoS ONE* **2014**, *9*, e90571. [CrossRef] [PubMed]

68.  Lee, A.; Rode, A.; Nicoll, A.; Maczurek, A.E.; Lim, L.; Lim, S.; Angus, P.; Kronborg, I.; Arachchi, N.; Gorelik, A.; *et al.* Circulating CD147 predicts mortality in advanced hepatocellular carcinoma. *J. Gastroenterol. Hepatol.* **2016**, *31*, 459–466. [CrossRef] [PubMed]

69.  Sidhu, S.S.; Mengistab, A.T.; Tauscher, A.N.; LaVail, J.; Basbaum, C. The microvesicle as a vehicle for emmprin in tumor-stromal interactions. *Oncogene* **2004**, *23*, 956–963. [CrossRef] [PubMed]

70.  Millimaggi, D.; Mari, M.; D'Ascenzo, S.; Carosa, E.; Jannini, E.A.; Zucker, S.; Carta, G.; Pavan, A.; Dolo, V. Tumor vesicle-associated CD147 modulates the angiogenic capability of endothelial cells. *Neoplasia* **2007**, *9*, 349–357. [CrossRef] [PubMed]

71.  Zhang, W.; Zhao, P.; Xu, X.L.; Cai, L.; Song, Z.S.; Cao, D.Y.; Tao, K.S.; Zhou, W.P.; Chen, Z.N.; Dou, K.F. Annexin A2 promotes the migration and invasion of human hepatocellular carcinoma cells *in vitro* by regulating the shedding of CD147-harboring microvesicles from tumor cells. *PLoS ONE* **2013**, *8*, e67268. [CrossRef] [PubMed]

72.  Kornek, M.; Lynch, M.; Mehta, S.H.; Lai, M.; Exley, M.; Afdhal, N.H.; Schuppan, D. Circulating microparticles as disease-specific biomarkers of severity of inflammation in patients with hepatitis c or nonalcoholic steatohepatitis. *Gastroenterology* **2012**, *143*, 448–458. [CrossRef] [PubMed]

73.  Baron, M.; Leroyer, A.S.; Majd, Z.; Lalloyer, F.; Vallez, E.; Bantubungi, K.; Chinetti-Gbaguidi, G.; Delerive, P.; Boulanger, C.M.; Staels, B.; *et al.* PPARα activation differently affects microparticle content in atherosclerotic lesions and liver of a mouse model of atherosclerosis and NASH. *Atherosclerosis* **2011**, *218*, 69–76. [CrossRef] [PubMed]

74.  Ajamieh, H.; Farrell, G.C.; McCuskey, R.S.; Yu, J.; Chu, E.; Wong, H.J.; Lam, W.; Teoh, N.C. Acute atorvastatin is hepatoprotective against ischaemia-reperfusion injury in mice by modulating enos and microparticle formation. *Liver Int.* **2015**, *35*, 2174–2186. [CrossRef] [PubMed]

75.  Povero, D.; Eguchi, A.; Li, H.; Johnson, C.D.; Papouchado, B.G.; Wree, A.; Messer, K.; Feldstein, A.E. Circulating extracellular vesicles with specific proteome and liver microRNAs are potential biomarkers for liver injury in experimental fatty liver disease. *PLoS ONE* **2014**, *9*, e113651. [CrossRef] [PubMed]

76.  Povero, D.; Eguchi, A.; Niesman, I.R.; Andronikou, N.; de Mollerat du Jeu, X.; Mulya, A.; Berk, M.; Lazic, M.; Thapaliya, S.; Parola, M.; *et al.* Lipid-induced toxicity stimulates hepatocytes to release angiogenic microparticles that require vanin-1 for uptake by endothelial cells. *Sci. Signal.* **2013**, *6*, ra88. [CrossRef] [PubMed]

77.  Csak, T.; Bala, S.; Lippai, D.; Satishchandran, A.; Catalano, D.; Kodys, K.; Szabo, G. MicroRNA-122 regulates hypoxia-inducible factor-1 and vimentin in hepatocytes and correlates with fibrosis in diet-induced steatohepatitis. *Liver Int.* **2015**, *35*, 532–541. [CrossRef] [PubMed]

78. Kranendonk, M.E.; Visseren, F.L.; van Herwaarden, J.A.; Nolte-'t Hoen, E.N.; de Jager, W.; Wauben, M.H.; Kalkhoven, E. Effect of extracellular vesicles of human adipose tissue on insulin signaling in liver and muscle cells. *Obesity* **2014**, *22*, 2216–2223. [CrossRef] [PubMed]

79. Deng, Z.B.; Liu, Y.; Liu, C.; Xiang, X.; Wang, J.; Cheng, Z.; Shah, S.V.; Zhang, S.; Zhang, L.; Zhuang, X.; *et al.* Immature myeloid cells induced by a high-fat diet contribute to liver inflammation. *Hepatology* **2009**, *50*, 1412–1420. [CrossRef] [PubMed]

80. Raubenheimer, P.J.; Nyirenda, M.J.; Walker, B.R. A choline-deficient diet exacerbates fatty liver but attenuates insulin resistance and glucose intolerance in mice fed a high-fat diet. *Diabetes* **2006**, *55*, 2015–2020. [CrossRef] [PubMed]

81. Anstee, Q.M.; Goldin, R.D. Mouse models in non-alcoholic fatty liver disease and steatohepatitis research. *Int. J. Exp. Pathol.* **2006**, *87*, 1–16. [CrossRef] [PubMed]

82. Murakami, Y.; Toyoda, H.; Tanahashi, T.; Tanaka, J.; Kumada, T.; Yoshioka, Y.; Kosaka, N.; Ochiya, T.; Taguchi, Y.H. Comprehensive miRNA expression analysis in peripheral blood can diagnose liver disease. *PLoS ONE* **2012**, *7*, e48366.

83. Lagos-Quintana, M.; Rauhut, R.; Yalcin, A.; Meyer, J.; Lendeckel, W.; Tuschl, T. Identification of tissue-specific microRNAs from mouse. *Curr. Biol. CB* **2002**, *12*, 735–739. [PubMed]

84. Barad, O.; Meiri, E.; Avniel, A.; Aharonov, R.; Barzilai, A.; Bentwich, I.; Einav, U.; Gilad, S.; Hurban, P.; Karov, Y.; *et al.* MicroRNA expression detected by oligonucleotide microarrays: System establishment and expression profiling in human tissues. *Gen. Res.* **2004**, *14*, 2486–2494. [CrossRef] [PubMed]

85. Yamada, H.; Ohashi, K.; Suzuki, K.; Munetsuna, E.; Ando, Y.; Yamazaki, M.; Ishikawa, H.; Ichino, N.; Teradaira, R.; Hashimoto, S. Longitudinal study of circulating miR-122 in a rat model of non-alcoholic fatty liver disease. *Clin. Chim. Acta Int. J. Clin. Chem.* **2015**, *446*, 267–271. [CrossRef] [PubMed]

86. Koeck, E.S.; Iordanskaia, T.; Sevilla, S.; Ferrante, S.C.; Hubal, M.J.; Freishtat, R.J.; Nadler, E.P. Adipocyte exosomes induce transforming growth factor β pathway dysregulation in hepatocytes: A novel paradigm for obesity-related liver disease. *J. Surg. Res.* **2014**, *192*, 268–275. [CrossRef] [PubMed]

87. Itagaki, H.; Shimizu, K.; Morikawa, S.; Ogawa, K.; Ezaki, T. Morphological and functional characterization of non-alcoholic fatty liver disease induced by a methionine-choline-deficient diet in c57bl/6 mice. *Int. J. Clin. Exp. Pathol.* **2013**, *6*, 2683–2696. [PubMed]

88. Verma, S.; Jensen, D.; Hart, J.; Mohanty, S.R. Predictive value of alt levels for non-alcoholic steatohepatitis (NASH) and advanced fibrosis in non-alcoholic fatty liver disease (NAFLD). *Liver Int.* **2013**, *33*, 1398–1405. [CrossRef] [PubMed]

89. Fraser, R.; Cogger, V.C.; Dobbs, B.; Jamieson, H.; Warren, A.; Hilmer, S.N.; le Couteur, D.G. The liver sieve and atherosclerosis. *Pathology* **2012**, *44*, 181–186. [CrossRef] [PubMed]

90. Redzic, J.S.; Kendrick, A.A.; Bahmed, K.; Dahl, K.D.; Pearson, C.G.; Robinson, W.A.; Robinson, S.E.; Graner, M.W.; Eisenmesser, E.Z. Extracellular vesicles secreted from cancer cell lines stimulate secretion of MMP-9, IL-6, TGF-β1 and emmprin. *PLoS ONE* **2013**, *8*, e71225. [CrossRef] [PubMed]

91. He, M.; Qin, H.; Poon, T.C.; Sze, S.C.; Ding, X.; Co, N.N.; Ngai, S.M.; Chan, T.F.; Wong, N. Hepatocellular carcinoma-derived exosomes promote motility of immortalized hepatocyte through transfer of oncogenic proteins and RNAs. *Carcinogenesis* **2015**, *36*, 1008–1018. [CrossRef] [PubMed]

92. Farazuddin, M.; Dua, B.; Zia, Q.; Khan, A.A.; Joshi, B.; Owais, M. Chemotherapeutic potential of curcumin-bearing microcells against hepatocellular carcinoma in model animals. *Int. J. Nanomed.* **2014**, *9*, 1139–1152.

93. Laakso, T.; Edman, P.; Brunk, U. Biodegradable microspheres VII: Alterations in mouse liver morphology after intravenous administration of polyacryl starch microparticles with different biodegradability. *J. Pharm. Sci.* **1988**, *77*, 138–144. [CrossRef] [PubMed]

# 6

# Gut Microbiota and Lifestyle Interventions in NAFLD

**David Houghton [1],\*, Christopher J. Stewart [2], Christopher P. Day [1,3] and Michael Trenell [1,\***

[1] Institute of Cellular Medicine, Newcastle University, Newcastle upon Tyne NE4 6BE, UK;
chris.day@newcastle.ac.uk

[2] Alkek Center for Metagenomics and Microbiome Research, Department of Molecular Virology and
Microbiology, Baylor College of Medicine, Houston, TX 77030, USA; Christopher.Stewart@bcm.edu

[3] Liver Unit, Newcastle upon Tyne Hospitals NHS Trust, Freeman Hospital,
Newcastle upon Tyne NE7 7DN, UK

\* Correspondence: david.houghton@ncl.ac.uk (D.H.); michael.trenell@newcastle.ac.uk (M.T.)

Academic Editors: Giovanni Targher and Amedeo Lonardo

**Abstract:** The human digestive system harbors a diverse and complex community of microorganisms that work in a symbiotic fashion with the host, contributing to metabolism, immune response and intestinal architecture. However, disruption of a stable and diverse community, termed "dysbiosis", has been shown to have a profound impact upon health and disease. Emerging data demonstrate dysbiosis of the gut microbiota to be linked with non-alcoholic fatty liver disease (NAFLD). Although the exact mechanism(s) remain unknown, inflammation, damage to the intestinal membrane, and translocation of bacteria have all been suggested. Lifestyle intervention is undoubtedly effective at improving NAFLD, however, not all patients respond to these in the same manner. Furthermore, studies investigating the effects of lifestyle interventions on the gut microbiota in NAFLD patients are lacking. A deeper understanding of how different aspects of lifestyle (diet/nutrition/exercise) affect the host–microbiome interaction may allow for a more tailored approach to lifestyle intervention. With gut microbiota representing a key element of personalized medicine and nutrition, we review the effects of lifestyle interventions (diet and physical activity/exercise) on gut microbiota and how this impacts upon NAFLD prognosis.

**Keywords:** NAFLD; gut microbiota; lifestyle; diet and exercise

## 1. Non-Alcoholic Fatty Liver Disease (NAFLD)

Non-alcoholic fatty liver disease (NAFLD) represents a spectrum of liver disease including simple steatosis, non-alcoholic steatohepatitis (NASH), fibrosis and cirrhosis, in the absence of excessive alcohol consumption [1]. NAFLD is the leading aetiology of liver disease [2], although factors leading to the development of NAFLD and progression to more advanced liver disease are poorly understood [3]. NAFLD is strongly associated with metabolic syndrome and its features including insulin resistance, obesity, hyperlipidemia, low high density lipoproteins (HDL), and hypertension and is considered the hepatic manifestation of the metabolic syndrome [4].

The incidence of NAFLD is closely associated with dietary intake and lack of physical activity, which typically manifests in obesity [5]. NAFLD is further accompanied by excess risk of type 2 diabetes mellitus (T2DM) and cardiovascular disease (CVD) [6]. The multifactorial aetiology of NAFLD is determined by both the patient's genetics and the environmental factors to which they are exposed, which may account for the substantial inter-patient variability common to the disease [7]. Although genetic polymorphisms have been attributed to account for a small portion of the patient inter-variability, there are additional contributing factors that have also been identified, spanning epigenetics, hormones, nutrition and physical inactivity [5,7]. Despite advances in NAFLD pathology, the reasons for the large inter-patient variability in progression remains incompletely understood. Consequently, a potential new diagnostic and therapeutic target receiving considerable attention is the collection of microorganisms that reside the gastrointestinal (GI) system. Despite humans being >99% identical genetically, the collection of bacteria, fungi, archea, virus, and phage are hugely diverse and highly individual from one person to the next. Termed the gut microbiota, bacteria in the gut alone accounts for around 70% of the total bacteria in the body and include 500–1000 different bacterial species [8–11].

Bacterial evolutionary linages are represented by phylogenetic trees, demonstrating the relatedness of bacteria to one another, classified from life, domain, kingdom, phylum, class, order, family, genus and finally species. The majority of research into gut microbiota has focused on phylum (Firmicutes, Bacteroidetes, *etc.*), genus (*Bacteroides, Lactobacillus, etc.*), and species (*Roseburia* spp. and *Eubacterium* spp.).

## 2. Gut Microbiota

Historical evidence spanning eight decades has demonstrated a link between the bacteria in the GI system and the liver, present from early fetal life and throughout life [8,12]. The gut microbiota in a healthy individual has been shown to be stable, absent of clinical manipulation (e.g., antibiotics), provided that a healthy diet and physical activity, combined with a healthy lifestyle (e.g., limited alcohol, not smoking, *etc.*) are maintained [13–18]. A healthy balance of bacteria in the GI system ensures that the gut microbiota works in a symbiotic nature with the host and its functions include maintaining a supply of essential nutrients, metabolism, immune response and intestinal architecture [19]. However, a change in the diversity leading to a reduced abundance of beneficial bacteria, with increased prevalence of potentially pathogenic bacteria can occur, which has been termed "dysbiosis" [17]. Dysbiosis of the gut microbiota has been associated with many disease states from early infancy [20], through childhood [21] and into adulthood [18]. Thus, manipulation of the gut microbiome to ensure a non-dysbiotic state offers attractive therapeutic for a range of conditions and overall health status.

Synonymous to NAFLD, inter-patient variability of the gut microbiota is well recognized, with each individual harboring a unique collection of microorganisms from the thousands that can potentially colonize, primarily from the phyla Firmicutes, Bacteroides and Actinobacteria [15,22]. Until recently, the majority of research published focused on these phyla, specifically the Firmicutes and Bacteroides, which are dominant in the gut microbiota from year three of life. However, recent advances in the throughput and affordability of deoxyribonucleic acid (DNA) sequencing technologies and associated bioinformatics [23] has facilitated an increased understanding of the pathophysiology of a number of diseases and adverse health conditions including obesity, metabolic syndrome, diabetes and cardiovascular disease [18,24–26], all of which are closely associated with NAFLD [4].

## 3. Gut Microbiota and NAFLD

NAFLD is a complex disease and with advances in the pathology of the disease new pharmacotherapy treatments are being developed [27,28]. However, lifestyle interventions accompanied by weight loss of between 5% and 10% remain the cornerstone of treatment [27,29]. The effectiveness of lifestyle changes are unprecedented with improvements in metabolic control and liver histology, and when accompanied by greater than 10% weight loss NASH resolution, fibrosis regression and reductions NAFLD activity score [30,31]. However, the difficulty in implementing and maintaining these lifestyle interventions in clinical practice in NAFLD is well documented, with randomized long-term studies lacking [32,33].

Due to the intimate relationship between liver and GI tract, it is unsurprising that gut microbiota dysbiosis has been linked with hepatic fat accumulation, and all stages of NAFLD in both animals and humans [7,34–41]. Although the exact mechanism linking the gut microbiota with NAFLD development and progression remains unknown, potential explanations include bacterial overgrowth, gut leakiness, increased endotoxemia absorption, and inflammation [3,36,42–45]. The increased knowledge of the gut microbiota in recent years has enhanced the understanding of the metabolic and immunological potential and microbial–host interactions, primarily in gut, but also in the liver and other organs. The role and identity of microbial produced metabolites and their direct function locally in the gut and also at other body sites remains unknown. However, increasing evidence suggests the gut microbiota as a genuine target for therapeutic interventions in the management of NAFLD (Figure 1) [8,19].

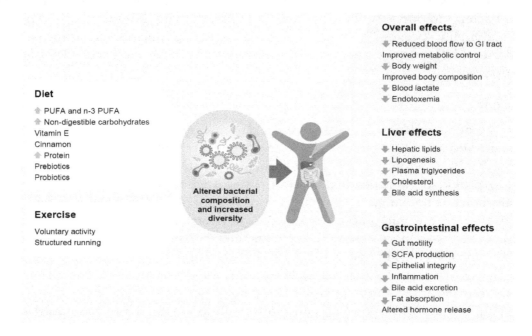

**Figure 1.** Impact of lifestyle interventions on gut microbiota and non-alcoholic fatty liver disease (NAFLD) and its risk factors (⬆ and ⬇ arrows denote increase or decrease in variables, respectively).

This review provides an overview of gut microbiota and its relationship with NAFLD by reviewing published data on how diet, nutrition and exercise modulate the gut microbiota and the liver. The purpose of this review is to assess the impact that lifestyle interventions (excluding pharmaceutical and surgical) have on gut microbiota and how this may interact with NAFLD development and progression.

## 4. Lifestyle Interventions in NAFLD

As the incidence of NAFLD increases [1], the individual and societal burden of its management weigh heavily on health care systems throughout the world, and the need for treatments to combat this is crucial [46]. Although the understanding of NAFLD has increased considerably in the last 20 years, the exact cause of why some people develop more severe forms of NAFLD is not fully understood. The development of NAFLD results from two key factors: (1) greater calories consumed compared to those expended; and (2) genetic susceptibility. Although genetic susceptibility cannot be altered (excluding epigenetic changes), calories consumed and expended can be modified, and has led to a large body of research undertaken investigating the impact of various lifestyle modification interventions [27,29]. Lifestyle interventions that lead to a reduction in weight and/or an increase in physical activity/exercise have consistently been shown to reduce hepatic lipids, improve glucose control and insulin sensitivity [29], and more recently improve liver histology [30,31]. The control of calories consumed *vs.* those expended may incorporate a number of interventions including exercise/physical activity independent of weight loss [47–49], diet modification [50–52] or diet and exercise/physical activity [30,31,53,54]. However, why some patients respond to interventions, and others do not is unknown. Modulation of the gut microbiota through the various lifestyle modifications discussed here may provide an insight into the inter-patient variability observed in NAFLD, and improve the number of people who may respond to specific lifestyle interventions to treat NAFLD.

## 5. Diet and Gut Microbiota

Exposure to environmental factors plays a significant role in the pathophysiology of NAFLD [6], particular dietary intake [55]. A regular healthy balanced diet has been shown to maintain a stable and healthy gut microbiota and reduce the risk of numerous diseases [56,57]. Recent evidence has emphasized the importance of calorie excess, in contrast to macronutrient content, as a major contributor to weight gain [58]. This is particularly important given the highly calorific content of the Western diet (high in fat and carbohydrates), which is associated with an altered gut microbiota and increased risk of developing obesity and NAFLD [35,46,59]. Although there are some conflicting findings, a strong association has been reported between obesity and changes in the gut microbiota, which may be responsible for enhanced energy harvest, weight gain and metabolic syndrome [60–62]. The link between the diet and the composition and function of the gut microbiota is unsurprising given that dietary components provide nutrients for bacteria, which then produce metabolites involved in energy balance, metabolism, immune response and the pathophysiology of NAFLD [63–65]. Indeed, bacteria in the gut are responsible for the digestion and production of many essential vitamins and minerals. The link between diet, gut microbiota, and health has been elegantly shown in animal models. Animals that were switched from low fat/fiber rich plant diets, to high fat/high sugar diets had significant increases in Bacilli and Erysipelotrichi from the Firmicutes phylum, which were associated with a significant decrease in the abundance of members of the Bacteroidetes phylum [66]. Furthermore, the role of the gut microbiome alone in causing obesity, independent of diet, was first demonstrated by Ley *et al.* [67] who showed mice transplanted an "obese microbiota" would have significantly greater weight gain than mice transplanted with a "lean microbiota". The substantial impact of the diet has also been shown in humans, where a rural African diet (high in fiber and vegetables) had a higher relative abundance of Bacteroidetes and a lower relative abundance of Firmicutes compared with the urban European diet (high in fat and sugar, low in fiber and vegetables). Even more interesting was that the samples from Africa had two bacterial species (*Prevottela* and *Xylanibacter*) that were not detectable in the European samples. Further evidence has been reported when comparing a control diet *vs.* diets high in non-digestible carbohydrates, where the authors reported that the non-digestible carbohydrates produce significant changes in the composition of the gut microbiota within a number of days [62].

Although there are contrasting results in the specific bacterial taxa that are modulated through the diet, the key message is that the diet is able to have a direct and long-term impact on the gut microbiota composition and function, which has a profound implication for health. Any modulation of the diet, such as an increase in non-digestible carbohydrates and/or weight loss has the potential to alter the gut microbiota and potentially disease phenotype, such as NAFLD. This approach of modulating the gut microbiota by modifying the dietary components (fats, proteins and carbohydrates), probiotics (living microorganisms that provide health effects on the host), and prebiotics (ingredients that are selectively fermented and modulate the changes in both the composition and activity of the gut microbiota) has been established for some time, although the links between specific bacteria with disease and mechanisms are often lacking [68]. This paper will now report the impact that macronutrients (fats, proteins and carbohydrates), probiotics and prebiotics manipulation has on the gut microbiota and the NAFLD phenotype.

## 6. Fat

Although the exact pathophysiology of NAFLD is unknown, the accumulation of lipids in the liver is a key pre-requisite for development and progression [69]. The cause of lipid accumulation in the liver is complex, but has been linked with an influx of fatty acids from fat depots, *de-novo* lipogenesis, and excess dietary fat intake, leading to steatosis. Increased fat intake is a common finding in NAFLD patients [70,71], thus regulation of fat intake has been highlighted as potential target for therapeutic intervention to reduce hepatic lipids [72]. Contrasting results have been reported in human studies that have used a high fat diet to increase hepatic lipid content [73,74], whereas others have reported no effect of a high fat diet on hepatic lipids [75,76]. The lack of consistency is likely to be due to the duration of the studies (10 days–3 weeks) and the various forms of fat used (saturated, polyunsaturated (PUFA) and mono-unsaturated (MUFA)). Furthermore, in a regular Western style diet the high fat content is normally supplemented by high carbohydrates and therefore it may be the combination of fat and carbohydrates that stimulate the development and progression of NAFLD [77]. The Western diet associated with NAFLD has also been associated with gut microbiota dysbiosis, which represents a potential source for the inter-patient variability observed in NAFLD, and progression from simple steatosis to NASH [36,78].

Although the exact mechanisms of how high fat diets lead to the development of NAFLD through gut microbiota modulation are unknown, research has predominantly focused on gut barrier function [77], leaky gut, endotoxemia, gut derived toxins and inflammation [45,79]. Despite the links between high fat diets, NAFLD, and the gut microbiota, there is a need to identify specific microbial changes that may be causative, which would highlight potential targets for diagnosis and treatment. The majority of studies investigating the impact that a high fat diet can have on the gut microbiota have been based around changes in the Firmicutes:Bacteroidetes ratio. This was firstly shown by Turnbaugh, *et al.* [80] in germ free mice that were fed a high fat diet and failed to develop obesity. Once inoculated with the microbiota from a mouse fed a high fat diet, the mice had increased weight, hepatic lipogenesis, fat deposition and insulin resistance, which was associated with an increase in Firmicutes and a subsequent decrease in Bacteroidetes [80]. This has subsequently been supported by decreases in *Eubacterium rectale*, *Blautia coccoides*, *Bifidobacteria* sp. and *Bacteroides* sp. [81–84]. Although these studies have identified that the gut microbiota is modulated with a high fat diet, the changes reported are limiting in their specificity (phylum changes rather than species), and the exact mechanism(s) linking these changes with NAFLD require further investigation.

There have been a number of mechanisms that have been identified to play a role in gut microbiota dysbiois associated with a high fat diet and the development of NAFLD including gut barrier dysfunction and translocation of microbes from the gut. Increased endotoxemia and inflammation in human [85–87] and animal studies [81,88–90] further suggests insulin resistance to be a key to the development of NAFLD and NASH [90,91]. High fat diets have also been shown to modulate the levels of Gammaproteobacteria and Erysipelotrichi, which have been shown to lead to choline deficiency, liver fat accumulation and NASH [65,92–94]. In addition, the ability of high fat diets to alter the gut microbiota and subsequently bile acids metabolism and synthesis by alleviating farnesoid X receptor (FXR) [95–97]. Although not exhaustive, the mechanisms discussed here have all been shown to have a direct impact upon the liver, therefore modulation of the gut microbiota in the presence of a high fat diet may offer the potential to reduce the risk and development of NAFLD.

The obvious treatment may be to put NAFLD patients on a low fat diet which have been shown to be effective in weight loss, reduce liver fat, improve metabolic control and modulate the gut microbiota [10,30,98]. However, managing and maintaining such diets can be difficult [32,33]. A number of alternative options for patients who may struggle with converting to a low fat diet include changing the form of fat consumed and increasing non-digestible carbohydrates. MUFA, PUFA and *n*-3 PUFA have been incorporated into dietary studies and shown to restore aspects of the high fat gut microbiota dysbiosis, including changes in Clostridia, Enterobacteriales, *Bifidobacterium* and *Lactobacillus casei* (Table 1) [99,100]. Although these studies do not report how these changes link with NAFLD, potential explanations may include reduced gut leakiness and inflammation, although these were not confirmed. In human studies, increases in MUFA, PUFA and *n*-3 PUFA have been shown to reduce hepatic lipid content and improve metabolic control in NAFLD patients [73,100], potentially due to increase fatty acid oxidation, redistribution of fatty acids and down regulation of gene expression of sterol regulatory element binding protein 1 (SREBP1-c) and factor for apoptosis (FAS). It is important to emphasize that the changes reported here did not influence weight, therefore suggesting the changes in the gut microbiota and hepatic lipids are diet driven rather than weight loss.

The use of non-digestible carbohydrates has been researched for a number of years and shown to be an effective treatment for increasing satiety, reducing blood glucose, insulin resistance, fat digestion and inducing weight loss [101]. Furthermore, non-digestible carbohydrates are effective in modulating gut microbiota and maintaining a healthy GI system [64]. However, the impact upon the gut microbiota in the presence of a high fat diet and mediators of NAFLD are lacking. Arabinoxylan and chitin-glucan have been shown to be effective at modulating the gut microbiota by increasing Bifidobacteria and restoring the abundance of *Bacteroides-Prevotella* spp., *Roseburia* spp., and *Clostridium* cluster fourteen a (XIVa) that were reduced following a high fat diet (Table 1). These changes in the gut microbiota were also supported by reductions in body fat, hepatic lipids, serum and hepatic cholesterol and insulin resistance, independent of calories consumed [102,103]. There is also evidence that, in the presence of high fat diets, chitosan and arabinoxylan are able to increase fat, bile acids and cholesterol in the feces. These studies suggest that non-digestible carbohydrates are able to modulate the gut microbiota, even in the presence of a high fat diet, potentially by binding to fat/cholesterol or inhibiting pancreatic lipase [101,104,105].

**Table 1.** Significant bacterial changes following dietary manipulation in the presence of high fat intake. XIV; fourteen, ↑ and ↓ denote increase or decrease in variable, respectively.

| Intervention/Treatment | Model Used | Non-Microbiome Changes | Bacterial Changes | Reference |
|---|---|---|---|---|
| Polyunsaturated fatty acids | Cells | Inhibit growth of mucus | ↑ *Lactobacillus casei* | [99] |
| Oleic acid and *n*-3 fatty acids (EPA and DHA) | Mice | ↓ Body Weight | ↑ *Clostridial* cluster XIV<br>↑ Enterobacteriales<br>↑ Firmicutes<br>↓ *Bifidobacterium* | [100] |
| Arabinoxylans | Mice | Improved gut barrier function<br>↓ Circulating inflammatory markers<br>↓ Adipocyte size<br>↓ Body weight gain<br>↓ Serum cholesterol<br>↓ Hepatic cholesterol<br>↓ Insulin resistance | ↑ *Prevotella* spp.<br>↑ *Roseburia* spp.<br>↑ *Bifidobacterium* | [102] |
| Chitin-Glucan | Mice | ↓ Body weight gain<br>↓ Fat Mass<br>↓ Fasting Glucose<br>↓ Hepatic Lipids<br>↓ Cholesterol | ↑ *Clostridial* cluster XIV | [103] |

Although a low fat diet may be preferable for patients with NAFLD, such a considerable change from an established lifestyle will be difficult for patients with NAFLD to incorporate. It is also important to recognize that, in general, a reduction in fat intake is typically accompanied by an increase in carbohydrate content. The data here suggest that changing the type of fat ingested and incorporating a larger proportion of non-digestible carbohydrates into the diet may be effective modulating the gut microbiota, reducing hepatic lipids and ameliorating risk factors associated with NAFLD. However, further work is required to assess the impact of diet on the gut microbiota specifically and further human intervention studies in patients with NAFLD are required to assess this.

## 7. Carbohydrates

Carbohydrates provide a crucial energy source for the host and gut microbiota [25]. Carbohydrate fermentation, specifically non-digestible carbohydrates, is a core activity of the human gut microbiota, driving the energy and carbon economy of the colon [106]. The move towards the Western style diet, which is high in processed carbohydrates and low in non-digestible carbohydrates, has been attributed to the rise and prevalence of obesity and NAFLD in these demographics [8,65,107]. This was recently confirmed in a meta-analysis where fructose was linked with poor liver health, although this was confounded by excessive energy intake, which is likely to be due to high fructose intake [108].

Excessive intake of calories in NAFLD is associated with sugar intake, with fructose being identified as having a crucial role to play (potentially due to altered hormone release). With regard to NAFLD, excess fructose, which is primarily metabolized in the liver, is linked to elevated steatosis [109–111]. Fructose has also been suggested to be a key driver in alteration of gut microbiota, potentially causing dysbiosis, as well as increased intestinal permeability and endotoxins in portal blood [112,113]. Notably, such factors have been previously reported in NAFLD [114]. Increased endotoxins and inflammatory cytokines have been identified to be part of the multiple hits hypothesis that exposes the liver to inflammation and injury [91]. Furthermore, endotoxemia is also linked with activation of Kupffer cells through toll like receptor dependent mechanisms, weight gain, poor metabolic control and increased plasma triglycerides, hepatic lipogenic enzymes and hepatic steatosis [111,113,115–118].

Replacing non-digestible carbohydrates with simple carbohydrates, such as fructose, will alter the substrate made available to the gut microbiota and ultimately affect the metabolic outputs and the microbial composition [67,106,119]. Numerous studies have reported that reducing non-digestible carbohydrates in the diet significantly reduces the levels of *Roseburia* spp. and *Eubacterium rectale* subgroup of cluster XIVa from the Firmicutes phylum and bifidobacteria from the Actinobacteria phylum [98,120]. More recently, the same group have also shown that increasing the levels of non-digestible carbohydrates can increase levels of *Ruminococcus bromii* (phylum:Firmicutes), however, these changes were dependent on the individuals initial microbiota profile [62]. These changes reflect the impact that non-digestible carbohydrates have on gut microbiota and subsequent health implications, although studies linking carbohydrates intake, such as non-digestible carbohydrates and fructose, with specific bacterial changes in NAFLD are lacking.

There are few studies investigating the effects of high carbohydrate intake similar to the Western diet on the gut microbiota composition. Ferrere, *et al.* [121] reported increased relative abundance of the class Erysipelotrichi (phylum:Firmicutes) following high fructose diet. Turnbaugh, Backhed, Fulton and Gordon [84] also reported that a high carbohydrate diet was able to increase the relative abundance of bacteria from the class Mollicutes (phylum:Firmicutes) and enrich genes that encode fructose metabolism, but reduce genes required for starch and sucrose metabolism. The authors suggested that the increase in Mollicutes might reduce microbial diversity, including a reduction in the relative abundance of the genus *Bacteroides* (phylum:Bacteroidetes), which is associated with poor health [61]. However, in humans Boursier, Mueller, Barret, Machado, Fizanne, Araujo-Perez, Guy, Seed, Rawls, David, Hunault, Oberti, Cales and Diehl [7] reported increased levels of *Bacteroides* in NASH patients compared to controls, which suggests that the data which we extrapolate from animal models require validation in human populations. Further studies should ascertain the effect of high fructose diets on specific bacteria to potentially identify targets for treatment.

The cornerstone of NAFLD treatment is weight loss, through diet and/or physical activity/exercise, which is effective in improving both liver histology [30] and modulating the gut microbiota [10,31]. In recent years a reduction in calories in the form of carbohydrates has been prevalent in many fad diets. Although initially effective for weight loss, such diets also have a substantial impact upon the gut microbiota and short chain fatty acids (SCFA) [98]. SCFA contribute around 10% of our daily energy requirements and provide a hospitable environment for cross feeding between microbial communities [108]. Specifically, a reduction in butyrate and butyrate producing bacteria has been shown in such diets, which may have detrimental effects on the GI structure and immune response [98,106,120]. An alternative would be to increase the amount of non-digestible carbohydrates consumed, which has been shown to be effective in maintaining a healthy gut microbiota [67] and ameliorating obesity and insulin resistance, which appear to be necessary for the development of NAFLD [122,123]. Furthermore, SCFA, including butyrate have been shown to contribute towards maintaining epithelial integrity, gut motility, hormone secretion, reducing appetite and inflammation [106], all of which are associated with NAFLD [122,123]. Increased intake of non-digestible carbohydrates has also been shown to improve glucose uptake, adipokine profile, and alter colonic fermentation, although the latter was only confirmed with breath tests [124]. Oligofructose specifically has also been shown to induce weight loss, reduce calories consumed and improved glucose uptake [125]. The authors also reported reductions in grehlin and increased peptide YY response, which have both been associated with changes in the gut microbiota following dietary intervention [126,127].

Further treatments to combat the detrimental effects of a high carbohydrate diet may involve increased protein intake, Vitamin E, and cinnamon [128–131]. All of which have been shown to be effective in reducing weight gain, body fat, adipocyte size, insulin resistance and hepatic steatosis. Although these all show promise, there are currently no data on whether these may be able to modulate the gut microbiota in NAFLD patients and should be explored further. Increased intake of carbohydrates, specifically fructose, is undoubtedly linked with NAFLD, due to either metabolism in the liver or through increasing calories consumed. Replacement of these simple carbohydrates with non-digestible carbohydrates provides potential to have a direct impact upon gut microbiota dysbiosis and have a positive effect on mediators of NAFLD.

## 8. Protein

Like carbohydrate, an increase in protein in the diet at the expense of carbohydrates and fat had been utilized in a number of fad diets to facilitate weight loss [132]. However, the effect that protein may have on the gut microbiota in humans, and specifically NAFLD are lacking. Furthermore, the small number of studies investigating the effects of high protein diets have predominantly focused on the products produced during fermentation [64]. This is surprising given the amount of protein that reaches the colon in a healthy diet (12–18 g), which would be expected to rise in a high protein diet [133], and provide nutrients for bacterial proliferation. Although an essential macronutrient, excess protein has been linked with potentially damaging effects on the gut microbiota and intestinal structure through toxic substances produced [64,133–135]. The small number of studies that have reported the impact that high protein diets have on the gut microbiota have reported high levels of *Clostridium* spp. and *Bacteroides* spp., with concurrent reductions in *Bifidobacterium* spp., *Roseburia* spp., and *Eubacterium* spp. [136,137]. The reductions in *Bifidobacterium* spp., *Roseburia* spp., and *Eubacterium* spp. bacterial species are associated with butyrate production, endotoxemia, mucus barrier function, and insulin sensitivity [81,136]. This suggests that the decreases in these bacteria may be detrimental to health and increase the risk of NAFLD [35–37,40,138,139].

Various animal models have been used to investigate the impact of protein on the gut microbiome with the main findings summarized in Table 2. In cats the authors utilized a high protein/low carbohydrate and a moderate protein and carbohydrate diet for eight weeks [140]. Ordination analysis of this data demonstrated that increases in the abundance of genre *Clostridium*, *Faecalibacterium*, *Ruminococcus*, *Blautia* and *Eubacterium* were clustered with plasma triglycerides. Contrastingly, piglets fed a high protein diet showed little microbial change, except reductions in *Faecalibacterium prausnitzii*, but were shown to have a higher increase in colonic permeability and higher cytokine secretion [141]. Whether this small change in bacteria can be directly attributed to the bacterial changes remains to be seen. However, the differing animal models and protein sources may account for the difference reported here. Further animal data from chickens and rats fed diets high in protein showed reductions in hepatic lipids and adipose tissue [142–144]. More recently, high protein diets have been shown to be effective for reducing hepatic lipids, blood lipids, body fat, CVD risk and improve insulin sensitivity and anti-oxidative potential [132,145–149]. Potential explanations for these results have been linked with increased satiety, increased energy expenditure, reduced hepatic lipid oxidation, cell death, hormone release in the GI system and bile acid metabolism [126,127,150], all of which are associated with the pathophysiology of NAFLD [123].

**Table 2.** Significant bacterial changes following high protein intake (↑ and ↓ denote increase or decrease in variable, respectively).

| Intervention/Treatment | Model Used | Non-Microbiome Changes | Bacterial Changes | Reference |
|---|---|---|---|---|
| High Protein/Moderate Carbohydrates High Protein/Low Carbohydrates | Obese Men | ↑ Branch chain amino acids<br>↑ Phenylacetic acid<br>↑ N-nitroso compounds<br>↓ Butyrate<br>↓ Phenolic acids | ↓ *Roseburia*<br>↓ *Eubacterium* | [137] |
| High Protein/Low Carbohydrates | Kittens | | ↑ *Clostridium*<br>↑ *Faecalibacterium*<br>↑ *Ruminococcus*<br>↑ *Blautia*<br>↑ *Eubacterium* | [140] |
| High Protein | Piglets | ↑ Branch chain amino acids<br>↑ Colonic Permeability<br>↑ Cytokine Secretion | ↓ *Faecalibacterium prausnitzii* | [141] |

Although there has been no direct link between the gut microbiota, NAFLD, and a high protein diet, there is evidence that an excess of 36 g/day of protein was identified as a risk factor for increasing the risk of NAFLD [111]. Furthermore, in T2DM an increase in protein intake resulted in reduced insulin sensitivity, increased gluconeogenesis and increase glucagon [151,152].

Overall, there are contrasting evidence on whether diets high in protein may be an effective treatment for gut microbiota modulation and NAFLD management. Discrepancies are likely due to differing study designs, including the source of protein (animal *vs.* plant protein), varying manipulations of the diets (protein to carbohydrate and fat ratios) populations sampled (Healthy, NAFLD, T2DM, obese, *etc.*) and study duration. The optimal benefits of diets high in protein to modulate the gut microbiota and aid with NAFLD management strategies should be explored further.

## 9. Prebiotics and Probiotics

Given the connection between the gut microbiota, diet, and health [65,84], coupled to issues with sustained dietary modification, an alternative approach utilizes pre- and probiotics to indirectly or directly confer beneficial colonizers of the GI, respectively [153]. Although there are various definitions, prebiotics is most commonly referred to as ingredients that are selectively fermented and modulate the changes in both the composition and activity of the gut microbiota [68,154]. Probiotics are different in that they are living (viable) microorganisms which have the ability to provide health effects on the host when provided in adequate amounts, similar to the bacteria that are already present [155].

## 10. Prebiotics

Fructans are the most extensively studied prebiotics and have been linked with modulation of the gut microbiota (summarized in Table 3), resulting in positive health benefits. In animal models, the administration of prebiotics increased 18 potentially beneficial species, notably *Bifidobacterium* spp. (Phylum: Actinobacteria) and Bacteroidetes [156–158]. Changes in gut microbiota are also associated with appetite regulation, improved glucose tolerance, increased satiety, reduced ghrelin, plasma triglycerides, oxidative stress and inflammation and calories consumed [82,158–160].

Further animal data have demonstrated that prebiotics are able to reduce hepatic lipids, cholesterol, plasma triglycerides and increase the SCFA propionate [161–163]. Daubioul, Rousseau, Demeure, Gallez, Taper, Declerck and Delzenne [161] suggested that the improved lipid profile and hepatic lipids were due to changes in the gut microbiota, which ultimately altered metabolites of fermentation. Alterations in the acetate:propionate ratio has been shown to reduce lipogenesis and account for the reductions in hepatic lipids. Although the authors suggest that the changes in SCFA are due to modulation of the gut microbiota, the authors failed to measure specific bacteria, focusing rather on the metabolites. It is intriguing that increased SCFA production, specifically butyrate and propionate, protect against diet-induced obesity in mice [164]. However, such studies underscore the need to understand the complex interplay between microbial–host interaction in gut and to which extent the bacterial community is causing the phenotypes observed.

In human cohorts, where systematic study is challenging, studies elucidating the exact effects and mechanisms of prebiotics on the gut microbiota and resulting microbial–host interaction are lacking. Studies in healthy and T2DM patients have provided similar results, reporting increased satiety and reduced ghrelin, body weight, glucose, and inflammation [125,157,165,166]. There is a need for studies investigating the effects of prebiotics in NAFLD. In a small pilot study in biopsy confirmed NASH patients, Daubioul, et al. [167] reported that prebiotics had a positive impact on liver aminotransferases and insulin, but no effects on plasma triglycerides. A recent study reported that prebiotics were effective at significantly reducing inflammatory cytokines, liver aminotransferases, insulin sensitivity and steatosis in NASH patients [168]. Notably, the study compares lifestyle alone with lifestyle and prebiotics, thus it is difficult to ascertain how much affect the prebiotics with no other lifestyle interventions alone would have. As with existing animal data, such studies lack analysis of the gut microbiota and thus relating potential mechanisms to changes in the gut microbiota is not possible.

A recent meta-analysis analyzing 26 randomized controlled trials concluded that prebiotics were effective in increasing satiety and improving insulin sensitivity [169]. While specific effects of prebiotics on the gut microbiota remain poorly understood, the majority of studies have reported increases in Bifidobacteria [170–173]. Dewulf, et al. [174] also reported an increase in Bifidobacteria, as well as increased levels of *Faecalibacterium prausnitzii* and reductions in *Bacteroides intestinalis*, *Bacteroides vulgatus* and *Propionibacterium*, which they associated with endotoxemia, although they failed to report any changes in plasma endotoxemia. Although these studies demonstrate promise that prebiotics may be used as a potential treatment for NAFLD, further work is required to investigate additional overall changes in the gut microbiome. Rapid advances in NGS and other 'omic technologies offer promise for more systematic understanding of entire treatment mechanisms. In addition, there are currently no studies that have reported the effects of prebiotics on hepatic lipids or liver histology, and evidence linking specific bacteria with the pathophysiology of NAFLD is lacking.

**Table 3.** Significant bacterial changes following prebiotic consumption (↑ and ↓ denote increase or decrease in variable, respectively).

| Intervention/Treatment | Model Used | Non-Microbiome Changes | Bacterial Changes | Reference |
|---|---|---|---|---|
| Prebiotic Diet | Mice | Improved Glucose Tolerance<br>Improved Leptin Sensitivity<br>↑ GLP-1<br>↑ L-cell GLP-1<br>↓ Fat Mass<br>↓ Oxidative Stress<br>↓ Inflammation | ↓ Firmicutes<br>↑ Bacteroidetes<br>Changed 102 taxa | [162] |
| Prebiotics—Xylo-oligosaccharide and inulin | Human | ↑ Butyrate<br>↑ Propionate<br>↓ Acetate<br>↓ P-creso<br>↓ Lipopolysaccharides | ↑ *Bifidobacterium* | [164] |
| Prebiotics—β2-1 Fructans | Human | | ↑ *Bifidobacterium* | [172] |
| Prebiotic—Galactooligosaccharides (GOSs) | Human | ↑ Phagocytosis<br>↑ Natural killer cells<br>↓ Inflammation | ↑ *Bifidobacterium* | [173] |
| Prebiotic—Galactooligosaccharides (GOSs) | Human | ↓ Inflammation<br>↓ IgA<br>↓ Calcoprotectin<br>↓ Cholesterol<br>↓ Insulin | ↑ *Bifidobacterium* | [174] |

**Table 3.** *Cont.*

| Intervention/Treatment | Model Used | Non-Microbiome Changes | Bacterial Changes | Reference |
|---|---|---|---|---|
| Prebiotics—Inulin type fructans | Human | ↓ Fat Mass<br>↓ Plasma Lactate<br>↓ Phosphatidylcholine | ↑ *Bifidobacterium*<br>↑ *Faecalibacterium prausnitzi*<br>↓ *Bacteroides intestinalis*<br>↓ *Bacteroides vulgatus*<br>↓ *Propionibacterium* | [175] |

## 11. Probiotics

Probiotics have been suggested as a potential treatment for patients with NAFLD, due to their apparent ability to modulate the gut microbiota (Table 4) and impact upon metabolic control, inflammation, lipid profile and intestinal permeability [155,175], and have been systematically reviewed in detail elsewhere [176]. However, the exact mechanisms of how probiotics are able to do this are not fully understood. Although not exhaustive, proposed mechanisms include direct microbe-to-microbe interaction and competition with pathogenic bacteria potentially leading to eradication and a healthy balance of gut microbiota [62,177]. Furthermore, probiotics have been shown to be effective at improving epithelial barrier integrity [178] and stimulating the host immune response [179,180].

One of the first studies to investigate the use of probiotics was conducted over 10 years ago in mice. The authors demonstrated that a course of a common brand of probiotics called VSL#3, which included *Streptococcus thermophiles, Lactobacillus (species: acidophilus, delbrueckii, casei* and *plantarum*) and *Bifidobacterium (species: breve, longum* and *infantis*) over four weeks was as effective as an anti-TNF antibody at improving liver histology, reducing hepatic lipids, and reducing serum alanine aminotransferase [181]. Importantly, the authors also reported a reduction in pro-inflammatory cytokines and hepatic insulin resistance resulting from modulation of the gut microbiota, although they failed to assess this. This early study into probiotics demonstrates potential for ameliorating multiple hits that are associated with the pathophysiology and development of NAFLD [69,91]. Subsequent to this pioneering study, further animal work has reported that probiotics are effective at reducing cholesterol, low density lipoproteins (LDL), very low density lipoproteins (VLDL), triglycerides [182,183], fat depots [184], hepatic lipid content [185–187], steatotic and peroxidase factors and liver aminotransferase [188,189]. There is also evidence demonstrating improvements in hepatic insulin resistance and metabolic control [81,186,190,191]

There is also a body of evidence that has reported reduced inflammation and endotoxemia following probiotic administration period. An exaggerated and damaging inflammatory response occurs in a range of conditions and current evidence associates dysbiosis of the gut microbiota with inflammation, although it is unclear if this is cause or effect. This is especially prevalent in the case of the mucosa and tight protein junctions, where pathogenic bacteria cause damage and increase gut permeability leading to chronic inflammation and endotoxemia [155,192]. Direct modulation of the gut microbiota with viable organisms in probiotics has been shown to reduce hepatic inflammation [188], circulating inflammatory markers [181,191,193], endotoxemia in portal blood [194] and provide essential nutrients for maintaining intestinal epithelium integrity [178,195].

Although these data do imply that probiotics may play a role in the therapeutic management of NAFLD, human data are lacking. In obese children who were non-compliant to lifestyle interventions, probiotics significantly reduced alanine aminotransferase (ALT) and anti-peptidoglycan-polysaccharide antibodies, but did not reduce liver fat [196]. In three well-designed randomized controlled studies, the authors observed that probiotics high in *Lactobacillus gasseri* reduced abdominal adiposity and serum lipids [197–199]. However, the duration of these studies was relatively short and the effects on liver steatosis and specific bacterial changes were not reported.

Similar results have been shown in patients with liver disease, where probiotics have been shown to be effective at restoring neutrophil phagocytic capacity in cirrhosis and reducing IL-10, IL-6 and TNF-α secretion and toll like receptor expression [200,201]. More specifically, in NAFLD, the administration of probiotics resulted in a significant reduction liver aminotransferase [202,203], although no changes in hepatic lipids, liver histology or gut microbiota were reported.

The majority of the studies discussed suggest that gut microbiota modulation following consumption of probiotics was responsible for the beneficial effects observed. Early animal data from Cani, Neyrinck, Fava, Knauf, Burcelin, Tuohy, Gibson and Delzenne [81] demonstrated that supplementing mice on a high fat diet with *Bifidobacterium* restored the levels of *Bifidobacterium* comparable to controls on a normal chow fed diet. More recently Bifidobacteria added to animal feed has been shown to increase the abundance of *Bifidobacterium* and *Clostridiaceae* and reduce the abundance of *Enterobacteria* and Eubacteriaceae [184,187,191,193,204]. The changes in bacterial diversity discussed here were also supported by reductions in inflammatory cytokines, endotoxemia, hepatic lipids and gut permeability.

**Table 4.** Significant bacterial changes following probiotic consumption (↑ and ↓ denote increase or decrease in variable, respectively).

| Intervention/Treatment | Model Used | Non-Microbiome Changes | Bacterial Changes | Reference |
|---|---|---|---|---|
| Probiotic—oligofructose and Bifidobacterium species | Mice | ↓ Endotoxemia<br>Improved glucose tolerance | ↑ *Bifidobacterium* | [81] |
| Probiotic—Bifidobacterium longum | Rat | ↓ Endotoxemia<br>↓ Inflammation<br>↓ Intestinal myeloperoxidase<br>↓ Body Weight<br>↓ Fat Depots<br>↓ Systolic Blood Pressure<br>Improve insulin sensitivity | ↑ *Bifidobacterium* | [185] |
| Probiotic—Bifidobacterium longum or Lactobacillus acidophilus | Rat | ↓ Hepatic Lipids | ↑ *Bifidobacterium longum*<br>↑ *Lactobacillus acidophilus* | [188] |
| Probiotic—Bifidobacterium pseudocatenulatum | Mice | ↓ Cholesterol<br>↓ Triglycerides<br>↓ Glucose levels<br>↓ Insulin resistance<br>↓ Leptin<br>↓ Inflammation<br>↓ Hepatic Lipids | ↑ *Bifidobacterium*<br>↓ Enterobacteria | [192] |
| Probiotic—Bifidobacterium pseudocatenulatum | Mice | ↓ Inflammation<br>↓ Endotoxemia<br>↓ B cells<br>↓ Macrophages<br>↓ Cholesterol<br>↓ Body Weight Gain<br>↓ Triglycerides<br>↓ Insulin resistance | ↓ *Firmicutes*<br>↓ *Proteobacteria* | [194] |
| Probiotic—Bifidobacterium breve | Mice | ↑ Propionate | ↑ *Clostridiaceae*<br>↓ *Eubacteriaceae* | [205] |

Although existing data suggest probiotics represent a safe and effective treatment option for NAFLD, there are instances where probiotics were ineffective, such as in Crohn's disease [205] and Helicobacter infections [206]. Such results may simply represent inefficiency of the probiotics selected for these studies and it is plausible different probiotic combinations may yield different results. It should be noted that probiotics are regarded as safe, with little data showing any adverse effects of supplementation. As each disease is uniquely complex, so too must the probiotic selected for treatment, with better characterization of the disease mechanism informing the specific probiotics to use [62]. Important considerations also include the route of administration, dosage, how often to take the treatment, and for how long. As we better understand the most effective means of administering probiotics as well as which specific combinations of bacteria to use, the efficacy of treatment should become apparent. In the era of personalized medicine it is feasible that each NAFLD patient can have their gut microbiota profile determined, allowing probiotics to be tailored to the individual.

## 12. Exercise

Exercise is well recognized for its health benefits and its ability to attenuate the risk of CVD, obesity, mental disorders, diabetes and intestinal diseases [207,208]. More specifically exercise has been shown to be effective at modulating hepatic steatosis and its mediators, improve body composition, liver and adipose tissue insulin sensitivity independent of weight loss [29,47–49,209]. Furthermore exercise (both endurance and high intensity) training has been shown to attenuate inflammation and improve insulin secretion by upregulating glucagon-like peptide-1 secretion in the GI tract and pancreas [209–211]. Despite the strong associations among exercise, liver health, metabolic control and inflammation, evidence linking exercise, the gut microbiota and NAFLD in humans is lacking. Understanding the interplay between the triad and resulting mechanisms in NAFLD will be fundamental to translating therapeutics into clinical practice.

In a recent study, Clarke, *et al.* [212] investigated the effects of effects of exercise in rugby players compared sedentary overweight and obese controls. The authors observed that the highly active rugby players had a significantly more diverse gut microbiota and lower levels of inflammatory and metabolic markers compared to the controls. Specifically, the authors identified increased relative abundance of Firmicutes, Proteobacteria and reduced relative abundance of Bacteroidetes. These observations are based on extremities of a population with vastly different diet and calorie consumption, thus linking findings directly to the gut microbiota is challenging [18,213]. The authors acknowledge these confounding variables, stating future studies must be well designed in an attempt to isolate the effects that exercise may have on the gut microbiota.

Although animal models do not offer a direct comparison with humans, the control over interventions allows an excellent model to develop disease states and may make it easier to tease out the impact that exercise alone may have on the gut microbiota. To date, there are no animal studies looking specifically at exercise and the gut microbiota in an animal model of NAFLD. There are, however, a number of other animal studies that have investigated the effects of exercise on the gut microbiota in type 2 diabetes [214], obesity, CVD [215], high fat intake [216,217] and low activity levels [218], which are all risk factors for the development and progression of NAFLD [5,6], summarized in Table 5.

**Table 5.** Significant bacterial changes following exercise (↑ and ↓ denote increase or decrease in variable, respectively).

| Intervention/Treatment | Model Used | Non-Microbiome Changes | Bacterial Changes | Reference |
|---|---|---|---|---|
| Controlled treadmill running | Mice | | ↑ *Lactobacillus* spp.<br>↑ *Clostridium leptum* (C-IV)<br>↓ *Clostridium* cluster (C-XI)<br>↓ *Bifidobacterium* spp | [215] |
| Controlled treadmill running | Rat | ↓ Blood Lactate | ↑ *Allocaculum*<br>↑ *Pseudomonas*<br>↑ *Lactobacillus*<br>↓ *Streptococcus*<br>↓ *Aggregatibacter*<br>↓ *Sutturella* | [216] |
| Voluntary wheel running | Mice | ↓ Body Weight<br>↓ Body Fat<br>↓ Blood glucose<br>↑ Heart:Body Weight | ↑ Bacteroidetes<br>↓ Firmicutes<br>↓ Actinobacteria | [217] |

**Table 5.** *Cont.*

| Intervention/Treatment | Model Used | Non-Microbiome Changes | Bacterial Changes | Reference |
|---|---|---|---|---|
| Controlled wheel running | Mice | | ↓ *Streptococcus*<br>↓ Bacteroidetes<br>↑ Firmicutes | [218] |
| Voluntary wheel running | Rat | ↓ Body Fat<br>↑ Lean Body Mass<br>↓ Non-esterified fatty acids<br>↓ Cholesterol | ↓ Firmicutes<br>↑ Cyanobacteria<br>↑ Proteobacteia | [219] |
| Voluntary wheel running | Rat | ↑ Cecal size and weight<br>↑ Butyrate production<br>↓ Body Weight | ↑ SM7/11<br>↑ T2-87 | [220] |
| Voluntary and forced treadmill running | Mice | ↓ Body Weight | ↑ *Dorea*<br>↑ *Anaerotruncus*<br>↑ *Nautilia*<br>↑ *Coprococcus*<br>↑ *Oscillospira*<br>↓ *Turicibacter*<br>↓ *Moryella*<br>↓ *Prevotella* | [221] |
| Voluntary wheel running | Mice | ↓ Body Weight | ↑ Enterococcsceae<br>↑ Staphylococcsceae<br>↓ Erysipelotrichaceae | [222] |
| Voluntary wheel running | Rat | ↑ Body Weight<br>↑ Serum Leptin<br>↓ Serum Ghrelin | ↑ *B. Coccoides-E Rectale*<br>↑ *Lactobacillus*<br>↓ *Clostridium*<br>↓ *Enteroccocus*<br>↓ *Prevotella*<br>↓ *Bacteroides* | [223] |
| Voluntary wheel running | Rat | ↑ Body Weight<br>↑ Lean Body Mass | ↓ *Rikenellaceae* g_AF12<br>↓ *Rikenellaceae* g<br>↓ *Desulfovibrio spp*<br>↑ *Blautia* spp<br>↑ *Turicibacter*<br>↑ *Anaerostipes spp*<br>↑ *Methanosphaera* | [224] |
| Single Peak Exercise Test | Human | ↑ Bacteria in blood | ↑ Actinobacteria<br>↑ Firmicutes | [225] |

The first animal study to investigate the effects of exercise on the gut microbiota was performed nearly a decade ago using rats who voluntarily exercised for five weeks [219]. Rats that exercised had a distinctly different bacterial cluster from the sedentary rats, with a significant increase in bacterial producing bacterium (SM7/11 and T2-87). The exercised mice also consumed fewer calories, had reduced body weight and an in increase in butyrate. Both voluntary and forced exercise has since been shown to elicit significant clustering and increased richness of the gut microbiota, with distinctive changes in the abundance of genus *Lactobacillus*, *Bifidobacterium*, *Dorea*, *Turicibacter*, *Anaerotruncus* and species *Enterococcus faecium* when compared with sedentary animals [220–222].

The role of genetic and epigenetic predisposition is unclear, but the gut microbiota evolves with the host from birth [8,12]. Therefore, early manipulation of the microbiota may have beneficial effects later in life. Genetically altered rats with low activity levels from birth had a greater shift in bacterial diversity when compare to the highly active rats [218]. Furthermore, this extenuated increase in bacterial diversity in the low activity rats was supported by a greater improvement in body composition and serum lipid profile, when compared with the highly active mice. The beneficial effects of exercise early in life suggests that even in those with a genetic predisposition to be sedentary may be able to modulate their gut microbiota and risk factors for NAFLD. Further evidence was presented when exercising juvenile and adults rats [223]. Juvenile rats had greater shifts in bacterial composition when compared with the exercising adult rats, which were closely related to body composition of the rats. These studies together suggest that early stimulus and the activity predisposition (low *vs.* high) may be involved in characterizing gut microbiota phenotypes.

Further exercise studies have investigated the effects of exercise on the gut microbiota in hypertension, obesity and diabetes, which are all closely associated with NAFLD [6]. Petriz, Castro,

Almeida, Gomes, Fernandes, Kruger, Pereira and Franco [215] exercised obese and hypertensive rats five times per week for four weeks and observed altered composition and diversity of the gut microbiota, with specific increases in *Allobaculum* in hypertensive rats, and *Pseudomonas* and *Lactobacillus* in the obese rats. In a similar exercise intervention, Lambert, Myslicki, Bomhof, Belke, Shearer and Reimer [214] exercised diabetic and control mice and compared them with matched sedentary controls. The authors observed a significant increase in the abundance of several Firmicutes species and reductions in the abundance of *Bacteroides* spp., which had previously been reported in humans [212]. The only human study to look at the acute effects of exercise on gut microbiota was performed in patients with myalgic encephalomyelitis/chronic fatigue syndrome compared to healthy controls [224]. The authors reported that following a single maximal exercise bout the gut microbiota of patients was significantly altered in comparison with controls. Furthermore the patients had a significantly larger level of bacteria recovered in the blood when compared with the healthy controls. Although the authors only conducted a single bout of exercise, they suggest that the altered gut microbiota led to an increase in bacterial translocation and may contribute to worsening myalgic encephalomyelitis/chronic fatigue syndrome. The increased bacteria in the blood may be due to an increase in inflammatory cytokines (IL-6, IL-8, IL-1β, and TNF-α), which have been shown to be required to initiate villus injury and reduce intestinal barrier function [210]. However, the authors failed to report on inflammation, and it must be pointed out that the exercise performed was maximal, which would not be routinely performed. Despite this there is a large body of evidence demonstrating that exercise is able to reduce inflammation [211], hepatic lipids [29], and improves metabolic control [47,209,225,226]. However, further work would need to compare different modalities of exercise and intensities to assess their impact on the gut microbiota, liver fat, metabolic control, inflammation and patients health.

Inter-study variability has been reported by Petriz, Castro, Almeida, Gomes, Fernandes, Kruger, Pereira and Franco [215], who reported increased relative abundance of *Allobaculum*, *Pseudomonas* and *Lactobacillus*. However, Liu, Park, Holscher, Padilla, Scroggins, Welly, Britton, Koch, Vieira-Potter and Swanson [218] reported increased relative abundance of Christensenellaceae, Helicobacteraceae and Desulfovibrionaccae, and Choi, Eum, Rampersaud, Daunert, Abreu and Toborek [221] reported increased relative abundance of the family Enterococcaceae and decreased relative abundance of Erysipelotrichaceae.

Possible reasons for discrepancy reported between studies may include; varying disease type and status amongst studies, exercise intervention duration and/or intensity, diet incorporated (ranging from high fat diet to regular animal chow) and body composition changes. Of particular note, the varying methods and technologies used to extract and sequence the 16S rRNA gene creates potential sources of bias between studies.

Exercise does appear to be able to modulate the gut microbiota and reduce the risk of NAFLD, however, the mechanism(s) remain unknown. Potential mechanisms include: (1) increased butyrate production, which is linked with colonic epithelial cell proliferation and modulation of mucosal immunity and exclusion of pathogens [215,219,227]; (2) increased primary bile acid secretion and cholesterol turnover [228]; (3) growth of beneficial bacteria [221]; and (4) increased core body temperature and reduced blood flow to the GI system reducing gut transit time and substrate delivery to the microbiota [218,229,230]. Although the exact mechanism remains elusive and methodological bias hinders direct cross-study comparisons, existing data indicate that exercise may be able to modulate the composition, diversity and relative abundance of the gut microbiota in NAFLD patients. Further investigation of the impact of exercise on gut microbiota is required and may address why some patients respond to exercise and some do not.

## 13. Conclusions

The gut microbiota has been studied for decades, however, recent developments in 16S rRNA gene sequencing, coupled to advances in computational processing of data has enhanced our understanding of the microbial–host interactions [23]. The gut microbiota has been associated with a range of diseases, from obesity, metabolic syndrome, diabetes, and cardiovascular disease [18,24–26] to NAFLD [7,34,36–41]. However, existing studies are largely focused on profiling the bacterial community and fail to provide functional information between the gut microbiota and the host. Ultimately, it still remains unknown whether the gut microbiome is *causing* the disease, or simply an *effect* of disease pathophysiology.

This review reveals that diet, pre/probiotics, and exercise play a significant role in the function and diversity of the gut microflora. To date, studies have predominantly focused on pre-clinical models, which have limitations in the transferability of their data to humans. Although much is known, significant questions about how lifestyle therapies may influence the gut microbiota as a therapeutic target for NAFLD care. However, the links between the gut microbiota and NAFLD should continue to be explored to:

(1)   better understand inter-patient variability;

(2)   develop potential biomarkers for NAFLD development and progression;

(3)   understand the mechanism(s) linking the gut microbiota and NAFLD;

(4)   develop an understanding of how aspects of lifestyle interventions interact with the gut microbiota and how this may impact upon health; and

(5)   tailor prebiotics and probiotics to influence health for each individual.

Furthermore, although these lifestyle interventions clearly impact upon NAFLD, understanding of how they interact with the gut microbiota and NAFLD is lacking and requires longitudinal studies with large sample sizes. For example, the diet has been shown to modulate the gut microbiota in days [62], but these changes are generally reversed in a similar time frame. Therefore, we need to understand the best mechanisms for modulating the long-term establishment of a healthy gut microbiota and the resulting health implications this may have.

As technologies are increasingly developed and the associated costs are reduced, there is huge potential to systematically determine the importance of both the presence of certain bacteria and their ultimate function is a given community. For understanding such complex processes and interaction at the microbe and host levels, there is a need to integrate multiple techniques in a systems biology approach. A focus on large-scale collaborative studies that explore many relevant biological samples to comprehensively determine disease mechanisms and therapeutic efficiency is necessary. This represents an important time for life sciences and the prospect of advances in diseases such as NAFLD is promising.

**Author Contributions:** David Houghton, Christopher J. Stewart, Christopher P. Day and Michael Trenell participated in the study concept and design. David Houghton and Christopher J. Stewart conducted the literature search and acquisition of the literature presented. David Houghton, Christopher J. Stewart, Christopher P. Day and Michael Trenell drafted the manuscript, read and approved the final manuscript.

## References

1.   Anstee, Q.M.; McPherson, S.; Day, C.P. How big a problem is non-alcoholic fatty liver disease? *BMJ* **2011**, *343*, d3897. [CrossRef] [PubMed]

2.   Harrison, S.A.; Day, C.P. Benefits of lifestyle modification in NAFLD. *Gut* **2007**, *56*, 1760–1769. [CrossRef] [PubMed]

3.   Henao-Mejia, J.; Elinav, E.; Jin, C.; Hao, L.; Mehal, W.Z.; Strowig, T.; Thaiss, C.A.; Kau, A.L.; Eisenbarth, S.C.; Jurczak, M.J.; *et al.* Inflammasome-mediated dysbiosis regulates progression of NAFLD and obesity. *Nature* **2012**, *482*, 179–185. [CrossRef] [PubMed]

4.   De Alwis, N.M.; Day, C.P. Non-alcoholic fatty liver disease: The mist gradually clears. *J. Hepatol.* **2008**, *48*, S104–S112. [CrossRef] [PubMed]

5.   Ratziu, V.; Sheikh, M.Y.; Sanyal, A.J.; Lim, J.K.; Conjeevaram, H.; Chalasani, N.; Abdelmalek, M.; Bakken, A.; Renou, C.; Palmer, M.; *et al.* A phase 2, randomized, double-blind, placebo-controlled study of GS-9450 in subjects with nonalcoholic steatohepatitis. *Hepatology* **2012**, *55*, 419–428. [CrossRef] [PubMed]

6.   Anstee, Q.M.; Targher, G.; Day, C.P. Progression of NAFLD to diabetes mellitus, cardiovascular disease or cirrhosis. *Nat. Rev. Gastroenterol. Hepatol.* **2013**, *10*, 330–344. [CrossRef] [PubMed]

7.   Boursier, J.; Mueller, O.; Barret, M.; Machado, M.; Fizanne, L.; Araujo-Perez, F.; Guy, C.D.; Seed, P.C.; Rawls, J.F.; David, L.A.; *et al.* The Severity of NAFLD Is Associated with Gut Dysbiosis and Shift in the Metabolic Function of the Gut Microbiota. Available online: http://www.mdlinx.com/gastroenterology/medical-news-article/2015/11/30/nafld-metabolic-function/6431385/ (accessed on 24 March 2016).

8.   Abu-Shanab, A.; Quigley, E.M. The role of the gut microbiota in nonalcoholic fatty liver disease. *Nat. Rev. Gastroenterol. Hepatol.* **2010**, *7*, 691–701. [CrossRef] [PubMed]

9.   Ley, R.E.; Peterson, D.A.; Gordon, J.I. Ecological and evolutionary forces shaping microbial diversity in the human intestine. *Cell* **2006**, *124*, 837–848. [CrossRef] [PubMed]

10.  Ley, R.E.; Turnbaugh, P.J.; Klein, S.; Gordon, J.I. Microbial ecology: Human gut microbes associated with obesity. *Nature* **2006**, *444*, 1022–1023. [CrossRef] [PubMed]

11.  Whitman, W.B.; Coleman, D.C.; Wiebe, W.J. Prokaryotes: The unseen majority. *Proc. Natl. Acad. Sci. USA* **1998**, *95*, 6578–6583. [CrossRef] [PubMed]

12.  Hoefert, B. Bacteria findings in duodenal juice of healthy and sick. *Zschr. Klin. Med.* **1921**, *92*, 221–235.

13.  Caballero, F.; Fernandez, A.; Matias, N.; Martinez, L.; Fucho, R.; Elena, M.; Caballeria, J.; Morales, A.; Fernandez-Checa, J.C.; Garcia-Ruiz, C. Specific contribution of methionine and choline in nutritional nonalcoholic steatohepatitis: Impact on mitochondrial S-adenosyl-L-methionine and glutathione. *J. Biol. Chem.* **2010**, *285*, 18528–18536. [CrossRef] [PubMed]

14.  Claesson, M.J.; Cusack, S.; O'Sullivan, O.; Greene-Diniz, R.; de Weerd, H.; Flannery, E.; Marchesi, J.R.; Falush, D.; Dinan, T.; Fitzgerald, G.; *et al.* Composition, variability, and temporal stability of the intestinal microbiota of the elderly. *Proc. Natl. Acad. Sci. USA* **2011**, *108*, 4586–4591. [CrossRef] [PubMed]

15.  Clemente, J.C.; Ursell, L.K.; Parfrey, L.W.; Knight, R. The impact of the gut microbiota on human health: An integrative view. *Cell* **2012**, *148*, 1258–1270. [CrossRef] [PubMed]

16.  Faith, J.J.; Guruge, J.L.; Charbonneau, M.; Subramanian, S.; Seedorf, H.; Goodman, A.L.; Clemente, J.C.; Knight, R.; Heath, A.C.; Leibel, R.L.; *et al.* The long-term stability of the human gut microbiota. *Science* **2013**, *341*, 1237439. [CrossRef] [PubMed]

17.  Holzapfel, W.H.; Haberer, P.; Snel, J.; Schillinger, U.; Huis in't Veld, J.H. Overview of gut flora and probiotics. *Int. J. Food Microbiol.* **1998**, *41*, 85–101. [CrossRef]

18.  Sommer, F.; Backhed, F. The gut microbiota—Masters of host development and physiology. *Nat. Rev. Microbiol.* **2013**, *11*, 227–238. [CrossRef] [PubMed]

19.  Hooper, L.V.; Gordon, J.I. Commensal host-bacterial relationships in the gut. *Science* **2001**, *292*, 1115–1118. [CrossRef] [PubMed]

20.  Stewart, C.J.; Marrs, E.C.; Nelson, A.; Lanyon, C.; Perry, J.D.; Embleton, N.D.; Cummings, S.P.; Berrington, J.E. Development of the preterm gut microbiome in twins at risk of necrotising enterocolitis and sepsis. *PLoS ONE* **2013**, *8*, e73465. [CrossRef] [PubMed]

21.  Stewart, J.A.; Chadwick, V.S.; Murray, A. Investigations into the influence of host genetics on the predominant eubacteria in the faecal microflora of children. *J. Med. Microbiol.* **2005**, *54*, 1239–1242. [CrossRef] [PubMed]

22.  Qin, J.; Li, R.; Raes, J.; Arumugam, M.; Burgdorf, K.S.; Manichanh, C.; Nielsen, T.; Pons, N.; Levenez, F.; Yamada, T.; *et al.* A human gut microbial gene catalogue established by metagenomic sequencing. *Nature* **2010**, *464*, 59–65. [CrossRef] [PubMed]

23.  Round, J.L.; Mazmanian, S.K. The gut microbiota shapes intestinal immune responses during health and disease. *Nat. Rev. Immunol.* **2009**, *9*, 313–323. [CrossRef] [PubMed]

24.  DuPont, A.W.; DuPont, H.L. The intestinal microbiota and chronic disorders of the gut. *Nat. Rev. Gastroenterol. Hepatol.* **2011**, *8*, 523–531. [CrossRef] [PubMed]

25.  Russell, W.R.; Duncan, S.H.; Flint, H.J. The gut microbial metabolome: Modulation of cancer risk in obese individuals. *Proc. Nutr. Soc.* **2013**, *72*, 178–188. [CrossRef] [PubMed]

26. Vrieze, A.; van Nood, E.; Holleman, F.; Salojarvi, J.; Kootte, R.S.; Bartelsman, J.F.; Dallinga-Thie, G.M.; Ackermans, M.T.; Serlie, M.J.; Oozeer, R.; *et al.* Transfer of intestinal microbiota from lean donors increases insulin sensitivity in individuals with metabolic syndrome. *Gastroenterology* **2012**, *143*, 913–916. [CrossRef] [PubMed]

27. Hardy, T.; Anstee, Q.M.; Day, C.P. Nonalcoholic fatty liver disease: New treatments. *Curr. Opin. Gastroenterol.* **2015**, *31*, 175–183. [CrossRef] [PubMed]

28. Taylor, R. Pathogenesis of type 2 diabetes: Tracing the reverse route from cure to cause. *Diabetologia* **2008**, *51*, 1781–1789. [CrossRef] [PubMed]

29. Thoma, C.; Day, C.P.; Trenell, M.I. Lifestyle interventions for the treatment of non-alcoholic fatty liver disease in adults: A systematic review. *J. Hepatol.* **2012**, *56*, 255–266. [CrossRef] [PubMed]

30. Vilar-Gomez, E.; Martinez-Perez, Y.; Calzadilla-Bertot, L.; Torres-Gonzalez, A.; Gra-Oramas, B.; Gonzalez-Fabian, L.; Friedman, S.L.; Diago, M.; Romero-Gomez, M. Weight loss via lifestyle modification significantly reduces features of nonalcoholic steatohepatitis. *Gastroenterology* **2015**, *149*, 367–378. [CrossRef] [PubMed]

31. Promrat, K.; Kleiner, D.E.; Niemeier, H.M.; Jackvony, E.; Kearns, M.; Wands, J.R.; Fava, J.L.; Wing, R.R. Randomized controlled trial testing the effects of weight loss on nonalcoholic steatohepatitis. *Hepatology* **2010**, *51*, 121–129. [CrossRef] [PubMed]

32. Dudekula, A.; Rachakonda, V.; Shaik, B.; Behari, J. Weight loss in nonalcoholic fatty liver disease patients in an ambulatory care setting is largely unsuccessful but correlates with frequency of clinic visits. *PLoS ONE* **2014**, *9*, e111808. [CrossRef] [PubMed]

33. Yamada, T.; Hara, K.; Svensson, A.K.; Shojima, N.; Hosoe, J.; Iwasaki, M.; Yamauchi, T.; Kadowaki, T. Successfully achieving target weight loss influences subsequent maintenance of lower weight and dropout from treatment. *Obesity* **2015**, *23*, 183–191. [CrossRef] [PubMed]

34. Bacchi, E.; Moghetti, P. Exercise for hepatic fat accumulation in type 2 diabetic subjects. *Int. J. Endocrinol.* **2013**, *2013*, 309191. [CrossRef] [PubMed]

35. Boursier, J.; Diehl, A.M. Implication of gut microbiota in nonalcoholic fatty liver disease. *PLoS Pathog.* **2015**, *11*, e1004559. [CrossRef] [PubMed]

36. Cani, P.D. When specific gut microbes reveal a possible link between hepatic steatosis and adipose tissue. *J. Hepatol.* **2014**, *61*, 5–6. [CrossRef] [PubMed]

37. Farhadi, A.; Gundlapalli, S.; Shaikh, M.; Frantzides, C.; Harrell, L.; Kwasny, M.M.; Keshavarzian, A. Susceptibility to gut leakiness: A possible mechanism for endotoxaemia in non-alcoholic steatohepatitis. *Liver Int.* **2008**, *28*, 1026–1033. [CrossRef] [PubMed]

38. Le Roy, T.; Llopis, M.; Lepage, P.; Bruneau, A.; Rabot, S.; Bevilacqua, C.; Martin, P.; Philippe, C.; Walker, F.; Bado, A.; *et al.* Intestinal microbiota determines development of non-alcoholic fatty liver disease in mice. *Gut* **2013**, *62*, 1787–1794. [CrossRef] [PubMed]

39. Mouzaki, M.; Comelli, E.M.; Arendt, B.M.; Bonengel, J.; Fung, S.K.; Fischer, S.E.; McGilvray, I.D.; Allard, J.P. Intestinal microbiota in patients with nonalcoholic fatty liver disease. *Hepatology* **2013**, *58*, 120–127. [CrossRef] [PubMed]

40. Wigg, A.J.; Roberts-Thomson, I.C.; Dymock, R.B.; McCarthy, P.J.; Grose, R.H.; Cummins, A.G. The role of small intestinal bacterial overgrowth, intestinal permeability, endotoxaemia, and tumour necrosis factor $\alpha$ in the pathogenesis of non-alcoholic steatohepatitis. *Gut* **2001**, *48*, 206–211. [CrossRef] [PubMed]

41. Zhu, L.; Baker, S.S.; Gill, C.; Liu, W.; Alkhouri, R.; Baker, R.D.; Gill, S.R. Characterization of gut microbiomes in nonalcoholic steatohepatitis (NASH) patients: A connection between endogenous alcohol and NASH. *Hepatology* **2013**, *57*, 601–609. [CrossRef] [PubMed]

42. Cani, P.D.; Osto, M.; Geurts, L.; Everard, A. Involvement of gut microbiota in the development of low-grade inflammation and type 2 diabetes associated with obesity. *Gut Microbes* **2012**, *3*, 279–288. [CrossRef] [PubMed]

43. Kirsch, R.; Clarkson, V.; Verdonk, R.C.; Marais, A.D.; Shephard, E.G.; Ryffel, B.; de la, M.H.P. Rodent nutritional model of steatohepatitis: Effects of endotoxin (lipopolysaccharide) and tumor necrosis factor $\alpha$ deficiency. *J. Gastroenterol. Hepatol.* **2006**, *21*, 174–182. [CrossRef] [PubMed]

44. Nolan, J.P. Intestinal endotoxins as mediators of hepatic injury—An idea whose time has come again. *Hepatology* **1989**, *10*, 887–891. [CrossRef] [PubMed]

45. Nolan, J.P.; Leibowitz, A.I. Endotoxins in liver disease. *Gastroenterology* **1978**, *75*, 765–766. [PubMed]

46.  Trenell, M.I. Sedentary behaviour, physical activity, and NAFLD: Curse of the chair. *J. Hepatol.* **2015**, *63*, 1064–1065. [CrossRef] [PubMed]

47.  Hallsworth, K.; Fattakhova, G.; Hollingsworth, K.G.; Thoma, C.; Moore, S.; Taylor, R.; Day, C.P.; Trenell, M.I. Resistance exercise reduces liver fat and its mediators in non-alcoholic fatty liver disease independent of weight loss. *Gut* **2011**, *60*, 1278–1283. [CrossRef] [PubMed]

48.  Hickman, I.J.; Byrne, N.M.; Croci, I.; Chachay, V.S.; Clouston, A.D.; Hills, A.P.; Bugianesi, B.; Whitehead, J.P.; Gastaldelli, A.; O'Moore-Sullivan, T.M.; *et al.* Randomised study of the metabolic and histological effects of exercise in non alcoholic steatohepatitis. *J. Diabetes Metab.* **2013**, *4*. [CrossRef]

49.  Johnson, N.A.; Sachinwalla, T.; Walton, D.W.; Smith, K.; Armstrong, A.; Thompson, M.W.; George, J. Aerobic exercise training reduces hepatic and visceral lipids in obese individuals without weight loss. *Hepatology* **2009**, *50*, 1105–1112. [CrossRef] [PubMed]

50.  Kirk, E.; Reeds, D.N.; Finck, B.N.; Mayurranjan, S.M.; Patterson, B.W.; Klein, S. Dietary fat and carbohydrates differentially alter insulin sensitivity during caloric restriction. *Gastroenterology* **2009**, *136*, 1552–1560. [CrossRef] [PubMed]

51.  Viljanen, A.P.; Iozzo, P.; Borra, R.; Kankaanpaa, M.; Karmi, A.; Lautamaki, R.; Jarvisalo, M.; Parkkola, R.; Ronnemaa, T.; Guiducci, L.; *et al.* Effect of weight loss on liver free fatty acid uptake and hepatic insulin resistance. *J. Clin. Endocrinol. Metab.* **2009**, *94*, 50–55. [CrossRef] [PubMed]

52.  Wong, V.W.; Chan, R.S.; Wong, G.L.; Cheung, B.H.; Chu, W.C.; Yeung, D.K.; Chim, A.M.; Lai, J.W.; Li, L.S.; Sea, M.M.; *et al.* Community-based lifestyle modification programme for non-alcoholic fatty liver disease: A randomized controlled trial. *J. Hepatol.* **2013**, *59*, 536–542. [CrossRef] [PubMed]

53.  Lazo, M.; Solga, S.F.; Horska, A.; Bonekamp, S.; Diehl, A.M.; Brancati, F.L.; Wagenknecht, L.E.; Pi-Sunyer, F.X.; Kahn, S.E.; Clark, J.M. Effect of a 12-month intensive lifestyle intervention on hepatic steatosis in adults with type 2 diabetes. *Diabetes Care* **2010**, *33*, 2156–2163. [CrossRef] [PubMed]

54.  Oza, N.; Eguchi, Y.; Mizuta, T.; Ishibashi, E.; Kitajima, Y.; Horie, H.; Ushirogawa, M.; Tsuzura, T.; Nakashita, S.; Takahashi, H.; *et al.* A pilot trial of body weight reduction for nonalcoholic fatty liver disease with a home-based lifestyle modification intervention delivered in collaboration with interdisciplinary medical staff. *J. Gastroenterol.* **2009**, *44*, 1203–1208. [CrossRef] [PubMed]

55.  Lim, J.S.; Mietus-Snyder, M.; Valente, A.; Schwarz, J.M.; Lustig, R.H. The role of fructose in the pathogenesis of NAFLD and the metabolic syndrome. *Nat. Rev. Gastroenterol. Hepatol.* **2010**, *7*, 251–264. [CrossRef] [PubMed]

56.  Costello, E.K.; Lauber, C.L.; Hamady, M.; Fierer, N.; Gordon, J.I.; Knight, R. Bacterial community variation in human body habitats across space and time. *Science* **2009**, *326*, 1694–1697. [CrossRef] [PubMed]

57.  Zoetendal, E.G.; Akkermans, A.D.; De Vos, W.M. Temperature gradient gel electrophoresis analysis of 16s rrna from human fecal samples reveals stable and host-specific communities of active bacteria. *Appl. Environ. Microbiol.* **1998**, *64*, 3854–3859. [PubMed]

58.  Sacks, F.M.; Bray, G.A.; Carey, V.J.; Smith, S.R.; Ryan, D.H.; Anton, S.D.; McManus, K.; Champagne, C.M.; Bishop, L.M.; Laranjo, N.; *et al.* Comparison of weight-loss diets with different compositions of fat, protein, and carbohydrates. *N. Engl. J. Med.* **2009**, *360*, 859–873. [CrossRef] [PubMed]

59.  Weinsier, R.L.; Hunter, G.R.; Heini, A.F.; Goran, M.I.; Sell, S.M. The etiology of obesity: Relative contribution of metabolic factors, diet, and physical activity. *Am. J. Med.* **1998**, *105*, 145–150. [CrossRef]

60.  Karlsson, F.; Tremaroli, V.; Nielsen, J.; Backhed, F. Assessing the human gut microbiota in metabolic diseases. *Diabetes* **2013**, *62*, 3341–3349. [CrossRef] [PubMed]

61.  Ley, R.E.; Backhed, F.; Turnbaugh, P.; Lozupone, C.A.; Knight, R.D.; Gordon, J.I. Obesity alters gut microbial ecology. *Proc. Natl. Acad. Sci. USA* **2005**, *102*, 11070–11075. [CrossRef] [PubMed]

62.  Walker, A.W.; Ince, J.; Duncan, S.H.; Webster, L.M.; Holtrop, G.; Ze, X.; Brown, D.; Stares, M.D.; Scott, P.; Bergerat, A.; *et al.* Dominant and diet-responsive groups of bacteria within the human colonic microbiota. *ISME J.* **2011**, *5*, 220–230. [CrossRef] [PubMed]

63.  Saghizadeh, M.; Ong, J.M.; Garvey, W.T.; Henry, R.R.; Kern, P.A. The expression of TNF $\alpha$ by human muscle. Relationship to insulin resistance. *J. Clin. Investig.* **1996**, *97*, 1111–1116. [CrossRef] [PubMed]

64.  Scott, K.P.; Gratz, S.W.; Sheridan, P.O.; Flint, H.J.; Duncan, S.H. The influence of diet on the gut microbiota. *Pharmacol. Res.* **2013**, *69*, 52–60. [CrossRef] [PubMed]

65.  Spencer, M.D.; Hamp, T.J.; Reid, R.W.; Fischer, L.M.; Zeisel, S.H.; Fodor, A.A. Association between composition of the human gastrointestinal microbiome and development of fatty liver with choline deficiency. *Gastroenterology* **2011**, *140*, 976–986. [CrossRef] [PubMed]

66.  Turnbaugh, P.J.; Ridaura, V.K.; Faith, J.J.; Rey, F.E.; Knight, R.; Gordon, J.I. The effect of diet on the human gut microbiome: A metagenomic analysis in humanized gnotobiotic mice. *Sci. Transl. Med.* **2009**, *1*, 6ra14. [CrossRef] [PubMed]

67.  De Filippo, C.; Cavalieri, D.; di Paola, M.; Ramazzotti, M.; Poullet, J.B.; Massart, S.; Collini, S.; Pieraccini, G.; Lionetti, P. Impact of diet in shaping gut microbiota revealed by a comparative study in children from europe and rural africa. *Proc. Natl. Acad. Sci. USA* **2010**, *107*, 14691–14696. [CrossRef] [PubMed]

68.  Gibson, G.R.; Roberfroid, M.B. Dietary modulation of the human colonic microbiota: Introducing the concept of prebiotics. *J. Nutr.* **1995**, *125*, 1401–1412. [PubMed]

69.  Day, C.P.; James, O.F. Steatohepatitis: A tale of two "hits"? *Gastroenterology* **1998**, *114*, 842–845. [CrossRef]

70.  Musso, G.; Gambino, R.; De Michieli, F.; Cassader, M.; Rizzetto, M.; Durazzo, M.; Faga, E.; Silli, B.; Pagano, G. Dietary habits and their relations to insulin resistance and postprandial lipemia in nonalcoholic steatohepatitis. *Hepatology* **2003**, *37*, 909–916. [CrossRef] [PubMed]

71.  Toshimitsu, K.; Matsuura, B.; Ohkubo, I.; Niiya, T.; Furukawa, S.; Hiasa, Y.; Kawamura, M.; Ebihara, K.; Onji, M. Dietary habits and nutrient intake in non-alcoholic steatohepatitis. *Nutrition* **2007**, *23*, 46–52. [CrossRef] [PubMed]

72.  Donnelly, K.L.; Smith, C.I.; Schwarzenberg, S.J.; Jessurun, J.; Boldt, M.D.; Parks, E.J. Sources of fatty acids stored in liver and secreted via lipoproteins in patients with nonalcoholic fatty liver disease. *J. Clin. Investig.* **2005**, *115*, 1343–1351. [CrossRef] [PubMed]

73.  Westerbacka, J.; Lammi, K.; Hakkinen, A.M.; Rissanen, A.; Salminen, I.; Aro, A.; Yki-Jarvinen, H. Dietary fat content modifies liver fat in overweight nondiabetic subjects. *J. Clin. Endocrinol. Metab.* **2005**, *90*, 2804–2809. [CrossRef] [PubMed]

74.  Van Herpen, N.A.; Schrauwen-Hinderling, V.B.; Schaart, G.; Mensink, R.P.; Schrauwen, P. Three weeks on a high-fat diet increases intrahepatic lipid accumulation and decreases metabolic flexibility in healthy overweight men. *J. Clin. Endocrinol. Metab.* **2011**, *96*, E691–E695. [CrossRef] [PubMed]

75.  Marina, A.; von Frankenberg, A.D.; Suvag, S.; Callahan, H.S.; Kratz, M.; Richards, T.L.; Utzschneider, K.M. Effects of dietary fat and saturated fat content on liver fat and markers of oxidative stress in overweight/obese men and women under weight-stable conditions. *Nutrients* **2014**, *6*, 4678–4690. [CrossRef] [PubMed]

76.  Utzschneider, K.M.; Bayer-Carter, J.L.; Arbuckle, M.D.; Tidwell, J.M.; Richards, T.L.; Craft, S. Beneficial effect of a weight-stable, low-fat/low-saturated fat/low-glycaemic index diet to reduce liver fat in older subjects. *Br. J. Nutr.* **2013**, *109*, 1096–1104. [CrossRef] [PubMed]

77.  Delarue, J.; Lalles, J.P. Nonalcoholic fatty liver disease: Roles of the gut and the liver and metabolic modulation by some dietary factors and especially long-chain *n*-3 PUFA. *Mol. Nutr. Food Res.* **2016**, *60*, 147–159. [CrossRef] [PubMed]

78.  Tilg, H.; Moschen, A.R. Insulin resistance, inflammation, and non-alcoholic fatty liver disease. *Trends Endocrinol. Metab.* **2008**, *19*, 371–379. [CrossRef] [PubMed]

79.  Cani, P.D.; Amar, J.; Iglesias, M.A.; Poggi, M.; Knauf, C.; Bastelica, D.; Neyrinck, A.M.; Fava, F.; Tuohy, K.M.; Chabo, C.; *et al.* Metabolic endotoxemia initiates obesity and insulin resistance. *Diabetes* **2007**, *56*, 1761–1772. [CrossRef] [PubMed]

80.  Turnbaugh, P.J.; Ley, R.E.; Mahowald, M.A.; Magrini, V.; Mardis, E.R.; Gordon, J.I. An obesity-associated gut microbiome with increased capacity for energy harvest. *Nature* **2006**, *444*, 1027–1031. [CrossRef] [PubMed]

81.  Cani, P.D.; Neyrinck, A.M.; Fava, F.; Knauf, C.; Burcelin, R.G.; Tuohy, K.M.; Gibson, G.R.; Delzenne, N.M. Selective increases of bifidobacteria in gut microflora improve high-fat-diet-induced diabetes in mice through a mechanism associated with endotoxaemia. *Diabetologia* **2007**, *50*, 2374–2383. [CrossRef] [PubMed]

82.  Hildebrandt, M.A.; Hoffmann, C.; Sherrill-Mix, S.A.; Keilbaugh, S.A.; Hamady, M.; Chen, Y.Y.; Knight, R.; Ahima, R.S.; Bushman, F.; Wu, G.D. High-fat diet determines the composition of the murine gut microbiome independently of obesity. *Gastroenterology* **2009**, *137*, 1716–1724. [CrossRef] [PubMed]

83.  Murphy, E.F.; Cotter, P.D.; Healy, S.; Marques, T.M.; O'Sullivan, O.; Fouhy, F.; Clarke, S.F.; O'Toole, P.W.; Quigley, E.M.; Stanton, C.; *et al.* Composition and energy harvesting capacity of the gut microbiota: Relationship to diet, obesity and time in mouse models. *Gut* **2010**, *59*, 1635–1642. [CrossRef] [PubMed]

84. Turnbaugh, P.J.; Backhed, F.; Fulton, L.; Gordon, J.I. Diet-induced obesity is linked to marked but reversible alterations in the mouse distal gut microbiome. *Cell Host Microbe* **2008**, *3*, 213–223. [CrossRef] [PubMed]

85. Ghanim, H.; Abuaysheh, S.; Sia, C.L.; Korzeniewski, K.; Chaudhuri, A.; Fernandez-Real, J.M.; Dandona, P. Increase in plasma endotoxin concentrations and the expression of toll-like receptors and suppressor of cytokine signaling-3 in mononuclear cells after a high-fat, high-carbohydrate meal: Implications for insulin resistance. *Diabetes Care* **2009**, *32*, 2281–2287. [CrossRef] [PubMed]

86. Pendyala, S.; Walker, J.M.; Holt, P.R. A high-fat diet is associated with endotoxemia that originates from the gut. *Gastroenterology* **2012**, *142*, 1100–1101. [CrossRef] [PubMed]

87. Pussinen, P.J.; Havulinna, A.S.; Lehto, M.; Sundvall, J.; Salomaa, V. Endotoxemia is associated with an increased risk of incident diabetes. *Diabetes Care* **2011**, *34*, 392–397. [CrossRef] [PubMed]

88. Amar, J.; Chabo, C.; Waget, A.; Klopp, P.; Vachoux, C.; Bermudez-Humaran, L.G.; Smirnova, N.; Berge, M.; Sulpice, T.; Lahtinen, S.; *et al.* Intestinal mucosal adherence and translocation of commensal bacteria at the early onset of type 2 diabetes: Molecular mechanisms and probiotic treatment. *EMBO Mol. Med.* **2011**, *3*, 559–572. [CrossRef] [PubMed]

89. Caesar, R.; Tremaroli, V.; Kovatcheva-Datchary, P.; Cani, P.D.; Backhed, F. Crosstalk between gut microbiota and dietary lipids aggravates wat inflammation through TLR signaling. *Cell Metab.* **2015**, *22*, 658–668. [CrossRef] [PubMed]

90. Su, L.; Wang, J.H.; Cong, X.; Wang, L.H.; Liu, F.; Xie, X.W.; Zhang, H.H.; Fei, R.; Liu, Y.L. Intestinal immune barrier integrity in rats with nonalcoholic hepatic steatosis and steatohepatitis. *Chin. Med. J.* **2012**, *125*, 306–311. [PubMed]

91. Tilg, H.; Moschen, A.R. Evolution of inflammation in nonalcoholic fatty liver disease: The multiple parallel hits hypothesis. *Hepatology* **2010**, *52*, 1836–1846. [CrossRef] [PubMed]

92. Corbin, K.D.; Zeisel, S.H. Choline metabolism provides novel insights into nonalcoholic fatty liver disease and its progression. *Curr. Opin. Gastroenterol.* **2012**, *28*, 159–165. [CrossRef] [PubMed]

93. Jiang, X.C.; Li, Z.; Liu, R.; Yang, X.P.; Pan, M.; Lagrost, L.; Fisher, E.A.; Williams, K.J. Phospholipid transfer protein deficiency impairs apolipoprotein-b secretion from hepatocytes by stimulating a proteolytic pathway through a relative deficiency of vitamin e and an increase in intracellular oxidants. *J. Biol. Chem.* **2005**, *280*, 18336–18340. [CrossRef] [PubMed]

94. Dumas, M.E.; Barton, R.H.; Toye, A.; Cloarec, O.; Blancher, C.; Rothwell, A.; Fearnside, J.; Tatoud, R.; Blanc, V.; Lindon, J.C.; *et al.* Metabolic profiling reveals a contribution of gut microbiota to fatty liver phenotype in insulin-resistant mice. *Proc. Natl. Acad. Sci. USA* **2006**, *103*, 12511–12516. [CrossRef] [PubMed]

95. Fukiya, S.; Arata, M.; Kawashima, H.; Yoshida, D.; Kaneko, M.; Minamida, K.; Watanabe, J.; Ogura, Y.; Uchida, K.; Itoh, K.; *et al.* Conversion of cholic acid and chenodeoxycholic acid into their 7-oxo derivatives by bacteroides intestinalis AM-1 isolated from human feces. *FEMS Microbiol. Lett.* **2009**, *293*, 263–270. [CrossRef] [PubMed]

96. Islam, K.B.; Fukiya, S.; Hagio, M.; Fujii, N.; Ishizuka, S.; Ooka, T.; Ogura, Y.; Hayashi, T.; Yokota, A. Bile acid is a host factor that regulates the composition of the cecal microbiota in rats. *Gastroenterology* **2011**, *141*, 1773–1781. [CrossRef] [PubMed]

97. Sayin, S.I.; Wahlstrom, A.; Felin, J.; Jantti, S.; Marschall, H.U.; Bamberg, K.; Angelin, B.; Hyotylainen, T.; Oresic, M.; Backhed, F. Gut microbiota regulates bile acid metabolism by reducing the levels of tauro-β-muricholic acid, a naturally occurring fxr antagonist. *Cell Metab.* **2013**, *17*, 225–235. [CrossRef] [PubMed]

98. Duncan, S.H.; Lobley, G.E.; Holtrop, G.; Ince, J.; Johnstone, A.M.; Louis, P.; Flint, H.J. Human colonic microbiota associated with diet, obesity and weight loss. *Int. J. Obes.* **2008**, *32*, 1720–1724. [CrossRef] [PubMed]

99. Kankaanpaa, P.E.; Salminen, S.J.; Isolauri, E.; Lee, Y.K. The influence of polyunsaturated fatty acids on probiotic growth and adhesion. *FEMS Microbiol. Lett.* **2001**, *194*, 149–153. [CrossRef] [PubMed]

100. Mujico, J.R.; Baccan, G.C.; Gheorghe, A.; Diaz, L.E.; Marcos, A. Changes in gut microbiota due to supplemented fatty acids in diet-induced obese mice. *Br. J. Nutr.* **2013**, *110*, 711–720. [CrossRef] [PubMed]

101. Bozzetto, L.; Prinster, A.; Annuzzi, G.; Costagliola, L.; Mangione, A.; Vitelli, A.; Mazzarella, R.; Longobardo, M.; Mancini, M.; Vigorito, C.; *et al.* Liver fat is reduced by an isoenergetic MUFA diet in a controlled randomized study in type 2 diabetic patients. *Diabetes Care* **2012**, *35*, 1429–1435. [CrossRef] [PubMed]

102. Houghton, D.; Wilcox, M.D.; Chater, P.I.; Brownlee, I.A.; Seal, C.J.; Pearson, J.P. Biological activity of alginate and its effect on pancreatic lipase inhibition as a potential treatment for obesity. *Food Hydrocoll.* **2015**, *49*, 18–24. [CrossRef] [PubMed]

103. Neyrinck, A.M.; Possemiers, S.; Druart, C.; van de Wiele, T.; De Backer, F.; Cani, P.D.; Larondelle, Y.; Delzenne, N.M. Prebiotic effects of wheat arabinoxylan related to the increase in *Bifidobacteria*, *Roseburia* and *Bacteroides/Prevotella* in diet-induced obese mice. *PLoS ONE* **2011**, *6*, e20944. [CrossRef] [PubMed]

104. Neyrinck, A.M.; Possemiers, S.; Verstraete, W.; De Backer, F.; Cani, P.D.; Delzenne, N.M. Dietary modulation of *Clostridial* cluster xiva gut bacteria (*Roseburia* spp.) by chitin-glucan fiber improves host metabolic alterations induced by high-fat diet in mice. *J. Nutr. Biochem.* **2012**, *23*, 51–59. [CrossRef] [PubMed]

105. Lopez, H.W.; Levrat, M.A.; Guy, C.; Messager, A.; Demigne, C.; Remesy, C. Effects of soluble corn bran arabinoxylans on cecal digestion, lipid metabolism, and mineral balance (Ca, Mg) in rats. *J. Nutr. Biochem.* **1999**, *10*, 500–509. [CrossRef]

106. Wydro, P.; Krajewska, B.; Hac-Wydro, K. Chitosan as a lipid binder: A langmuir monolayer study of chitosan-lipid interactions. *Biomacromolecules* **2007**, *8*, 2611–2617. [CrossRef] [PubMed]

107. Flint, H.J.; Scott, K.P.; Louis, P.; Duncan, S.H. The role of the gut microbiota in nutrition and health. *Nat. Rev. Gastroenterol. Hepatol.* **2012**, *9*, 577–589. [CrossRef] [PubMed]

108. David, L.A.; Maurice, C.F.; Carmody, R.N.; Gootenberg, D.B.; Button, J.E.; Wolfe, B.E.; Ling, A.V.; Devlin, A.S.; Varma, Y.; Fischbach, M.A.; *et al.* Diet rapidly and reproducibly alters the human gut microbiome. *Nature* **2014**, *505*, 559–563. [CrossRef] [PubMed]

109. Chung, M.; Ma, J.T.; Patel, K.; Berger, S.; Lau, J.; Lichtenstein, A.H. Fructose, high-fructose corn syrup, sucrose, and nonalcoholic fatty liver disease or indexes of liver health: A systematic review and meta-analysis. *Am. J. Clin. Nutr.* **2014**, *100*, 833–849. [CrossRef] [PubMed]

110. Collison, K.S.; Saleh, S.M.; Bakheet, R.H.; Al-Rabiah, R.K.; Inglis, A.L.; Makhoul, N.J.; Maqbool, Z.M.; Zaidi, M.Z.; Al-Johi, M.A.; Al-Mohanna, F.A. Diabetes of the liver: The link between nonalcoholic fatty liver disease and HFCS-55. *Obesity* **2009**, *17*, 2003–2013. [CrossRef] [PubMed]

111. Saad, M.F.; Khan, A.; Sharma, A.; Michael, R.; Riad-Gabriel, M.G.; Boyadjian, R.; Jinagouda, S.D.; Steil, G.M.; Kamdar, V. Physiological insulinemia acutely modulates plasma leptin. *Diabetes* **1998**, *47*, 544–549. [CrossRef] [PubMed]

112. Zelber-Sagi, S.; Nitzan-Kaluski, D.; Goldsmith, R.; Webb, M.; Blendis, L.; Halpern, Z.; Oren, R. Long term nutritional intake and the risk for non-alcoholic fatty liver disease (NAFLD): A population based study. *J. Hepatol.* **2007**, *47*, 711–717. [CrossRef] [PubMed]

113. Bergheim, I.; Weber, S.; Vos, M.; Kramer, S.; Volynets, V.; Kaserouni, S.; McClain, C.J.; Bischoff, S.C. Antibiotics protect against fructose-induced hepatic lipid accumulation in mice: Role of endotoxin. *J. Hepatol.* **2008**, *48*, 983–992. [CrossRef] [PubMed]

114. Spruss, A.; Kanuri, G.; Wagnerberger, S.; Haub, S.; Bischoff, S.C.; Bergheim, I. Toll-like receptor 4 is involved in the development of fructose-induced hepatic steatosis in mice. *Hepatology* **2009**, *50*, 1094–1104. [CrossRef] [PubMed]

115. Thuy, S.; Ladurner, R.; Volynets, V.; Wagner, S.; Strahl, S.; Konigsrainer, A.; Maier, K.P.; Bischoff, S.C.; Bergheim, I. Nonalcoholic fatty liver disease in humans is associated with increased plasma endotoxin and plasminogen activator inhibitor 1 concentrations and with fructose intake. *J. Nutr.* **2008**, *138*, 1452–1455. [PubMed]

116. Bizeau, M.E.; Pagliassotti, M.J. Hepatic adaptations to sucrose and fructose. *Metabolism* **2005**, *54*, 1189–1201. [CrossRef] [PubMed]

117. Pagliassotti, M.J.; Prach, P.A.; Koppenhafer, T.A.; Pan, D.A. Changes in insulin action, triglycerides, and lipid composition during sucrose feeding in rats. *Am. J. Physiol.* **1996**, *271*, R1319–R1326. [PubMed]

118. Poulsom, R. Morphological changes of organs after sucrose or fructose feeding. *Prog. Biochem. Pharmacol.* **1986**, *21*, 104–134. [PubMed]

119. Spruss, A.; Kanuri, G.; Stahl, C.; Bischoff, S.C.; Bergheim, I. Metformin protects against the development of fructose-induced steatosis in mice: Role of the intestinal barrier function. *Lab. Investig.* **2012**, *92*, 1020–1032. [CrossRef] [PubMed]

120. Walker, A.W.; Duncan, S.H.; McWilliam Leitch, E.C.; Child, M.W.; Flint, H.J. Ph and peptide supply can radically alter bacterial populations and short-chain fatty acid ratios within microbial communities from the human colon. *Appl. Environ. Microbiol.* **2005**, *71*, 3692–3700. [CrossRef] [PubMed]

121. Duncan, S.H.; Belenguer, A.; Holtrop, G.; Johnstone, A.M.; Flint, H.J.; Lobley, G.E. Reduced dietary intake of carbohydrates by obese subjects results in decreased concentrations of butyrate and butyrate-producing bacteria in feces. *Appl. Environ. Microbiol.* **2007**, *73*, 1073–1078. [CrossRef] [PubMed]

122. Ferrere, G.; Leroux, A.; Wrzosek, L.; Puchois, V.; Gaudin, F.; Ciocan, D.; Renoud, M.L.; Naveau, S.; Perlemuter, G.; Cassard, A.M. Activation of kupffer cells is associated with a specific dysbiosis induced by fructose or high fat diet in mice. *PLoS ONE* **2016**, *11*, e0146177. [CrossRef] [PubMed]

123. Pagano, G.; Pacini, G.; Musso, G.; Gambino, R.; Mecca, F.; Depetris, N.; Cassader, M.; David, E.; Cavallo-Perin, P.; Rizzetto, M. Nonalcoholic steatohepatitis, insulin resistance, and metabolic syndrome: Further evidence for an etiologic association. *Hepatology* **2002**, *35*, 367–372. [CrossRef] [PubMed]

124. Vrieze, A.; Holleman, F.; Zoetendal, E.G.; de Vos, W.M.; Hoekstra, J.B.; Nieuwdorp, M. The environment within: How gut microbiota may influence metabolism and body composition. *Diabetologia* **2010**, *53*, 606–613. [CrossRef] [PubMed]

125. Nilsson, A.C.; Ostman, E.M.; Holst, J.J.; Bjorck, I.M. Including indigestible carbohydrates in the evening meal of healthy subjects improves glucose tolerance, lowers inflammatory markers, and increases satiety after a subsequent standardized breakfast. *J. Nutr.* **2008**, *138*, 732–739. [PubMed]

126. Parnell, J.A.; Reimer, R.A. Weight loss during oligofructose supplementation is associated with decreased ghrelin and increased peptide YY in overweight and obese adults. *Am. J. Clin. Nutr.* **2009**, *89*, 1751–1759. [CrossRef] [PubMed]

127. Hashidume, T.; Sasaki, T.; Inoue, J.; Sato, R. Consumption of soy protein isolate reduces hepatic srebp-1c and lipogenic gene expression in wild-type mice, but not in FXR-deficient mice. *Biosci. Biotechnol. Biochem.* **2011**, *75*, 1702–1707. [CrossRef] [PubMed]

128. Jakubowicz, D.; Froy, O. Biochemical and metabolic mechanisms by which dietary whey protein may combat obesity and type 2 diabetes. *J. Nutr. Biochem.* **2013**, *24*, 1–5. [CrossRef] [PubMed]

129. Faure, P.; Rossini, E.; Lafond, J.L.; Richard, M.J.; Favier, A.; Halimi, S. Vitamin e improves the free radical defense system potential and insulin sensitivity of rats fed high fructose diets. *J. Nutr.* **1997**, *127*, 103–107. [PubMed]

130. Noguchi, Y.; Nishikata, N.; Shikata, N.; Kimura, Y.; Aleman, J.O.; Young, J.D.; Koyama, N.; Kelleher, J.K.; Takahashi, M.; Stephanopoulos, G. Ketogenic essential amino acids modulate lipid synthetic pathways and prevent hepatic steatosis in mice. *PLoS ONE* **2010**, *5*, e12057. [CrossRef] [PubMed]

131. Pichon, L.; Huneau, J.F.; Fromentin, G.; Tome, D. A high-protein, high-fat, carbohydrate-free diet reduces energy intake, hepatic lipogenesis, and adiposity in rats. *J. Nutr.* **2006**, *136*, 1256–1260. [PubMed]

132. Qin, B.; Nagasaki, M.; Ren, M.; Bajotto, G.; Oshida, Y.; Sato, Y. Cinnamon extract prevents the insulin resistance induced by a high-fructose diet. *Horm. Metab. Res.* **2004**, *36*, 119–125. [PubMed]

133. Halton, T.L.; Hu, F.B. The effects of high protein diets on thermogenesis, satiety and weight loss: A critical review. *J. Am. Coll. Nutr.* **2004**, *23*, 373–385. [CrossRef] [PubMed]

134. Cummings, J.H. Carbohydrate and protein digestion: The substrate available for fermentation. In *The Large Intestine in Nutrition and Disease*; Danone Institute: Brussels, Belgium, 1997; pp. 15–42.

135. Smith, E.A.; Macfarlane, G.T. Enumeration of human colonic bacteria producing phenolic and indolic compounds: Effects of pH, carbohydrate availability and retention time on dissimilatory aromatic amino acid metabolism. *J. Appl. Bacteriol.* **1996**, *81*, 288–302. [CrossRef] [PubMed]

136. Smith, E.A.; Macfarlane, G.T. Studies on amine production in the human colon: Enumeration of amine forming bacteria and physiological effects of carbohydrate and pH. *Anaerobe* **1996**, *2*, 285–297.

137. Russell, W.R.; Gratz, S.W.; Duncan, S.H.; Holtrop, G.; Ince, J.; Scobbie, L.; Duncan, G.; Johnstone, A.M.; Lobley, G.E.; Wallace, R.J.; *et al.* High-protein, reduced-carbohydrate weight-loss diets promote metabolite profiles likely to be detrimental to colonic health. *Am. J. Clin. Nutr.* **2011**, *93*, 1062–1072. [PubMed]

138. Shen, Q.; Chen, Y.A.; Tuohy, K.M. A comparative *in vitro* investigation into the effects of cooked meats on the human faecal microbiota. *Anaerobe* **2010**, *16*, 572–577. [PubMed]

139. Aron-Wisnewsky, J.; Gaborit, B.; Dutour, A.; Clement, K. Gut microbiota and non-alcoholic fatty liver disease: New insights. *Clin. Microbiol. Infect.* **2013**, *19*, 338–348. [PubMed]

140. Schnabl, B.; Brenner, D.A. Interactions between the intestinal microbiome and liver diseases. *Gastroenterology* **2014**, *146*, 1513–1524. [PubMed]

141. Hooda, S.; Vester Boler, B.M.; Kerr, K.R.; Dowd, S.E.; Swanson, K.S. The gut microbiome of kittens is affected by dietary protein: Carbohydrate ratio and associated with blood metabolite and hormone concentrations. *Br. J. Nutr.* **2013**, *109*, 1637–1646. [PubMed]

142. Boudry, G.; Jamin, A.; Chatelais, L.; Gras-Le Guen, C.; Michel, C.; Le Huerou-Luron, I. Dietary protein excess during neonatal life alters colonic microbiota and mucosal response to inflammatory mediators later in life in female pigs. *J. Nutr.* **2013**, *143*, 1225–1232. [CrossRef] [PubMed]

143. Cohen, A.M.; Teitelbaum, A. Effect of different levels of protein in sucrose and starch diets on lipid synthesis in the rat. *Isr. J. Med. Sci.* **1966**, *2*, 727–732. [PubMed]

144. Masoro, E.J.; Chaikoff, I.L.; Chernick, S.S.; Felts, J.M. Previous nutritional state and glucose conversion to fatty acids in liver slices. *J. Biol. Chem.* **1950**, *185*, 845–856. [PubMed]

145. Yeh, Y.Y.; Leveille, G.A. Effect of dietary protein on hepatic lipogenesis in the growing chick. *J. Nutr.* **1969**, *98*, 356–366. [PubMed]

146. Bortolotti, M.; Maiolo, E.; Corazza, M.; van Dijke, E.; Schneiter, P.; Boss, A.; Carrel, G.; Giusti, V.; Le, K.A.; Quo Chong, D.G.; *et al.* Effects of a whey protein supplementation on intrahepatocellular lipids in obese female patients. *Clin. Nutr.* **2011**, *30*, 494–498. [CrossRef] [PubMed]

147. Farnsworth, E.; Luscombe, N.D.; Noakes, M.; Wittert, G.; Argyiou, E.; Clifton, P.M. Effect of a high-protein, energy-restricted diet on body composition, glycemic control, and lipid concentrations in overweight and obese hyperinsulinemic men and women. *Am. J. Clin. Nutr.* **2003**, *78*, 31–39. [PubMed]

148. Jenkins, D.J.; Kendall, C.W.; Vidgen, E.; Augustin, L.S.; van Erk, M.; Geelen, A.; Parker, T.; Faulkner, D.; Vuksan, V.; Josse, R.G.; *et al.* High-protein diets in hyperlipidemia: Effect of wheat gluten on serum lipids, uric acid, and renal function. *Am. J. Clin. Nutr.* **2001**, *74*, 57–63. [PubMed]

149. Samaha, F.F.; Iqbal, N.; Seshadri, P.; Chicano, K.L.; Daily, D.A.; McGrory, J.; Williams, T.; Williams, M.; Gracely, E.J.; Stern, L. A low-carbohydrate as compared with a low-fat diet in severe obesity. *N. Engl. J. Med.* **2003**, *348*, 2074–2081. [CrossRef] [PubMed]

150. Yang, H.Y.; Tzeng, Y.H.; Chai, C.Y.; Hsieh, A.T.; Chen, J.R.; Chang, L.S.; Yang, S.S. Soy protein retards the progression of non-alcoholic steatohepatitis via improvement of insulin resistance and steatosis. *Nutrition* **2011**, *27*, 943–948. [CrossRef] [PubMed]

151. Gentile, C.L.; Nivala, A.M.; Gonzales, J.C.; Pfaffenbach, K.T.; Wang, D.; Wei, Y.; Jiang, H.; Orlicky, D.J.; Petersen, D.R.; Pagliassotti, M.J.; *et al.* Experimental evidence for therapeutic potential of taurine in the treatment of nonalcoholic fatty liver disease. *Am. J. Physiol. Regul. Integr. Comp. Physiol.* **2011**, *301*, R1710–R1722. [CrossRef] [PubMed]

152. Linn, T.; Geyer, R.; Prassek, S.; Laube, H. Effect of dietary protein intake on insulin secretion and glucose metabolism in insulin-dependent diabetes mellitus. *J. Clin. Endocrinol. Metab.* **1996**, *81*, 3938–3943. [PubMed]

153. Linn, T.; Santosa, B.; Gronemeyer, D.; Aygen, S.; Scholz, N.; Busch, M.; Bretzel, R.G. Effect of long-term dietary protein intake on glucose metabolism in humans. *Diabetologia* **2000**, *43*, 1257–1265. [CrossRef] [PubMed]

154. Delzenne, N.M.; Neyrinck, A.M.; Backhed, F.; Cani, P.D. Targeting gut microbiota in obesity: Effects of prebiotics and probiotics. *Nat. Rev. Endocrinol.* **2011**, *7*, 639–646. [CrossRef] [PubMed]

155. Slavin, J. Fiber and prebiotics: Mechanisms and health benefits. *Nutrients* **2013**, *5*, 1417–1435. [CrossRef] [PubMed]

156. Moschen, A.R.; Kaser, S.; Tilg, H. Non-alcoholic steatohepatitis: A microbiota-driven disease. *Trends Endocrinol. Metab.* **2013**, *24*, 537–545. [CrossRef] [PubMed]

157. Cani, P.D.; Joly, E.; Horsmans, Y.; Delzenne, N.M. Oligofructose promotes satiety in healthy human: A pilot study. *Eur. J. Clin. Nutr.* **2006**, *60*, 567–572. [CrossRef] [PubMed]

158. Cani, P.D.; Knauf, C.; Iglesias, M.A.; Drucker, D.J.; Delzenne, N.M.; Burcelin, R. Improvement of glucose tolerance and hepatic insulin sensitivity by oligofructose requires a functional glucagon-like peptide 1 receptor. *Diabetes* **2006**, *55*, 1484–1490. [CrossRef] [PubMed]

159. Everard, A.; Lazarevic, V.; Derrien, M.; Girard, M.; Muccioli, G.G.; Neyrinck, A.M.; Possemiers, S.; van Holle, A.; Francois, P.; de Vos, W.M.; *et al.* Responses of gut microbiota and glucose and lipid metabolism to prebiotics in genetic obese and diet-induced leptin-resistant mice. *Diabetes* **2011**, *60*, 2775–2786. [CrossRef] [PubMed]

160. Cani, P.D.; Dewever, C.; Delzenne, N.M. Inulin-type fructans modulate gastrointestinal peptides involved in appetite regulation (glucagon-like peptide-1 and ghrelin) in rats. *Br. J. Nutr.* **2004**, *92*, 521–526. [CrossRef] [PubMed]

161. Sugatani, J.; Wada, T.; Osabe, M.; Yamakawa, K.; Yoshinari, K.; Miwa, M. Dietary inulin alleviates hepatic steatosis and xenobiotics-induced liver injury in rats fed a high-fat and high-sucrose diet: Association with the suppression of hepatic cytochrome p450 and hepatocyte nuclear factor 4α expression. *Drug Metab. Dispos.* **2006**, *34*, 1677–1687. [CrossRef] [PubMed]

162. Daubioul, C.; Rousseau, N.; Demeure, R.; Gallez, B.; Taper, H.; Declerck, B.; Delzenne, N. Dietary fructans, but not cellulose, decrease triglyceride accumulation in the liver of obese zucker FA/FA rats. *J. Nutr.* **2002**, *132*, 967–973. [PubMed]

163. Fiordaliso, M.; Kok, N.; Desager, J.P.; Goethals, F.; Deboyser, D.; Roberfroid, M.; Delzenne, N. Dietary oligofructose lowers triglycerides, phospholipids and cholesterol in serum and very low density lipoproteins of rats. *Lipids* **1995**, *30*, 163–167. [CrossRef] [PubMed]

164. Parnell, J.A.; Reimer, R.A. Effect of prebiotic fibre supplementation on hepatic gene expression and serum lipids: A dose-response study in JCR:LA-cp rats. *Br. J. Nutr.* **2010**, *103*, 1577–1584. [CrossRef] [PubMed]

165. Lin, H.V.; Frassetto, A.; Kowalik, E.J., Jr.; Nawrocki, A.R.; Lu, M.M.; Kosinski, J.R.; Hubert, J.A.; Szeto, D.; Yao, X.; Forrest, G.; et al. Butyrate and propionate protect against diet-induced obesity and regulate gut hormones via free fatty acid receptor 3-independent mechanisms. *PLoS ONE* **2012**, *7*, e35240. [CrossRef] [PubMed]

166. Archer, B.J.; Johnson, S.K.; Devereux, H.M.; Baxter, A.L. Effect of fat replacement by inulin or lupin-kernel fibre on sausage patty acceptability, post-meal perceptions of satiety and food intake in men. *Br. J. Nutr.* **2004**, *91*, 591–599. [CrossRef] [PubMed]

167. Dehghan, P.; Pourghassem Gargari, B.; Asghari Jafar-abadi, M. Oligofructose-enriched inulin improves some inflammatory markers and metabolic endotoxemia in women with type 2 diabetes mellitus: A randomized controlled clinical trial. *Nutrition* **2014**, *30*, 418–423. [CrossRef] [PubMed]

168. Daubioul, C.; Horsmans, Y.; Lambert, P.; Danse, E.; Delzenne, N.M. Effects of oligofructose on glucose and lipid metabolism in patients with nonalcoholic steatohepatitis: Results of a pilot study. *Eur. J. Clin. Nutr.* **2005**, *59*, 723–726. [CrossRef] [PubMed]

169. Malaguarnera, M.; Vacante, M.; Antic, T.; Giordano, M.; Chisari, G.; Acquaviva, R.; Mastrojeni, S.; Malaguarnera, G.; Mistretta, A.; Li Volti, G.; et al. *Bifidobacterium longum* with fructo-oligosaccharides in patients with non alcoholic steatohepatitis. *Dig. Dis. Sci.* **2012**, *57*, 545–553. [CrossRef] [PubMed]

170. Kellow, N.J.; Coughlan, M.T.; Reid, C.M. Metabolic benefits of dietary prebiotics in human subjects: A systematic review of randomised controlled trials. *Br. J. Nutr.* **2014**, *111*, 1147–1161. [CrossRef] [PubMed]

171. Lecerf, J.M.; Depeint, F.; Clerc, E.; Dugenet, Y.; Niamba, C.N.; Rhazi, L.; Cayzeele, A.; Abdelnour, G.; Jaruga, A.; Younes, H.; et al. Xylo-oligosaccharide (XOS) in combination with inulin modulates both the intestinal environment and immune status in healthy subjects, while XOS alone only shows prebiotic properties. *Br. J. Nutr.* **2012**, *108*, 1847–1858. [CrossRef] [PubMed]

172. Lomax, A.R.; Cheung, L.V.; Tuohy, K.M.; Noakes, P.S.; Miles, E.A.; Calder, P.C. B2-1 fructans have a bifidogenic effect in healthy middle-aged human subjects but do not alter immune responses examined in the absence of an *in vivo* immune challenge: Results from a randomised controlled trial. *Br. J. Nutr.* **2012**, *108*, 1818–1828. [CrossRef] [PubMed]

173. Vulevic, J.; Drakoularakou, A.; Yaqoob, P.; Tzortzis, G.; Gibson, G.R. Modulation of the fecal microflora profile and immune function by a novel trans-galactooligosaccharide mixture (B-GOS) in healthy elderly volunteers. *Am. J. Clin. Nutr.* **2008**, *88*, 1438–1446. [PubMed]

174. Vulevic, J.; Juric, A.; Tzortzis, G.; Gibson, G.R. A mixture of trans-galactooligosaccharides reduces markers of metabolic syndrome and modulates the fecal microbiota and immune function of overweight adults. *J. Nutr.* **2013**, *143*, 324–331. [CrossRef] [PubMed]

175. Dewulf, E.M.; Cani, P.D.; Claus, S.P.; Fuentes, S.; Puylaert, P.G.; Neyrinck, A.M.; Bindels, L.B.; de Vos, W.M.; Gibson, G.R.; Thissen, J.P.; et al. Insight into the prebiotic concept: Lessons from an exploratory, double blind intervention study with inulin-type fructans in obese women. *Gut* **2013**, *62*, 1112–1121. [CrossRef] [PubMed]

176. Lirussi, F.; Mastropasqua, E.; Orando, S.; Orlando, R. Probiotics for non-alcoholic fatty liver disease and/or steatohepatitis. *Cochrane Database Syst. Rev.* **2007**, *1*, CD005165. [PubMed]

177. Tarantino, G.; Finelli, C. Systematic review on intervention with prebiotics/probiotics in patients with obesity-related nonalcoholic fatty liver disease. *Future Microbiol.* **2015**, *10*, 889–902. [CrossRef] [PubMed]

178. Solga, S.F.; Diehl, A.M. Non-alcoholic fatty liver disease: Lumen-liver interactions and possible role for probiotics. *J. Hepatol.* **2003**, *38*, 681–687. [CrossRef]

179. Wang, Y.; Liu, Y.; Sidhu, A.; Ma, Z.; McClain, C.; Feng, W. *Lactobacillus rhamnosus* GG culture supernatant ameliorates acute alcohol-induced intestinal permeability and liver injury. *Am. J. Physiol. Gastrointest. Liver Physiol.* **2012**, *303*, G32–G41. [CrossRef] [PubMed]

180. Spruss, A.; Bergheim, I. Dietary fructose and intestinal barrier: Potential risk factor in the pathogenesis of nonalcoholic fatty liver disease. *J. Nutr. Biochem.* **2009**, *20*, 657–662. [CrossRef] [PubMed]

181. Reid, G.; Younes, J.A.; Van der Mei, H.C.; Gloor, G.B.; Knight, R.; Busscher, H.J. Microbiota restoration: Natural and supplemented recovery of human microbial communities. *Nat. Rev. Microbiol.* **2011**, *9*, 27–38. [CrossRef] [PubMed]

182. Li, Z.; Yang, S.; Lin, H.; Huang, J.; Watkins, P.A.; Moser, A.B.; Desimone, C.; Song, X.Y.; Diehl, A.M. Probiotics and antibodies to TNF inhibit inflammatory activity and improve nonalcoholic fatty liver disease. *Hepatology* **2003**, *37*, 343–350. [CrossRef] [PubMed]

183. Paik, H.D.; Park, J.S.; Park, E. Effects of bacillus polyfermenticus scd on lipid and antioxidant metabolisms in rats fed a high-fat and high-cholesterol diet. *Biol. Pharm. Bull.* **2005**, *28*, 1270–1274. [CrossRef] [PubMed]

184. Yadav, H.; Jain, S.; Sinha, P.R. Oral administration of dahi containing probiotic *Lactobacillus acidophilus* and *Lactobacillus casei* delayed the progression of streptozotocin-induced diabetes in rats. *J. Dairy Res.* **2008**, *75*, 189–195. [CrossRef] [PubMed]

185. Chen, J.J.; Wang, R.; Li, X.F.; Wang, R.L. *Bifidobacterium longum* supplementation improved high-fat-fed-induced metabolic syndrome and promoted intestinal reg i gene expression. *Exp. Biol. Med.* **2011**, *236*, 823–831. [CrossRef] [PubMed]

186. Lee, H.Y.; Park, J.H.; Seok, S.H.; Baek, M.W.; Kim, D.J.; Lee, K.E.; Paek, K.S.; Lee, Y. Human originated bacteria, *Lactobacillus rhamnosus* PL60, produce conjugated linoleic acid and show anti-obesity effects in diet-induced obese mice. *Biochim. Biophys. Acta* **2006**, *1761*, 736–744. [CrossRef] [PubMed]

187. Ma, X.; Hua, J.; Li, Z. Probiotics improve high fat diet-induced hepatic steatosis and insulin resistance by increasing hepatic nkt cells. *J. Hepatol.* **2008**, *49*, 821–830. [CrossRef] [PubMed]

188. Xu, R.Y.; Wan, Y.P.; Fang, Q.Y.; Lu, W.; Cai, W. Supplementation with probiotics modifies gut flora and attenuates liver fat accumulation in rat nonalcoholic fatty liver disease model. *J. Clin. Biochem. Nutr.* **2012**, *50*, 72–77. [CrossRef] [PubMed]

189. Esposito, E.; Iacono, A.; Bianco, G.; Autore, G.; Cuzzocrea, S.; Vajro, P.; Canani, R.B.; Calignano, A.; Raso, G.M.; Meli, R. Probiotics reduce the inflammatory response induced by a high-fat diet in the liver of young rats. *J. Nutr.* **2009**, *139*, 905–911. [CrossRef] [PubMed]

190. Velayudham, A.; Dolganiuc, A.; Ellis, M.; Petrasek, J.; Kodys, K.; Mandrekar, P.; Szabo, G. VSL#3 probiotic treatment attenuates fibrosis without changes in steatohepatitis in a diet-induced nonalcoholic steatohepatitis model in mice. *Hepatology* **2009**, *49*, 989–997. [PubMed]

191. Al-Salami, H.; Butt, G.; Fawcett, J.P.; Tucker, I.G.; Golocorbin-Kon, S.; Mikov, M. Probiotic treatment reduces blood glucose levels and increases systemic absorption of gliclazide in diabetic rats. *Eur. J. Drug Metab. Pharmacokinet.* **2008**, *33*, 101–106. [CrossRef] [PubMed]

192. Cano, P.G.; Santacruz, A.; Trejo, F.M.; Sanz, Y. Bifidobacterium cect 7765 improves metabolic and immunological alterations associated with obesity in high-fat diet-fed mice. *Obesity* **2013**, *21*, 2310–2321. [CrossRef] [PubMed]

193. Eslamparast, T.; Eghtesad, S.; Hekmatdoost, A.; Poustchi, H. Probiotics and nonalcoholic fatty liver disease. *Middle East J. Dig. Dis.* **2013**, *5*, 129–136. [PubMed]

194. Moya-Perez, A.; Neef, A.; Sanz, Y. Bifidobacterium pseudocatenulatum cect 7765 reduces obesity-associated inflammation by restoring the lymphocyte-macrophage balance and gut microbiota structure in high-fat diet-fed mice. *PLoS ONE* **2015**, *10*, e0126976.

195. Fan, J.G.; Xu, Z.J.; Wang, G.L. Effect of lactulose on establishment of a rat non-alcoholic steatohepatitis model. *World J. Gastroenterol.* **2005**, *11*, 5053–5056. [CrossRef] [PubMed]

196. Kanauchi, O.; Fujiyama, Y.; Mitsuyama, K.; Araki, Y.; Ishii, T.; Nakamura, T.; Hitomi, Y.; Agata, K.; Saiki, T.; Andoh, A.; *et al.* Increased growth of bifidobacterium and eubacterium by germinated barley foodstuff,

accompanied by enhanced butyrate production in healthy volunteers. *Int. J. Mol. Med.* **1999**, *3*, 175–179. [CrossRef] [PubMed]

197. Vajro, P.; Mandato, C.; Licenziati, M.R.; Franzese, A.; Vitale, D.F.; Lenta, S.; Caropreso, M.; Vallone, G.; Meli, R. Effects of *Lactobacillus rhamnosus* strain GG in pediatric obesity-related liver disease. *J. Pediatr. Gastroenterol. Nutr.* **2011**, *52*, 740–743. [CrossRef] [PubMed]

198. Kadooka, Y.; Sato, M.; Imaizumi, K.; Ogawa, A.; Ikuyama, K.; Akai, Y.; Okano, M.; Kagoshima, M.; Tsuchida, T. Regulation of abdominal adiposity by probiotics (*Lactobacillus gasseri* SBT2055) in adults with obese tendencies in a randomized controlled trial. *Eur. J. Clin. Nutr.* **2010**, *64*, 636–643. [CrossRef] [PubMed]

199. Kadooka, Y.; Sato, M.; Ogawa, A.; Miyoshi, M.; Uenishi, H.; Ogawa, H.; Ikuyama, K.; Kagoshima, M.; Tsuchida, T. Effect of *Lactobacillus gasseri* SBT2055 in fermented milk on abdominal adiposity in adults in a randomised controlled trial. *Br. J. Nutr.* **2013**, *110*, 1696–1703. [CrossRef] [PubMed]

200. Osawa, K.; Miyoshi, T.; Yamauchi, K.; Koyama, Y.; Nakamura, K.; Sato, S.; Kanazawa, S.; Ito, H. Nonalcoholic hepatic steatosis is a strong predictor of high-risk coronary-artery plaques as determined by multidetector ct. *PLoS ONE* **2015**, *10*, e0131138. [CrossRef] [PubMed]

201. Loguercio, C.; Federico, A.; Tuccillo, C.; Terracciano, F.; D'Auria, M.V.; De Simone, C.; del Vecchio Blanco, C. Beneficial effects of a probiotic vsl#3 on parameters of liver dysfunction in chronic liver diseases. *J. Clin. Gastroenterol.* **2005**, *39*, 540–543. [PubMed]

202. Stadlbauer, V.; Mookerjee, R.P.; Hodges, S.; Wright, G.A.; Davies, N.A.; Jalan, R. Effect of probiotic treatment on deranged neutrophil function and cytokine responses in patients with compensated alcoholic cirrhosis. *J. Hepatol.* **2008**, *48*, 945–951. [CrossRef] [PubMed]

203. Aller, R.; De Luis, D.A.; Izaola, O.; Conde, R.; Gonzalez Sagrado, M.; Primo, D.; de La Fuente, B.; Gonzalez, J. Effect of a probiotic on liver aminotransferases in nonalcoholic fatty liver disease patients: A double blind randomized clinical trial. *Eur. Rev. Med. Pharmacol. Sci.* **2011**, *15*, 1090–1095. [PubMed]

204. Loguercio, C.; De Simone, T.; Federico, A.; Terracciano, F.; Tuccillo, C.; Di Chicco, M.; Carteni, M. Gut-liver axis: A new point of attack to treat chronic liver damage? *Am. J. Gastroenterol.* **2002**, *97*, 2144–2146. [CrossRef] [PubMed]

205. Wall, R.; Marques, T.M.; O'Sullivan, O.; Ross, R.P.; Shanahan, F.; Quigley, E.; Dinan, T.G.; Kiely, B.; Fitzgerald, G.F.; Cotter, P.D.; *et al.* Contrasting effects of *Bifidobacterium breve* NCIMB 702258 and *Bifidobacterium breve* DPC 6330 on the composition of murine brain fatty acids and gut microbiota. *Am. J. Clin. Nutr.* **2012**, *95*, 1278–1287. [CrossRef] [PubMed]

206. Shen, J.; Ran, H.Z.; Yin, M.H.; Zhou, T.X.; Xiao, D.S. Meta-analysis: The effect and adverse events of *lactobacilli* versus placebo in maintenance therapy for crohn disease. *Intern. Med. J.* **2009**, *39*, 103–109. [CrossRef] [PubMed]

207. Lionetti, E.; Indrio, F.; Pavone, L.; Borrelli, G.; Cavallo, L.; Francavilla, R. Role of probiotics in pediatric patients with *Helicobacter pylori* infection: A comprehensive review of the literature. *Helicobacter* **2010**, *15*, 79–87. [CrossRef] [PubMed]

208. Friedenreich, C.; Norat, T.; Steindorf, K.; Boutron-Ruault, M.C.; Pischon, T.; Mazuir, M.; Clavel-Chapelon, F.; Linseisen, J.; Boeing, H.; Bergman, M.; *et al.* Physical activity and risk of colon and rectal cancers: The european prospective investigation into cancer and nutrition. *Cancer Epidemiol. Biomark. Prev.* **2006**, *15*, 2398–2407. [CrossRef] [PubMed]

209. Warburton, D.E.; Nicol, C.W.; Bredin, S.S. Health benefits of physical activity: The evidence. *CMAJ* **2006**, *174*, 801–809. [CrossRef] [PubMed]

210. Marcinko, K.; Sikkema, S.R.; Samaan, M.C.; Kemp, B.E.; Fullerton, M.D.; Steinberg, G.R. High intensity interval training improves liver and adipose tissue insulin sensitivity. *Mol. Metab.* **2015**, *4*, 903–915. [CrossRef] [PubMed]

211. Ellingsgaard, H.; Hauselmann, I.; Schuler, B.; Habib, A.M.; Baggio, L.L.; Meier, D.T.; Eppler, E.; Bouzakri, K.; Wueest, S.; Muller, Y.D.; *et al.* Interleukin-6 enhances insulin secretion by increasing glucagon-like peptide-1 secretion from l cells and α cells. *Nat. Med.* **2011**, *17*, 1481–1489. [CrossRef] [PubMed]

212. Petersen, A.M.; Pedersen, B.K. The anti-inflammatory effect of exercise. *J. Appl. Physiol.* **2005**, *98*, 1154–1162. [CrossRef] [PubMed]

213. Clarke, S.F.; Murphy, E.F.; O'Sullivan, O.; Lucey, A.J.; Humphreys, M.; Hogan, A.; Hayes, P.; O'Reilly, M.; Jeffery, I.B.; Wood-Martin, R.; *et al.* Exercise and associated dietary extremes impact on gut microbial diversity. *Gut* **2014**, *63*, 1913–1920. [CrossRef] [PubMed]

214. Maslowski, K.M.; Mackay, C.R. Diet, gut microbiota and immune responses. *Nat. Immunol.* **2011**, *12*, 5–9. [CrossRef] [PubMed]

215. Lambert, J.E.; Myslicki, J.P.; Bomhof, M.R.; Belke, D.D.; Shearer, J.; Reimer, R.A. Exercise training modifies gut microbiota in normal and diabetic mice. *Appl. Physiol. Nutr. Metab.* **2015**, *40*, 749–752. [CrossRef] [PubMed]

216. Petriz, B.A.; Castro, A.P.; Almeida, J.A.; Gomes, C.P.; Fernandes, G.R.; Kruger, R.H.; Pereira, R.W.; Franco, O.L. Exercise induction of gut microbiota modifications in obese, non-obese and hypertensive rats. *BMC Genom.* **2014**, *15*, 511. [CrossRef] [PubMed]

217. Evans, C.C.; LePard, K.J.; Kwak, J.W.; Stancukas, M.C.; Laskowski, S.; Dougherty, J.; Moulton, L.; Glawe, A.; Wang, Y.; Leone, V.; *et al.* Exercise prevents weight gain and alters the gut microbiota in a mouse model of high fat diet-induced obesity. *PLoS ONE* **2014**, *9*, e92193. [CrossRef] [PubMed]

218. Kang, S.S.; Jeraldo, P.R.; Kurti, A.; Miller, M.E.; Cook, M.D.; Whitlock, K.; Goldenfeld, N.; Woods, J.A.; White, B.A.; Chia, N.; *et al.* Diet and exercise orthogonally alter the gut microbiome and reveal independent associations with anxiety and cognition. *Mol. Neurodegener.* **2014**, *9*, 36. [CrossRef] [PubMed]

219. Liu, T.W.; Park, Y.M.; Holscher, H.D.; Padilla, J.; Scroggins, R.J.; Welly, R.; Britton, S.L.; Koch, L.G.; Vieira-Potter, V.J.; Swanson, K.S. Physical activity differentially affects the cecal microbiota of ovariectomized female rats selectively bred for high and low aerobic capacity. *PLoS ONE* **2015**, *10*, e0136150. [CrossRef] [PubMed]

220. Matsumoto, M.; Inoue, R.; Tsukahara, T.; Ushida, K.; Chiji, H.; Matsubara, N.; Hara, H. Voluntary running exercise alters microbiota composition and increases n-butyrate concentration in the rat cecum. *Biosci. Biotechnol. Biochem.* **2008**, *72*, 572–576. [CrossRef] [PubMed]

221. Allen, J.M.; Berg Miller, M.E.; Pence, B.D.; Whitlock, K.; Nehra, V.; Gaskins, H.R.; White, B.A.; Fryer, J.D.; Woods, J.A. Voluntary and forced exercise differentially alters the gut microbiome in C57BL/6J mice. *J. Appl. Physiol.* **2015**, *118*, 1059–1066. [CrossRef] [PubMed]

222. Choi, J.J.; Eum, S.Y.; Rampersaud, E.; Daunert, S.; Abreu, M.T.; Toborek, M. Exercise attenuates PCB-induced changes in the mouse gut microbiome. *Environ. Health Perspect.* **2013**, *121*, 725–730. [CrossRef] [PubMed]

223. Queipo-Ortuno, M.I.; Seoane, L.M.; Murri, M.; Pardo, M.; Gomez-Zumaquero, J.M.; Cardona, F.; Casanueva, F.; Tinahones, F.J. Gut microbiota composition in male rat models under different nutritional status and physical activity and its association with serum leptin and ghrelin levels. *PLoS ONE* **2013**, *8*, e65465.

224. Mika, A.; Van Treuren, W.; Gonzalez, A.; Herrera, J.J.; Knight, R.; Fleshner, M. Exercise is more effective at altering gut microbial composition and producing stable changes in lean mass in juvenile versus adult male F344 rats. *PLoS ONE* **2015**, *10*, e0125889. [CrossRef] [PubMed]

225. Shukla, S.K.; Cook, D.; Meyer, J.; Vernon, S.D.; Le, T.; Clevidence, D.; Robertson, C.E.; Schrodi, S.J.; Yale, S.; Frank, D.N. Changes in gut and plasma microbiome following exercise challenge in myalgic encephalomyelitis/chronic fatigue syndrome (ME/CFS). *PLoS ONE* **2015**, *10*, e0145453. [CrossRef] [PubMed]

226. Cassidy, S.; Thoma, C.; Hallsworth, K.; Parikh, J.; Hollingsworth, K.G.; Taylor, R.; Jakovljevic, D.G.; Trenell, M.I. High intensity intermittent exercise improves cardiac structure and function and reduces liver fat in patients with type 2 diabetes: A randomised controlled trial. *Diabetologia* **2016**, *59*, 56–66. [CrossRef] [PubMed]

227. Hallsworth, K.; Thoma, C.; Hollingsworth, K.G.; Cassidy, S.; Anstee, Q.M.; Day, C.P.; Trenell, M.I. Modified high-intensity interval training reduces liver fat and improves cardiac function in non-alcoholic fatty liver disease: A randomised controlled trial. *Clin. Sci.* **2015**, *129*, 1097–1105. [CrossRef] [PubMed]

228. Schwiertz, A.; Taras, D.; Schafer, K.; Beijer, S.; Bos, N.A.; Donus, C.; Hardt, P.D. Microbiota and SCFA in lean and overweight healthy subjects. *Obesity* **2010**, *18*, 190–195. [CrossRef] [PubMed]

229. Meissner, M.; Lombardo, E.; Havinga, R.; Tietge, U.J.F.; Kuipers, F.; Groen, A.K. Voluntary wheel running increases bile acid as well as cholesterol excretion and decreases atherosclerosis in hypercholesterolemic mice. *Atherosclerosis* **2011**, *218*, 323–329. [CrossRef] [PubMed]

230. Rowell, L.B.; Detry, J.R.; Profant, G.R.; Wyss, C. Splanchnic vasoconstriction in hyperthermic man—Role of falling blood pressure. *J. Appl. Physiol.* **1971**, *31*, 864–869. [PubMed]

# 7

# Definitions of Normal Liver Fat and the Association of Insulin Sensitivity with Acquired and Genetic NAFLD

**Elina M. Petäjä** [1,2,*] **and Hannele Yki-Järvinen** [1,2]

[1]  Minerva Foundation Institute for Medical Research, 00290 Helsinki, Finland;
   hannele.yki-jarvinen@helsinki.fi

[2]  Department of Medicine, University of Helsinki and Helsinki University Central Hospital,
   00290 Helsinki, Finland

*  Correspondence: elina.petaja@helsinki.fi

Academic Editors: Amedeo Lonardo and Giovanni Targher

**Abstract:** Non-alcoholic fatty liver disease (NAFLD) covers a spectrum of disease ranging from simple steatosis (NAFL) to non-alcoholic steatohepatitis (NASH) and fibrosis. "Obese/Metabolic NAFLD" is closely associated with obesity and insulin resistance and therefore predisposes to type 2 diabetes and cardiovascular disease. NAFLD can also be caused by common genetic variants, the patatin-like phospholipase domain-containing 3 (PNPLA3) or the transmembrane 6 superfamily member 2 (TM6SF2). Since NAFL, irrespective of its cause, can progress to NASH and liver fibrosis, its definition is of interest. We reviewed the literature to identify data on definition of normal liver fat using liver histology and different imaging tools, and analyzed whether NAFLD caused by the gene variants is associated with insulin resistance. Histologically, normal liver fat content in liver biopsies is most commonly defined as macroscopic steatosis in less than 5% of hepatocytes. In the population-based Dallas Heart Study, the upper 95th percentile of liver fat measured by proton magnetic spectroscopy ($^1$H-MRS) in healthy subjects was 5.6%, which corresponds to approximately 15% histological liver fat. When measured by magnetic resonance imaging (MRI)-based techniques such as the proton density fat fraction (PDFF), 5% macroscopic steatosis corresponds to a PDFF of 6% to 6.4%. In contrast to "Obese/metabolic NAFLD", NAFLD caused by genetic variants is not associated with insulin resistance. This implies that NAFLD is heterogeneous and that "Obese/Metabolic NAFLD" but not NAFLD due to the PNPLA3 or TM6SF2 genetic variants predisposes to type 2 diabetes and cardiovascular disease.

**Keywords:** insulin resistance; liver fat; obesity; PNPLA3; TM6SF2

## 1. Introduction

Non-alcoholic fatty liver disease (NAFLD) is defined as steatosis not caused by excess alcohol intake (>30 g/day in men and >20 g/day in women), hepatitis B or C, autoimmune hepatitis, iron overload, drugs or toxins [1]. It covers a spectrum from simple steatosis (NAFL) to non-alcoholic steatohepatitis (NASH) and cirrhosis [1,2]. NASH is characterized, in addition to steatosis, by ballooning necrosis, mild inflammation and possibly fibrosis, and can only be diagnosed using a liver biopsy [3].

Several longitudinal studies have shown that NAFLD increases the risk of and mortality from type 2 diabetes and cardiovascular disease [4]. Fibrosis stage is considered to be the most important histological feature predicting advanced liver disease [5,6]. It has been recently shown, however, that NAFL defined as macroscopic steatosis in more than 5% of hepatocytes progresses to

NASH and fibrosis [7–9], as hypothesized by earlier indirect evidence [10]. Thus, NAFL predicts both metabolic and liver complications of NAFLD. It is therefore of interest to define normal liver fat content in humans.

Although NAFLD commonly coexists with obesity, insulin resistance and type 2 diabetes [11], common genetic causes also exist. A variant in patatin-like phospholipase domain-containing 3 (PNPLA3) (rs738409 [G], encoding I148M) confers susceptibility to NAFL, NASH and fibrosis ("PNPLA3 NAFLD") [12]. Genetic variation in transmembrane 6 superfamily member 2 (TM6SF2) (rs58542926 [T], encoding E167K) is also increases liver fat and the risk of NASH ("TM6SF2 NAFLD") [13]. These two conditions do not appear to be characterized by insulin resistance, although both genetic and metabolic causes of NAFLD may exist in the same person [14]. If so, then these types of NAFLD would not predispose to type 2 diabetes and cardiovascular disease.

The ensuing review will focus on defining normal liver fat content and discussing how liver fat content is related to insulin sensitivity in "Obese/Metabolic NAFLD" and the common genetic forms of NAFLD.

## 2. Definitions of Normal Liver Fat

### 2.1. Biochemical and Histologic Definitions

The biochemical standard for normal triglyceride content in the human liver is 5.5% of triglyceride of wet liver tissue weight [15,16]. Histologically, the liver is considered steatotic when ≥5% of hepatocytes in a tissue section stained with hematoxylin and eosin contain macrovesicular steatosis [17–20]. Steatosis is graded by the pathologist from 0 to 3 based on its severity: grade 0 (normal) = <5%, grade 1 (mild) = 5%–33%, grade 2 (moderate) = 34%–66%, and grade 3 (severe) = ≥67% of hepatocytes characterized by macroscopic steatosis [17]. As discussed below, these percentages seem quite different from those obtained by proton magnetic resonance spectroscopy ($^1$H-MRS) (Table 1).

**Table 1.** Definitions of normal liver fat using different approaches.

| Study | Year | N | Subjects | Normal Value |
|---|---|---|---|---|
| | | | *Biochemical* | |
| Laurell S [21] | 1971 | 3 | Healthy subjects | 2.0 g/100 g of dry tissue weight |
| Donhoffer H [15] | 1974 | 107 | Unselected cadavers | 5.5 g/100 g of wet tissue weight |
| | | | *Histology* | |
| Kleiner DE [17] | 2005 | 576 + 162 | Adults and children | Macroscopic fat in <5% of hepatocytes |
| Brunt EM [3] | 2011 | 976 | Adults | Macroscopic fat in <5% of hepatocytes |
| Bedossa P [19] | 2012 | 679 | Morbidly obese adults | Macroscopic fat in <5% of hepatocytes |
| | | | *CT* | |
| Piekarski J [22] | 1980 | 100 | Healthy subjects | 50–57 HU or 8–10 HU higher than spleen |
| | | | *$^1$H-MRS* | |
| Szczepaniak LS [23] | 2005 | 345 | Population-based, healthy subjects | <5.56% |
| Petersen KF [24] | 2006 | 170 | Healthy subjects | <3.0% |
| | | | *MRI-PDFF* | |
| Fishbein MH [25] | 1998 | 28 | Healthy subjects | <9.0% |
| | | | *US* | |
| Joseph AE [26] | 1978 | 60 | Adults referred to gastroenterologist | Absense of echogenicity or brightness of the liver |
| Saveymuttu SH [27] | 1985 | 490 | Adults referred to gastroenterologist | Absense of echogenicity or brightness of the liver |

$^1$H-MRS, proton magnetic resonance spectroscopy; CT, computed tomography; HU, Houndsfield Unit; MRI-PDFF, magnetic resonance imaging-determined proton density fat fraction; US, ultrasound.

## 2.2. Proton Magnetic Resonance Spectroscopy ($^1$H-MRS)

Steatosis can most accurately be measured using $^1$H-MRS [28]. This technique enables sampling of a large volume fraction of the liver compared to a biopsy [29,30] and provides an accurate and reproducible measurement of liver fat content [30]. However, $^1$H-MRS is expensive, as it requires use of magnetic resonance imaging (MRI) scanner and special expertise to perform proton magnetic resonance spectroscopy ($^1$H-MRS) at the time of MRI scanning. $^1$H-MRS has been used in one population-based study, the Dallas Heart Study (DHS), to define normal liver fat content [23]. In this study, $^1$H-MRS was performed on 2349 subjects, of which 345 were considered healthy based on the following criteria: no history of liver disease or risk factors for hepatic steatosis (alcohol consumption $\leqslant$30 g/day in men, $\leqslant$20 g/day in women, body mass index (BMI) <25 kg/m$^2$, normal fasting serum glucose, non-diabetic and normal serum alanine aminotransferase (ALT) ($\leqslant$30 IU/L in men, $\leqslant$19 IU/L in women)). The upper limit of normal liver fat content was defined based on the upper 95th percentile in the healthy subjects and was 5.56% [23].

The $^1$H-MRS studies determine the hepatic triglyceride content rather than the percentage of hepatocytes with macroscopic lipid droplets. The relationship between $^1$H-MRS and histological liver fat content has been analyzed in two small studies, which included 13 [31], 12 [32] and 50 [33] subjects. In the first two studies, the $^1$H-MRS-determined normal liver fat in the DHS, *i.e.*, the 5.56% value corresponded to 15.7% [31] and 13.9% [32] of hepatocytes with macroscopic steatosis. On the third study, histological grade 1 (5%–33% macroscopic liver fat) corresponded to 11% (7%–14%), grade 2 (33%–66%) to 18% (14%–23%) and grade 3 (>66%) to 25% (10%–28%) $^1$H-MRS liver fat [33]. $^1$H-MRS-measured liver fat corresponds well to triglyceride content measured in a liver biopsy ($r = 0.90$, $p < 0.001$) [34]. These data show that the technique used to define normal liver fat influences the normal value.

## 2.3. Magnetic Resonance Imaging (MRI)

Hepatic steatosis can be diagnosed with MRI using an out-of-phase and in-phase imaging technique developed by Dixon WT *et al.* [35]. This method involves acquisition of MR images at echo times in which fat proton and water proton signals are either out-of-phase (water and fat signals cancel) or in-phase (water and fat signals add up) [35–37]. Once the out-of-phase and in-phase images are acquired by using constant calibration and other scanner settings, a quantitative fat signal fraction can be calculated from the hepatic signal [38]. Modified versions of the early Dixon method have been introduced. These include the hepatic fat fraction by Fishbein MH *et al.* which uses fast gradient echo techniques [25,39] and correlates well with histological liver fat content ($r = 0.77$, $p < 0.001$). The newer MRI-determined proton density fat fraction (PDFF) technique provides a quantitative, standardized and objective MRI measurement of hepatic fat based upon inherent tissue properties [40,41]. The MRI-PDFF method is reproducible and correlates closely with $^1$H-MRS ($r = 0.99$) [33,42] and liver histology (8.9%–9.4% at grade 1, 15.8%–16.3% at grade 2, and 22.1%–25.0% at grade 3, $p < 0.0001$) [33,43,44]. With this technique, the 5% macroscopic liver fat determined by histology corresponds to a PDFF value of 6% to 6.4% [45,46].

## 2.4. Ultrasound (US)

Ultrasound (US) is an inexpensive and widely available tool to visualize the liver and its fat content. Hepatic steatosis appears as a diffuse increase in parenchymal brightness and echogenicity on US images, and is often compared to hypoechogenity of the kidney cortex. Most studies score steatosis semiquantitatively as "mild", "moderate" and "severe" based upon the visual assessment of hepatic echogenicity [27,47–49]. Lack of standardization precludes accurate comparison of data acquired by different machines and investigators. US lacks sensitivity in obese subjects [50] and in subjects with low liver fat content [51]. The sensitivity of diagnosing fatty liver increases from 55% to 80% when liver fat increases from 10%–20% to over 30% [51]. A recent study [52] suggested that the optimum sensitivity for US was achieved at a $^1$H-MRS-measured liver fat content greater than 12.5%. A meta-analysis of 44 studies comprising 4720 subjects concluded that US has a sensitivity of 85% and a specificity of 94% for detecting 20%–30% macroscopic steatosis [53]. The sensitivity and specificity were 65% and 81% for detecting 0%–5% steatosis and 93% and 88%, respectively, for detecting >10% steatosis.

Xia MF *et al.* created an equation for accurate quantification of liver fat content using US in Chinese subjects [54]. A tissue-mimicking phantom was used as a standard and the US hepatic/renal ratio was measured to calculate liver fat content in 127 subjects, in whom liver fat was also measured using $^1$H-MRS. The adjusted $R^2$ for the model was 80%. The optimal cut-off for the US-measured liver fat content to diagnose hepatic steatosis was 9.15%, which yielded a sensitivity and specificity of 95% and 100%, respectively. The utility of this technique in other ethnic groups which are more obese than the Chinese in the face of a similar amount of liver fat [55,56] remains to be tested.

## 2.5. Computed Tomography (CT)

Hepatic steatosis can also be assessed by using computed tomography (CT) by comparing attenuation of the liver parenchyma to that of the spleen [57]. Tissue fat deposition lowers attenuation, hence fatty areas are less dense and appear darker than the non-fatty tissues [22]. The attenuation value in the healthy liver is 50 to 57 Houndsfield Units (HU) and 8 to 10 HU higher than that of spleen [22]. It decreases by 1.6 HU for every 1 mg of triglycerides per gram of liver tissue [58]. In subjects with steatosis, the mean attenuation value of the liver is lower than that of the spleen, and the liver appears darker than the spleen. Attenuation values less than 40 HU in the liver or 10 HU less in the liver than in the spleen are indicative of marked hepatic steatosis (>30%). Smaller fractions of fatty infiltration cannot be accurately and reliably assessed [59,60].

## 3. Non-Alcoholic Fatty Liver Disease (NAFLD) and Insulin Sensitivity

### 3.1. Insulin Resistance in "Obese/Metabolic NAFLD"

In subjects with NAFLD and the metabolic syndrome (MetS), *i.e.*, in "Obese/Metabolic NAFLD", liver fat is closely correlated with direct measures of insulin resistance such as the inability of insulin to suppress hepatic glucose production [61], and indirect measures such as fasting serum insulin and the product of fasting insulin and glucose (Homeostasis model assessment for insulin resistance [HOMA-IR]) [62]. Indeed, liver fat correlates better with fasting insulin than with liver enzymes such as serum ALT and aspartate aminotransferase (AST) [63,64]. This close association between fasting insulin and liver fat is physiologically feasible as the main action of insulin after an overnight fast is to restrain hepatic glucose production. The inability of insulin to suppress hepatic glucose production increases fasting glucose, which stimulates insulin secretion leading to hyperglycemia and hyperinsulinemia.

Lipolysis is the main source of fatty acids used for synthesis of intrahepatocellular triglycerides [65,66]. Liver fat is closely correlated with the ability of insulin to suppress lipolysis [67,68]. The ability of insulin to suppress very low density lipoprotein (VLDL) production is also impaired in NAFLD, which contributes to hypertriglyceridemia and a low high density lipoprotein (HDL) cholesterol concentration. Damaged hepatocytes release increased amounts of C-reactive protein (CRP) and coagulation factors, which could contribute to increased risk of cardiovascular disease and atherothrombotic vascular disease (Figure 1).

Any obese person with NAFLD and features of the MetS can be considered to have "Obese/Metabolic NAFLD" irrespective of genetic risk factors. The most recent proposal defines the MetS in 10 different ways [69]. The presence of any three out of five features (hypertriglyceridemia, low HDL cholesterol, hyperglycemia, hypertension, increased waist circumference) is required for diagnosis of the MetS [69]. For clinical practice, this definition still remains the best tool to diagnose insulin resistance, although the extent to which the 10 different definitions increase the risk of endpoints such as type 2 diabetes and cardiovascular disease is unclear. Measurement of fasting insulin and glucose concentrations and their calculation of their product HOMA-IR might seem more attractive direct tools to measure insulin sensitivity in subjects with NAFLD. The problem with this approach is that insulin assays are not internationally standardized and give highly variable results [70].

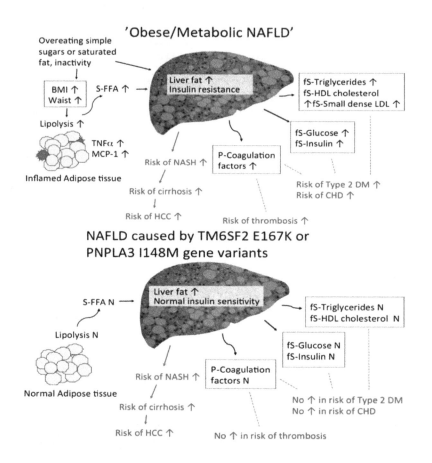

**Figure 1.** Schematic representation of causes and consequences of "Obese/Metabolic NAFLD" (**top**) and "TM6SF2 NAFLD" and "PNPLA3 NAFLD" (**bottom**). Abbreviations: BMI, body mass index; CHD, coronary heart disease; DM, diabetes mellitus; FFA, free fatty acids; fS, fasting serum; HCC, hepatocellular carcinoma; HDL, high density lipoprotein; MCP-1, monocyte chemoattractant protein-1; NAFLD, non-alcoholic fatty liver disease; NASH, non-alcoholic steatohepatits; LDL, low density lipoprotein; P, plasma; PNPLA3, patatin-like phospholipase domain-containing 3; S, serum; TM6SF2, transmembrane 6 superfamily member 2; TNF-α, tumor necrosis factor-α.

### 3.2. "Patatin-Like Phospholipase Domain-Containing 3 (PNPLA3) NAFLD" and Insulin Sensitivity

Approximately 30% of Europids and several other ethnic groups carry the PNPLA3 I148M variant [12]. The association between the PNPLA3 gene variant and NAFLD [12] has been replicated in over 50 studies, including eight genome wide association studies [71–73]. In a meta-analysis carriers of the I148M variant had 73% more liver fat, a 3.2-fold higher risk of necro-inflammation and a 3.2-fold greater risk of developing fibrosis than the non-carriers [71]. In a meta-analysis comprising 12 Asian studies, the risk of NAFLD was 1.9-fold increased in carriers compared to non-carriers [72]. Recent meta-analyses have also shown that this gene variant increases the risk of cirrhosis by 1.9-fold [74] and hepatocellular carcinoma (HCC) by 1.8-fold [75].

*In vitro*, the PNPLA3 I148M gene variant abolishes intrahepatocellular lipolysis [76,77] and by acting as a lysophosphatidic acid acyl transferase stimulates triglyceride synthesis from long unsaturated fatty acids containing coenzyme A (CoA) more than from saturated fatty acid CoAs [78]. The contribution of each these mechanisms to function of the PNPLA3 gene variant in the human liver is uncertain. It is clear, however, that the human liver lipidome markedly differs between "Obese/Metabolic NAFLD" and "PNPLA3 NAFLD" [14]. The increase in liver fat in the carriers of the PNPLA3 I148M gene variant is due to polyunsaturated triglycerides, whereas in "Obese/Metabolic NAFLD" the concentration of saturated triglycerides and insulin resistance-inducing ceramides is increased [14].

Table 2 summarizes the 14 studies that include data on insulin sensitivity in carriers and non-carriers of the I148M variant [12,79–91]. Carriers of the PNPLA3 I148M variant had more liver fat in their liver than non-carriers. Insulin sensitivity as evaluated by HOMA-IR [62], the hyperinsulinemic clamp technique, fasting or post-glucose insulin and glucose concentrations did not, however, differ between carriers and non-carriers of the gene variant. These studies included obese and non-obese, diabetic and non-diabetic as well as pediatric cohorts. Serum triglycerides were either similar or lower in variant allele carriers as compared to non-carriers, consistent with lack of insulin resistance (Table 2).

### 3.3. "Transmembrane 6 Superfamily Member 2 (TM6SF2) NAFLD" and Insulin Sensitivity

Approximately 7% of all subjects carry the TM6SF2 E167K variant. This gene variant increases the risk of NAFLD, independent of genetic variation in PNPLA3 at rs738409, obesity and alcohol intake [92]. A recent meta-analysis reported that carriers of the TM6SF2 E167K gene variant have a 2.1-fold higher risk of NAFLD than non-carriers [93]. They also had lower circulating total and low density lipoprotein (LDL) cholesterol, and triglyceride concentrations than non-carriers [93].

Four *in vitro* studies have examined the mechanism by which the TM6SF2 E167K gene variant could increase liver fat. Recombinant adeno-associated viral vectors expressing short hairpin RNAs were used to reduce *Tm6sf2* transcripts in the mouse liver, which increased hepatic triglyceride content three-fold [92]. TM6SF2 knock-out mice developed hepatic steatosis and had a three-fold reduced plasma VLDL triglyceride levels due to decreased lipidation [94]. In another study, TM6SF2 small interfering RNA inhibition also decreased export of triglyceride-rich lipoproteins and lipid droplet content in human hepatoma cell lines (Huh7 and HepG2) [95]. Overexpression of TM6SF2 in Huh7 cells reduced cellular triglyceride content [96]. Transient overexpression of human TM6SF2 in mice using a liver-targeting adenovirus containing the human TM6SF2 coding region increased, while knockdown of endogenous TM6SF2 decreased circulating total cholesterol [96]. In the latter study, no change in hepatic fat content was observed. This was hypothetized to be due to the transient exposure, compared to the lifetime exposure of humans carrying the gene variant [96].

Table 3 summarizes seven studies that have reported data on liver fat content and insulin sensitivity in carriers and non-carriers of TM6SF2 E167K gene variant [13,81,92,97–100]. In all but one of these studies, carriers had a significantly higher liver fat content as determined by [1]H-MRS, MRI, histology or US [13,92,97–100] than non-carriers. Insulin sensitivity, as determined by HOMA-IR or from oral glucose tolerance test measures did not differ between carriers and non-carriers. Triglyceride concentrations were either lower [81,98,100] or similar [13,97,99] but also in one study higher [92] in TM6SF2 E167K variant allele carriers compared to non-carriers.

**Table 2.** Insulin sensitivity in studies comparing liver fat between PNPLA3 I148M carriers and non-carriers.

| Cohort | N | BMI (kg/m²) | | | Liver Fat | | | Insulin Sensitivity (HOMA-IR) | | | S-Triglycerides (mmol/L) | | |
|---|---|---|---|---|---|---|---|---|---|---|---|---|---|
| | | I148II | I148IM | I148MM | I148II | I148IM | I148MM | I148II | I148IM | I148MM | I148II | I148IM | I148MM |
| Multiethnic¹ [12] | 2111 | 30.4 | 31.1 | 30.0 | 3.7%ᵃ | 4.6%ᵃ | 7.7%***,ᵃ | 3.3 | 3.5 | 3.3 | 1.32 | 1.35 | 1.41 |
| | | 31.6 | 32.0 | 32.2 | 3.1% | 4.8% | 4.8%*** | 3.3 | 3.3 | 4.4 | 0.97 | 0.97 | 1.02 |
| | | 29.2 | 28.8 | 28.8 | 3.5% | 3.7% | 3.5%*** | 2.3 | 2.4 | 2.0 | 1.25 | 1.21 | 0.90 |
| Germany [79] | 330 | 29.9 | 29.1 | 28.7 | 5.4%ᵃ | 6.0%ᵃ | 7.2%***,ᵃ | 12.6 ʸᶻ | 12.9 ʸᶻ | 12.9 ʸᶻ | NA | NA | NA |
| Finnish [80] | 291 | 30.5 | 30.0 | 32.2 | 9.0%ᵃ | 10.4%*,ᵃ | 14.1%**,ᵃ | 72 ʸᶻ | 70 ʸᶻ | 74 ʸᶻ | 1.82 | 1.60 | 1.52 |
| British [81] | 98 | 34.6 | 33.2 | 31.7 | 26.7%ᵃ | 28.8%ᵃ | 33.5%ᵃ | 2.4 | 3.1 | 2.6 | 1.60 | 1.70 | 1.40 |
| Multiethnic² [82] | 1214 | NAˣ | NAˣ | NAˣ | 57ᵇ | 55ᵇ | 46***,ᵇ | NAˣ | NAˣ | NAˣ | NAˣ | NAˣ | NAˣ |
| | | | | | 55 | 51 | 47*** | | | | | | |
| Dutch [83] | 470 | 37.7 | 37.6 | 37.6 | 66%ᶜ | 78%ᶜ | 100%***,ᶜ | 2.7 | 2.8 | 2.9 | 1.42 | 1.47 | 1.46 |
| Italian [84] | 61 | 25.7 | 25.9 | | 16%ᵈ | 32%*,ᵈ | | 3.4 | 4.7 | | 1.13 | 1.15 | |
| Italian [85] | 253 | 30.7 | 30.7 | 29.8 | 44%ᶜ | 48%ᶜ | 63%**,ᶜ | 3.9 | 4 | 5.2 | 1.64 | 1.85 | 1.79 |
| Italian [86] | 211 | 32.1 | 30.4 | 31.7 | 4ᵉ | 4ᵉ | 4ᵉ | 3.5 | 3.5 | 2.8 | 1.77 | 1.59 | 1.26** |
| Taiwanese [87] | 879 | 23.3 | 23.6 | 23.6 | 13%ᶠ | 19%ᶠ | 23%*,ᶠ | 1.4 | 1.5 | 1.5 | 1.11 | 1.16 | 1.38* |
| South Korean [88] | 1363 | 24.7 | 24.4 | 23.9** | 38%ᶠ | 45%ᶠ | 54%*,ᶠ | 2.3 | 2.1 | 1.6** | 1.54 | 1.38 | 1.31** |
| Taiwanese, pediatric [89] | 520 | 26.3 | 26.2 | 25.9 | 21%ᶠ | 13%ᶠ | 30%**,ᶠ | 2.4 | 2.5 | 1.7 | 1.11 | 1.03 | 0.94 |
| Italian, pediatric [90] | 475 | NA | NA | NA | 13%ᶠ | 19%ᶠ | 41%*,ᶠ | 3.3 | 3.0 | 3.0 | 0.56 | 0.56 | 0.53 |
| Italian, pediatric [91] | 149 | 95.2 ° | 95.0 ° | 94.1 ° | 70%ᵍ | 7%ᵍ | 4%***,ᵍ | 2.5 | 2.7 | 2.4 | 1.28 | 1.19 | 1.39 |
| | | | | | 30% | 78% | 4% | | | | | | |
| | | | | | 0% | 15% | 92% | | | | | | |

BMI, body mass index; CT, computed tomography; HOMA-IR, Homeostasis model assessment of insulin resistance [62]; HU, Houndsfield Unit; MRI, magnetic resonance imaging; NA, not available; OGTT, oral glucose tolerance test; US, ultrasound. * Significant difference between groups in ANOVA or t test. * $p < 0.05$; ** $p < 0.01$; *** $p < 0.0001$. Data are presented as mean or median. ¹ Caucasian, African and Hispanic Americans; ² Hispanic and African Americas. ° BMI centiles; ᵃ ¹H-MRS (liver fat content,%); ᵇ CT (liver density, HU); ᶜ Histology (prevalence of steatosis, %); ᵈ Histology (% hepatocytes steatotic); ᵉ US (severity of steatosis by Hamaguchi score, 3–4 = moderate); ᶠ US (prevalence of steatosis, %); ᵍ Histology (severity of steatosis, grade 1/2/3); ᶻ fasting serum insulin (pmol/L); ʸ hyperinsulinemic clamp was also performed, data not shown in the table; ᶻ fasting serum insulin (pmol/L); ʸ OGTT (arbitrary unit); ᶻ Histology (severity of steatosis, grade 1/2/3); ˣ Data not shown, but it was reported that genetic variation at rs738409 did not correlate with HOMA-IR, insulin sensitivity index, BMI or S-triglycerides.

**Table 3.** Insulin sensitivity in studies comparing liver fat between TM6SF2 E167K carriers and non-carriers.

| Cohort | N | BMI (kg/m²) | | Liver Fat | | Insulin Sensitivity (HOMA-IR) | | S-Triglycerides (mmol/L) | |
|---|---|---|---|---|---|---|---|---|---|
| | | EE | EK + KK | EE | EK + KK | EE | EK + KK | EE | EK + KK |
| Multiethnic [1] [92] | 4587 | 29.6 | 28.5/31.8 | 3.5% [a] | 4.4%/15.7% ***,[a] | 3.0 | 2.9/4.6 | 1.39 | 1.33/1.47 * |
| Finns [97] | 300 | 33.7 | 32.5 | 6.8% [a] | 11.2% *,[a] | 3.0 | 2.9 | 1.40 | 1.50 |
| British [81] | 98 | 32.6 | 35.4 | 28.5% [a] | 29.0% [a] | 2.7 | 4.0 | 1.60 | 1.50 * |
| Argentineans [13] | 361 | 29.8 | 30.2 | NA | NA | 3.1 | 3.0 | 1.87 | 1.31 |
| Multiethnic [2] [98] | 502 | 32.2 | 31.2/30.8 | S0: 3% [b]<br>S1: 50%<br>S2: 27%<br>S3: 20% | S0: 0%/0% [b]<br>S1: 35%/45%<br>S2: 40%/20%<br>S3: 25%/35% * | 3.5 | 2.8/2.8 | 1.70 | 1.36/1.08 ** |
| Multiethnic [1], pediatric [99] | 957[^] | 33.0 | 32.6 | 6.7% [c],[^] | 11.1% **,[c],[^] | 1.9 [x] | 2.0 [x] | 1.20 | 1.21 |
| Italian, pediatric [100] | 1010 | 2.9 [°] | 2.9 [°] | 47% [d] | 89% **,[d] | 5.6 | 4.6 | 1.12 | 1.02 * |

BMI, body mass index; BMI-SDS, body mass index standard deviation score; HOMA-IR, Homeostasis model assessment of insulin resistance [62]; MRI-PDFF, magnetic resonance imaging-measured proton density fat fraction; NA, not available; OGTT, oral glucose tolerance test; US, ultrasound; WBISI, whole body insulin sensitivity index. Significant difference between groups in ANOVA or $t$ test, * $p < 0.05$; ** $p < 0.01$; *** $p < 0.0001$. Data are presented as mean or median. [1] Caucasian, African and Hispanic Americans; [2] Caucasian, Asian, Hispanic; International Liver Disease Genetics Consortium; [^] Liver fat content available on 454 subjects, BMI, insulin sensitivity and S-triglycerides on 957 subjects; [°] BMI-SDS; [a] $^1$H-MRS (liver fat content, %); [b] Histology. prevalence of each steatosis grade; [c] MRI-PDFF, liver fat, %; ([^] ($n = 454$); [d] US (prevalence of steatosis, %); [x] OGTT (WBISI).

## 4. Materials and Methods

We performed a systematic search using PubMed and Medline on two topics. For definitions of normal liver fat, we used the following search terms and their combinations: "normal liver fat", "liver histology", "liver biopsy" and "liver triglycerides", "liver H-MRS", "liver MRI", "liver MRI-PDFF", "liver CT", "liver ultrasound" and received 526 matches. Thirty-three studies included data on normal liver fat content or compared liver fat measured using different techniques. To review the association between insulin resistance and genetic NAFLD, we searched for studies using the following search terms: "PNPLA3" or "TM6SF2" and "insulin resistance", "euglycemic (hyperinsulinemic) clamp", "fasting glucose", "fasting insulin", "HOMA-IR", "oral glucose tolerance test" and included studies which compared results between carriers and non-carriers of PNPLA3 I148M or TM6SF2 E167K gene variants. A total of 124 matched were found. Of these, 22 studies were informative with respect to liver fat content and insulin resistance between genotypes, and were thus included.

## 5. Conclusions

Normal liver fat content based on liver histology can be defined as macroscopic steatosis in less than 5% of hepatocytes. With $^1$H-MRS, normal liver fat in the population-based DHS was defined as less or equal than 5.56% [23], which corresponds to histologic liver fat of approximately 15% [31,32]. Definitions of normal liver fat content thus depend on the method used. There is also no prospective evidence that these normal values are of clinical relevance with respect to the development of liver fibrosis.

Although NAFLD has often been regarded simply as the hepatic manifestation of the MetS, it is now clear that NAFLD is heterogeneous. While "Obese/Metabolic NAFLD" is associated with NAFLD and features of the MetS and an increased risk of type 2 diabetes and cardiovascular disease, NAFLD caused by I148M variant in PNPLA3 and the E167K variant in TM6SF2 is not accompanied by insulin resistance. Thus, lack of insulin resistance does not exclude NAFLD and not all patients with NAFLD are at increased risk of type 2 diabetes and cardiovascular disease. Given that both the MetS and the genetic variants in PNPLA3 and TM6SF2 are common, there are also many individuals with "double trouble NAFLD" [14].

*Future Research and Uncertainties*

Although NAFL defined as macroscopic steatosis affecting >5% of hepatocytes predicts fibrosis [7–9], it is unknown how various degrees of steatosis predict liver outcomes. Such information would help the clinician to decide which patients to refer to the hepatologist. The same applies to the non-invasive markers of NAFL proposed to be used by the recent European NAFLD guideline if imaging tools are not available [101]. This guideline also recommended testing for the I148M gene variant in "selected cases and in clinical trials". The latter might be helpful in identifying patients with NAFLD who are at risk for advanced liver disease but who lack features of the MetS and are therefore not at risk for cardiovascular disease or type 2 diabetes. A cost–benefit analysis of this suggestion is warranted.

**Acknowledgments:** This study was supported by research grants from the Academy of Finland (Hannele Yki-Järvinen), EU H2020 EPoS 634413 (Hannele Yki-Järvinen), the Sigrid Juselius (Hannele Yki-Järvinen), State Research Funding (EVO) (Hannele Yki-Järvinen), the Novo Nordisk (Hannele Yki-Järvinen) Foundations and personal grants from the Finnish Medical Association (Elina M. Petäjä) and the Paulo Foundation (Elina M. Petäjä).

**Author Contributions:** Elina M. Petäjä and Hannele Yki-Järvinen have reviewed the literature and written the review.

## Abbreviations

| | |
|---|---|
| $^1$H-MRS | proton magnetic resonance spectroscopy |
| ALT | alanine aminotransferase |
| AST | aspartate aminotransferase |
| BMI | body mass index |
| BMI-SDS | body mass index standard deviation score |
| CHD | coronary heart disease |
| CoA | coenzyme A |
| CT | computed tomography |
| DM | diabetes mellitus |
| DHS | Dallas Heart Study |
| FFA | free fatty acids |
| fS | fasting serum |
| HDL | high density lipoprotein |
| MCP-1 | monocyte chemoattractant protein-1 |
| HCC | hepatocellular carcinoma |
| HDL | high density lipoprotein |
| HOMA-IR | homeostasis model assessment for insulin resistance |
| LDL | low density lipoprotein |
| MetS | metabolic syndrome |
| MRI | magnetic resonance imaging |
| NAFL | non-alcoholic fatty liver |
| NAFLD | non-alcoholic fatty liver disease |
| NASH | non-alcoholic steatohepatitis |
| OGTT | oral glucose tolerance test |
| P | plasma |
| PDFF | proton density fat fraction |
| PNPLA3 | patatin-like phospholipase domain-containing 3 |
| TM6SF2 | transmembrane 6 superfamily member 2 |
| TNF-$\alpha$ | tumor necrosis factor-$\alpha$ |
| US | ultrasound |
| VLDL | very low density lipoprotein |

## References

1.  Chalasani, N.; Younossi, Z.; Lavine, J.E.; Diehl, A.M.; Brunt, E.M.; Cusi, K.; Charlton, M.; Sanyal, A.J. The diagnosis and management of non-alcoholic fatty liver disease: Practice guideline by the American Association for the Study of Liver Diseases, American College of Gastroenterology, and the American Gastroenterological Association. *Am. J. Gastroenterol.* **2012**, *107*, 811–826. [CrossRef] [PubMed]

2.  Neuschwander-Tetri, B.A. Hepatic lipotoxicity and the pathogenesis of nonalcoholic steatohepatitis: The central role of nontriglyceride fatty acid metabolites. *Hepatology* **2010**, *52*, 774–788. [CrossRef] [PubMed]

3.  Brunt, E.M.; Kleiner, D.E.; Wilson, L.A.; Belt, P.; Neuschwander-Tetri, B.A. The NAS and the histopathologic diagnosis in NAFLD: Distinct clinicopathologic meanings. *Hepatology* **2011**, *53*, 810–820. [CrossRef] [PubMed]

4.  Anstee, Q.M.; Day, C.P. Progression of NAFLD to diabetes mellitus, cardiovascular disease or cirrhosis. *Nat. Rev. Gastroenterol. Hepatol.* **2013**, *10*, 330–344. [CrossRef] [PubMed]

5.  Angulo, P.; Kleiner, D.E.; Dam-Larsen, S.; Adams, L.A.; Bjornsson, E.S.; Charatcharoenwitthaya, P.; Mills, P.R.; Keach, J.C.; Lafferty, H.D.; Stahler, A.; *et al.* Liver fibrosis, but no other histologic features, is associated with long-term outcomes of patients with nonalcoholic fatty liver disease. *Gastroenterology* **2015**, *149*, 389–397. [CrossRef] [PubMed]

6.  Ekstedt, M.; Hagstrom, H.; Nasr, P.; Fredrikson, M.; Stal, P.; Kechagias, S.; Hultcrantz, R. Fibrosis stage is the strongest predictor for disease-specific mortality in NAFLD after up to 33 years of follow-up. *Hepatology* **2015**, *61*, 1547–1554. [CrossRef] [PubMed]

7.    McPherson, S.; Hardy, T.; Henderson, E.; Burt, A.D.; Day, C.P.; Anstee, Q.M. Evidence of NAFLD progression from steatosis to fibrosing-steatohepatitis using paired biopsies: Implications for prognosis and clinical management. *J. Hepatol.* **2015**, *62*, 1148–1155. [CrossRef] [PubMed]

8.    Pais, R.; Charlotte, F.; Fedchuk, L.; Bedossa, P.; Lebray, P.; Poynard, T.; Ratziu, V.; LIDO Study Group. A systematic review of follow-up biopsies reveals disease progression in patients with non-alcoholic fatty liver. *J. Hepatol.* **2013**, *59*, 550–556. [CrossRef] [PubMed]

9.    Wong, V.W.-S.; Wong, G.L.-H.; Choi, P.C.-L.; Chan, A.W.-H.; Li, M.K.-P.; Chan, H.-Y.; Chim, A.M.-L.; Yu, J.; Sung, J.J.-Y.; Chan, H.L.-Y. Disease progression of non-alcoholic fatty liver disease: A prospective study with paired liver biopsies at 3 years. *Gut* **2010**, *59*, 969–974. [CrossRef] [PubMed]

10.   Tarantino, G.; Conca, P.; Riccio, A.; Tarantino, M.; di Minno, M.N.; Chianese, D.; Pasanisi, F.; Contaldo, F.; Scopacasa, F.; Capone, D. Enhanced serum concentrations of transforming growth factor-beta1 in simple fatty liver: Is it really benign? *J. Transl. Med.* **2008**, *6*. [CrossRef] [PubMed]

11.   Yki-Järvinen, H. Non-alcoholic fatty liver disease as a cause and a consequence of metabolic syndrome. *Lancet Diabetes Endocrinol.* **2014**, *2*, 901–910. [CrossRef]

12.   Romeo, S.; Kozlitina, J.; Xing, C.; Pertsemlidis, A.; Cox, D.; Pennacchio, L.A.; Boerwinkle, E.; Cohen, J.C.; Hobbs, H.H. Genetic variation in PNPLA3 confers susceptibility to nonalcoholic fatty liver disease. *Nat. Genet.* **2008**, *40*, 1461–1465. [CrossRef] [PubMed]

13.   Sookoian, S.; Castaño, G.O.; Scian, R.; Mallardi, P.; Fernández Gianotti, T.; Burgueño, A.L.; San Martino, J.; Pirola, C.J. Genetic variation in transmembrane 6 superfamily member 2 and the risk of nonalcoholic fatty liver disease and histological disease severity. *Hepatology* **2015**, *61*, 515–525. [CrossRef] [PubMed]

14.   Luukkonen, P.K.; Zhou, Y.; Sädevirta, S.; Leivonen, M.; Arola, J.; Orešič, M.; Hyötyläinen, T.; Yki-Järvinen, H. Hepatic ceramides dissociate steatosis and insulin resistance in patients with non-alcoholic fatty liver disease. *J. Hepatol.* **2016**, *64*, 1167–1175. [CrossRef] [PubMed]

15.   Donhoffer, H. Quantitative estimation of lipids in needle biopsy sized specimens of cadaver liver. *Acta Med. Acad. Sci. Hung* **1974**, *31*, 47–49. [PubMed]

16.   Hoyumpa, D.A.M., Jr.; Greene, H.L.; Dunn, G.D.; Schenker, S. Fatty liver: Biochemical and clinical considerations. *Dig. Dis. Sci.* **1975**, *20*, 1142–1170. [CrossRef]

17.   Kleiner, D.E.; Brunt, E.M.; van Natta, M.; Behling, C.; Contos, M.J.; Cummings, O.W.; Ferrell, L.D.; Liu, Y.-C.; Torbenson, M.S.; Unalp-Arida, A.; *et al.* Nonalcoholic steatohepatitis clinical research network design and validation of a histological scoring system for nonalcoholic fatty liver disease. *Hepatology* **2005**, *41*, 1313–1321. [CrossRef] [PubMed]

18.   Brunt, E.M.; Tiniakos, D.G. Histopathology of nonalcoholic fatty liver disease. *World J. Gastroenterol.* **2010**, *16*, 5286–5296. [CrossRef] [PubMed]

19.   Bedossa, P.; Poitou, C.; Veyrie, N.; Bouillot, J.-L.; Basdevant, A.; Paradis, V.; Tordjman, J.; Clément, K. Histopathological algorithm and scoring system for evaluation of liver lesions in morbidly obese patients. *Hepatology* **2012**, *56*, 1751–1759. [CrossRef] [PubMed]

20.   Korenblat, K.M.; Fabbrini, E.; Mohammed, B.S.; Klein, S. Liver, muscle, and adipose tissue insulin action is directly related to intrahepatic triglyceride content in obese subjects. *Gastroenterology* **2008**, *134*, 1369–1375. [CrossRef] [PubMed]

21.   Laurell, S.; Lundquist, A. Lipid composition of human liver biopsy specimens. *Acta Med. Scand.* **1971**, *189*, 65–68. [CrossRef] [PubMed]

22.   Piekarski, J.; Goldberg, H.I.; Royal, S.A.; Axel, L.; Moss, A.A. Difference between liver and spleen CT numbers in the normal adult: Its usefulness in predicting the presence of diffuse liver disease. *Radiology* **1980**, *137*, 727–729. [CrossRef] [PubMed]

23.   Szczepaniak, L.S.; Nurenberg, P.; Leonard, D.; Browning, J.D.; Reingold, J.S.; Grundy, S.; Hobbs, H.H.; Dobbins, R.L. Magnetic resonance spectroscopy to measure hepatic triglyceride content: Prevalence of hepatic steatosis in the general population. *Am. J. Physiol. Endocrinol. Metab.* **2005**, *288*, E462–E468. [CrossRef] [PubMed]

24.   Petersen, K.F.; Dufour, S.; Feng, J.; Befroy, D.; Dziura, J.; Dalla Man, C.; Cobelli, C.; Shulman, G.I. Increased prevalence of insulin resistance and nonalcoholic fatty liver disease in Asian-Indian men. *Proc. Natl. Acad. Sci. USA* **2006**, *103*, 18273–18277. [CrossRef] [PubMed]

25.   Fishbein, M.H.; Gardner, K.G.; Potter, C.J.; Schmalbrock, P.; Smith, M.A. Introduction of fast MR imaging in the assessment of hepatic steatosis. *Magn. Reson. Imaging* **1997**, *15*, 287–293. [CrossRef]

26. Joseph, A.E.A.; Dewbury, K.C.; McGuire, P.G. Ultrasound in the detection of chronic liver disease (the "bright liver"). *Br. J. Radiol.* **1978**, *52*, 184–188. [CrossRef] [PubMed]

27. Saverymuttu, S.H.; Joseph, A.E.; Maxwell, J.D. Ultrasound scanning in the detection of hepatic fibrosis and steatosis. *Br. Med. J. (Clin. Res. Ed.)* **1986**, *292*, 13–15. [CrossRef]

28. Bohte, A.E.; van Werven, J.R.; Bipat, S.; Stoker, J. The diagnostic accuracy of US, CT, MRI and 1H-MRS for the evaluation of hepatic steatosis compared with liver biopsy: A meta-analysis. *Eur. Radiol.* **2011**, *21*, 87–97. [CrossRef] [PubMed]

29. Longo, R.; Ricci, C.; Masutti, F.; Vidimari, R.; Crocé, L.S.; Bercich, L.; Tiribelli, C.; Dalla Palma, L. Fatty infiltration of the liver: Quantification by 1H localized magnetic resonance spectroscopy and comparison with computed tomography. *Investig. Radiol.* **1993**, *28*, 297–302. [CrossRef]

30. Szczepaniak, L.S.; Babcock, E.E.; Schick, F.; Dobbins, R.L.; Garg, A.; Burns, D.K.; McGarry, J.D.; Stein, D.T. Measurement of intracellular triglyceride stores by H spectroscopy: Validation *in vivo*. *Am. J. Physiol. Endocrinol. Metab.* **1999**, *276*, E977–E989.

31. Kotronen, A.; Vehkavaara, S.; Seppälä-Lindroos, A.; Bergholm, R.; Yki-Järvinen, H. Effect of liver fat on insulin clearance. *Am. J. Physiol. Endocrinol. Metab.* **2007**, *293*, E1709–E1715. [CrossRef] [PubMed]

32. Cowin, G.J.; Jonsson, J.R.; Bauer, J.D.; Ash, S.; Ali, A.; Osland, E.J.; Purdie, D.M.; Clouston, A.D.; Powell, E.E.; Galloway, G.J. Magnetic resonance imaging and spectroscopy for monitoring liver steatosis. *J. Magn. Reson. Imaging* **2008**, *28*, 937–945. [CrossRef] [PubMed]

33. Noureddin, M.; Lam, J.; Peterson, M.R.; Middleton, M.; Hamilton, G.; Le, T.-A.; Bettencourt, R.; Changchien, C.; Brenner, D.A.; Sirlin, C.; *et al.* Utility of magnetic resonance imaging *versus* histology for quantifying changes in liver fat in nonalcoholic fatty liver disease trials. *Hepatology* **2013**, *58*, 1930–1940. [CrossRef] [PubMed]

34. Thomsen, C.; Becker, U.; Winkler, K.; Christoffersen, P.; Jensen, M.; Henriksen, O. Quantification of liver fat using magnetic resonance spectroscopy. *Magn. Reson. Imaging* **1994**, *12*, 487–495. [CrossRef]

35. Dixon, W.T. Simple proton spectroscopic imaging. *Radiology* **1984**, *153*, 189–194. [CrossRef] [PubMed]

36. Rofsky, N.M.; Weinreb, J.C.; Ambrosino, M.M.; Safir, J.; Krinsky, G. Comparison between in-phase and opposed-phase T1-weighted breath-hold FLASH sequences for hepatic imaging. *J. Comput. Assist. Tomogr.* **1996**, *20*, 230–235. [CrossRef] [PubMed]

37. Cassidy, F.H.; Yokoo, T.; Aganovic, L.; Hanna, R.F.; Bydder, M.; Middleton, M.S.; Hamilton, G.; Chavez, A.D.; Schwimmer, J.B.; Sirlin, C.B. Fatty liver disease: MR Imaging techniques for the detection and quantification of liver steatosis1. *Radiographics* **2009**, *29*, 231–260. [CrossRef] [PubMed]

38. Hussain, H.K.; Chenevert, T.L.; Londy, F.J.; Gulani, V.; Swanson, S.D.; McKenna, B.J.; Appelman, H.D.; Adusumilli, S.; Greenson, J.K.; Conjeevaram, H.S. Hepatic fat fraction: MR imaging for quantitative measurement and display—Early experience 1. *Radiology* **2005**, *237*, 1048–1055. [CrossRef] [PubMed]

39. Fishbein, M.H.; Stevens, W.R. Rapid MRI using a modified Dixon technique: A non-invasive and effective method for detection and monitoring of fatty metamorphosis of the liver. *Pediatr. Radiol.* **2001**, *31*, 806–809. [CrossRef] [PubMed]

40. Hines, C.D.G.; Frydrychowicz, A.; Hamilton, G.; Tudorascu, D.L.; Vigen, K.K.; Yu, H.; McKenzie, C.A.; Sirlin, C.B.; Brittain, J.H.; Reeder, S.B. $T_1$ independent, $T_2$* corrected chemical shift based fat-water separation with multi-peak fat spectral modeling is an accurate and precise measure of hepatic steatosis. *J. Magn. Reson. Imaging* **2011**, *33*, 873–881. [CrossRef] [PubMed]

41. Meisamy, S.; Hines, C.D.G.; Hamilton, G.; Sirlin, C.B.; McKenzie, C.A.; Yu, H.; Brittain, J.H.; Reeder, S.B. Quantification of hepatic steatosis with T1-independent, T2*-corrected MR imaging with spectral modeling of fat: blinded comparison with MR spectroscopy. *Radiology* **2011**, *258*, 767–775. [CrossRef] [PubMed]

42. Kang, G.H.; Cruite, I.; Shiehmorteza, M.; Wolfson, T.; Gamst, A.C.; Hamilton, G.; Bydder, M.; Middleton, M.S.; Sirlin, C.B. Reproducibility of MRI-determined proton density fat fraction across two different MR scanner platforms. *J. Magn. Reson. Imaging* **2011**, *34*, 928–934. [CrossRef] [PubMed]

43. Permutt, Z.; Le, T.A.; Peterson, M.R.; Seki, E.; Brenner, D.A.; Sirlin, C.; Loomba, R. Correlation between liver histology and novel magnetic resonance imaging in adult patients with non-alcoholic fatty liver disease—MRI accurately quantifies hepatic steatosis in NAFLD. *Aliment. Pharmacol. Ther.* **2012**, *36*, 22–29. [CrossRef] [PubMed]

44.  Patel, N.S.; Peterson, M.R.; Brenner, D.A.; Heba, E.; Sirlin, C.; Loomba, R. Association between novel MRI-estimated pancreatic fat and liver histology-determined steatosis and fibrosis in non-alcoholic fatty liver disease. *Aliment. Pharmacol. Ther.* **2013**, *37*, 630–639. [CrossRef] [PubMed]

45.  Idilman, I.S.; Aniktar, H.; Idilman, R.; Kabacam, G.; Savas, B. Hepatic steatosis: Quantification by proton density fat fraction with MR imaging *versus* liver biopsy. *Radiology* **2013**, *267*, 767–775. [CrossRef] [PubMed]

46.  Tang, A.; Tan, J.; Sun, M.; Hamilton, G.; Bydder, M.; Wolfson, T.; Gamst, A.C.; Middleton, M.; Brunt, E.M.; Loomba, R.; *et al.* Nonalcoholic fatty liver disease: MR imaging of liver proton density fat fraction to assess hepatic steatosis. *Radiology* **2013**, *267*, 422–431. [CrossRef] [PubMed]

47.  Needleman, L.; Kurtz, A.B.; Rifkin, M.D.; Cooper, H.S.; Pasto, M.E.; Goldberg, B.B. Sonography of diffuse benign liver-disease—Accuracy of pattern-recognition and grading. *Am. J. Roentgenol.* **1986**, *146*, 1011–1015. [CrossRef] [PubMed]

48.  Joseph, A.E.A.; Saverymuttu, S.H.; Al-Sam, S.; Cook, M.G.; Maxwell, J.D. Comparison of liver histology with ultrasonography in assessing diffuse parenchymal liver disease. *Clin. Radiol.* **1991**, *43*, 26–31. [CrossRef]

49.  Foster, K.J.; Dewbury, K.C.; Griffith, A.H.; Wright, R. The accuracy of ultrasound in the detection of fatty infiltration of the liver. *Br. J. Radiol.* **1979**, *53*, 440–442. [CrossRef] [PubMed]

50.  Mottin, C.C.; Moretto, M.; Padoin, A.V.; Swarowsky, A.M.; Toneto, M.G.; Glock, L.; Repetto, G. The role of ultrasound in the diagnosis of hepatic steatosis in morbidly obese patients. *Obes. Surg.* **2004**, *14*, 635–637. [CrossRef] [PubMed]

51.  Ryan, C.K.; Johnson, L.A.; Germin, B.I.; Marcos, A. One hundred consecutive hepatic biopsies in the workup of living donors for right lobe liver transplantation. *Liver Transpl.* **2002**, *8*, 1114–1122. [CrossRef] [PubMed]

52.  Bril, F.; Ortiz Lopez, C.; Lomonaco, R.; Orsak, B.; Freckleton, M.; Chintapalli, K.; Hardies, J.; Lai, S.; Solano, F.; Tio, F.; *et al.* Clinical value of liver ultrasound for the diagnosis of nonalcoholic fatty liver disease in overweight and obese patients. *Liver Int.* **2015**, *35*, 2139–2146. [CrossRef] [PubMed]

53.  Hernaez, R.; Lazo, M.; Bonekamp, S.; Kamel, I.; Brancati, F.L.; Guallar, E.; Clark, J.M. Diagnostic accuracy and reliability of ultrasonography for the detection of fatty liver: A meta-analysis. *Hepatology* **2011**, *54*, 1082–1090. [CrossRef] [PubMed]

54.  Xia, M.F.; Yan, H.M.; He, W.Y.; Li, X.M.; Li, C.L.; Yao, X.Z.; Li, R.K.; Zeng, M.S.; Gao, X. Standardized ultrasound hepatic/renal ratio and hepatic attenuation rate to quantify liver fat content: An improvement method. *Obesity (Silver Spring)* **2012**, *20*, 444–452. [CrossRef] [PubMed]

55.  Loomba, R.; Sanyal, A.J. The global NAFLD epidemic. *Nat. Rev. Gastroenterol. Hepatol.* **2013**, *10*, 686–690. [CrossRef] [PubMed]

56.  Wong, R.J.; Ahmed, A. Obesity and non-alcoholic fatty liver disease: Disparate associations among Asian populations. *World J. Hepatol.* **2014**, *6*, 263–273. [CrossRef] [PubMed]

57.  Schwenzer, N.F.; Springer, F.; Schraml, C.; Stefan, N.; Machann, J.; Schick, F. Non-invasive assessment and quantification of liver steatosis by ultrasound, computed tomography and magnetic resonance. *J. Hepatol.* **2009**, *51*, 433–445. [CrossRef] [PubMed]

58.  Bydder, G.M.; Chapman, R.W.G.; Harry, D.; Bassan, L.; Sherlock, S.; Kreel, L. Computed tomography attenuation values in fatty liver. *J. Comput. Tomogr.* **1981**, *5*, 33–35. [CrossRef]

59.  Park, S.H.; Kim, P.N.; Kim, K.W.; Lee, S.W.; Yoon, S.E.; Park, S.W.; Ha, H.K.; Lee, M.-G.; Hwang, S.; Lee, S.-G.; *et al.* Macrovesicular hepatic steatosis in living liver donors: Use of CT for quantitative and qualitative assessment1. *Radiology* **2006**, *239*, 105–112. [CrossRef] [PubMed]

60.  Kodama, Y.; Ng, C.S.; Wu, T.T.; Ayers, G.D.; Curley, S.A.; Abdalla, E.K.; Vauthey, J.N.; Charnsangavej, C. Comparison of CT methods for determining the fat content of the liver. *AJR Am. J. Roentgenol.* **2007**, *188*, 1307–1312. [CrossRef] [PubMed]

61.  Seppälä-Lindroos, A.; Vehkavaara, S.; Häkkinen, A.-M.; Goto, T.; Westerbacka, J.; Sovijärvi, A.; Halavaara, J.; Yki-Järvinen, H. Fat accumulation in the liver is associated with defects in insulin suppression of glucose production and serum free fatty acids independent of obesity in normal men. *J. Clin. Endocrinol. Metab.* **2002**, *87*, 3023–3028. [CrossRef] [PubMed]

62.  Matthews, D.R.; Hosker, J.P.; Rudenski, A.S.; Naylor, B.A.; Treacher, D.F.; Turner, R.C. Homeostasis model assessment: Insulin resistance and beta-cell function from fasting plasma glucose and insulin concentrations in man. *Diabetologia* **1985**, *28*, 412–419. [CrossRef] [PubMed]

63.  Kotronen, A.; Westerbacka, J.; Bergholm, R.; Yki-Järvinen, H. Liver fat in the metabolic syndrome. *J. Clin. Endocrinol. Metab.* **2007**, *92*, 3490–3497. [CrossRef] [PubMed]

64. Gastaldelli, A.; Kozakova, M.; Højlund, K.; Flyvbjerg, A.; Favuzzi, A.; Mitrakou, A.; Balkau, B. Fatty liver is associated with insulin resistance, risk of coronary heart disease, and early atherosclerosis in a large European population. *Hepatology* **2009**, *49*, 1537–1544. [CrossRef] [PubMed]

65. Donnelly, K.L.; Smith, C.I.; Schwarzenberg, S.J.; Jessurun, J.; Boldt, M.D.; Parks, E.J. Sources of fatty acids stored in liver and secreted via lipoproteins in patients with nonalcoholic fatty liver disease. *J. Clin. Investig.* **2005**, *115*, 1343–1351. [CrossRef] [PubMed]

66. Lambert, J.E.; Ramos-Roman, M.A.; Browning, J.D.; Parks, E.J. Increased *de novo* lipogenesis is a distinct characteristic of individuals with nonalcoholic fatty liver disease. *Gastroenterology* **2014**, *146*, 726–735. [CrossRef] [PubMed]

67. Kotronen, A.; Vehkavaara, S.; Yki-Järvinen, H. Increased liver fat, impaired insulin clearance, and hepatic and adipose tissue insulin resistance in type 2 diabetes. *Gastroenterology* **2008**, *135*, 122–130. [CrossRef] [PubMed]

68. Gastaldelli, A.; Cusi, K.; Pettiti, M.; Hardies, J.; Miyazaki, Y.; Berria, R.; Buzzigoli, E.; Sironi, A.M.; Cersosimo, E.; Ferrannini, E.; *et al.* Relationship between hepatic/visceral fat and hepatic insulin resistance in nondiabetic and type 2 diabetic subjects. *Gastroenterology* **2007**, *133*, 496–506. [CrossRef] [PubMed]

69. Alberti, K.G.M.M.; Eckel, R.H.; Grundy, S.M.; Zimmet, P.Z.; Cleeman, J.I.; Donato, K.A.; Fruchart, J.-C.; James, W.P.T.; Loria, C.M.; Smith, S.C.; *et al.* Harmonizing the metabolic syndrome: A joint interim statement of the international diabetes federation task force on epidemiology and prevention; national heart, lung, and blood institute; American heart association; world heart federation; international atherosclerosis society; and international association for the study of obesity. *Circulation* **2009**, *120*, 1640–1645. [PubMed]

70. Manley, S.E.; Stratton, I.M.; Clark, P.M.; Luzio, S.D. Comparison of 11 human insulin assays: Implications for clinical investigation and research. *Clin. Chem.* **2007**, *53*, 922–932. [CrossRef] [PubMed]

71. Sookoian, S.; Pirola, C.J. Meta-analysis of the influence of I148M variant of patatin-like phospholipase domain containing 3 gene (PNPLA3) on the susceptibility and histological severity of nonalcoholic fatty liver disease. *Hepatology* **2011**, *53*, 1883–1894. [CrossRef] [PubMed]

72. Zhang, L.; You, W.; Zhang, H.; Peng, R.; Zhu, Q.; Yao, A.; Li, X.; Zhou, Y.; Wang, X.; Pu, L.; *et al.* PNPLA3 polymorphisms (rs738409) and non-alcoholic fatty liver disease risk and related phenotypes: A meta-analysis. *J. Gastroenterol. Hepatol.* **2015**, *30*, 821–829. [CrossRef] [PubMed]

73. Xu, R.; Tao, A.; Zhang, S.; Deng, Y.; Chen, G. Association between patatin-like phospholipase domain containing 3 gene (PNPLA3) polymorphisms and nonalcoholic fatty liver disease: A HuGE review and meta-analysis. *Sci. Rep.* **2015**, *5*. [CrossRef]

74. Shen, J.-H.; Li, Y.-L.; Li, D.; Wang, N.-N.; Jing, L.; Huang, Y.-H. The rs738409 (I148M) variant of the PNPLA3 gene and cirrhosis: A meta-analysis. *J. Lipid Res.* **2015**, *56*, 167–175. [CrossRef]

75. Trépo, E.; Nahon, P.; Bontempi, G.; Valenti, L.; Falleti, E.; Nischalke, H.D.; Hamza, S.; Corradini, S.G.; Burza, M.A.; Guyot, E.; *et al.* Association between the PNPLA3 (rs738409 C>G) variant and hepatocellular carcinoma: Evidence from a meta-analysis of individual participant data. *Hepatology* **2014**, *59*, 2170–2177. [CrossRef]

76. He, S.; McPhaul, C.; Li, J.Z.; Garuti, R.; Kinch, L.; Grishin, N.V.; Hobbs, H.H. A sequence variation (I148M) in PNPLA3 associated with nonalcoholic fatty liver disease disrupts triglyceride hydrolysis. *J. Biol. Chem.* **2010**, *285*, 6706–6715. [CrossRef]

77. Huang, Y.; Cohen, J.C.; Hobbs, H.H. Expression and characterization of a PNPLA3 protein isoform (I148M) associated with nonalcoholic fatty liver disease. *J. Biol. Chem.* **2011**, *286*, 37085–37093. [CrossRef] [PubMed]

78. Kumari, M.; Schoiswohl, G.; Chitraju, C.; Paar, M.; Cornaciu, I.; Rangrez, A.Y.; Wongsiriroj, N.; Nagy, H.M.; Ivanova, P.T.; Scott, S.A.; *et al.* Adiponutrin functions as a nutritionally regulated lysophosphatidic acid acyltransferase. *Cell Metab.* **2012**, *15*, 691–702. [CrossRef] [PubMed]

79. Kantartzis, K.; Peter, A.; Machicao, F.; Machann, J.; Wagner, S.; Königsrainer, I.; Königsrainer, A.; Schick, F.; Fritsche, A.; Haring, H.-U.; *et al.* Dissociation between fatty liver and insulin resistance in humans carrying a variant of the patatin-like phospholipase 3 gene. *Diabetes* **2009**, *58*, 2616–2623. [CrossRef] [PubMed]

80. Kotronen, A.; Johansson, L.E.; Johansson, L.M.; Roos, C.; Westerbacka, J.; Hamsten, A.; Bergholm, R.; Arkkila, P.; Arola, J.; Kiviluoto, T.; *et al.* A common variant in PNPLA3, which encodes adiponutrin, is associated with liver fat content in humans. *Diabetologia* **2009**, *52*, 1056–1060. [CrossRef] [PubMed]

81.    Scorletti, E.; West, A.L.; Bhatia, L.; Hoile, S.P.; McCormick, K.G.; Burdge, G.C.; Lillycrop, K.A.; Clough, G.F.; Calder, P.C.; Byrne, C.D. Treating liver fat and serum triglyceride levels in NAFLD, effects of PNPLA3 and TM6SF2 genotypes: Results from the WELCOME trial. *J. Hepatol.* **2015**, *63*, 1476–1483. [CrossRef] [PubMed]

82.    Wagenknecht, L.E.; Palmer, N.D.; Bowden, D.W.; Rotter, J.I.; Norris, J.M.; Ziegler, J.; Chen, Y.D.I.; Haffner, S.; Scherzinger, A.; Langefeld, C.D. Association of PNPLA3 with non-alcoholic fatty liver disease in a minority cohort: The insulin resistance atherosclerosis family study. *Liver Int.* **2011**, *31*, 412–416. [CrossRef] [PubMed]

83.    Verrijken, A.; Beckers, S.; Francque, S.; Hilden, H.; Caron, S.; Zegers, D.; Ruppert, M.; Hubens, G.; Marck, E.; Michielsen, P.; et al. A gene variant of PNPLA3, but not of APOC3, is associated with histological parameters of NAFLD in an obese population. *Obesity (Silver Spring)* **2013**, *21*, 2138–2145. [CrossRef] [PubMed]

84.    Musso, G.; Cassader, M.; Gambino, R. PNPLA3 rs738409 and TM6SF2 rs58542926 gene variants affect renal disease and function in nonalcoholic fatty liver disease. *Hepatology* **2015**, *62*, 658–659. [CrossRef] [PubMed]

85.    Valenti, L.; Al-Serri, A.; Daly, A.K.; Galmozzi, E.; Rametta, R.; Dongiovanni, P.; Nobili, V.; Mozzi, E.; Roviaro, G.; Vanni, E.; et al. Homozygosity for the patatin-like phospholipase-3/adiponutrin I148M polymorphism influences liver fibrosis in patients with nonalcoholic fatty liver disease. *Hepatology* **2010**, *51*, 1209–1217. [CrossRef] [PubMed]

86.    Del Ben, M.; Polimeni, L.; Brancorsini, M.; di Costanzo, A.; D'Erasmo, L.; Baratta, F.; Loffredo, L.; Pastori, D.; Pignatelli, P.; Violi, F.; et al. Non-alcoholic fatty liver disease, metabolic syndrome and patatin-like phospholipase domain-containing protein3 gene variants. *Eur. J. Intern. Med.* **2014**, *25*, 566–570. [CrossRef] [PubMed]

87.    Wang, C.W.; Lin, H.Y.; Shin, S.J.; Yu, M.-L.; Lin, Z.-Y.; Dai, C.-Y.; Huang, J.-F.; Chen, S.-C.; Li, S.S.L.; Chuang, W.-L. The PNPLA3 I148M polymorphism is associated with insulin resistance and nonalcoholic fatty liver disease in a normoglycaemic population. *Liver Int.* **2011**, *31*, 1326–1331. [CrossRef] [PubMed]

88.    Park, J.H.; Cho, B.; Kwon, H.; Prilutsky, D.; Yun, J.M.; Choi, H.C.; Hwang, K.B.; Lee, I.H.; Kim, J.I.; Kong, S.W. I148M variant in PNPLA3 reduces central adiposity and metabolic disease risks while increasing nonalcoholic fatty liver disease. *Liver Int.* **2015**, *35*, 2537–2546. [CrossRef] [PubMed]

89.    Lin, Y.-C.; Chang, P.-F.; Hu, F.-C.; Yang, W.-S.; Chang, M.-H.; Ni, Y.-H. A Common variant in the PNPLA3 gene is a risk factor for Non-alcoholic fatty liver disease in obese Taiwanese children. *J. Pediatr.* **2011**, *158*, 740–744. [CrossRef] [PubMed]

90.    Romeo, S.; Sentinelli, F.; Cambuli, V.M.; Incani, M.; Congiu, T.; Matta, V.; Pilia, S.; Huang-Doran, I.; Cossu, E.; Loche, S.; et al. The 148M allele of the PNPLA3 gene is associated with indices of liver damage early in life. *J. Hepatol.* **2010**, *53*, 335–338. [CrossRef] [PubMed]

91.    Valenti, L.; Alisi, A.; Galmozzi, E.; Bartuli, A.; del Menico, B.; Alterio, A.; Dongiovanni, P.; Fargion, S.; Nobili, V. I148M patatin-like phospholipase domain-containing 3 gene variant and severity of pediatric nonalcoholic fatty liver disease. *Hepatology* **2010**, *52*, 1274–1280. [CrossRef] [PubMed]

92.    Kozlitina, J.; Smagris, E.; Stender, S.; Nordestgaard, B.G.; Zhou, H.H.; Tybjærg-Hansen, A.; Vogt, T.F.; Hobbs, H.H.; Cohen, J.C. Exome-wide association study identifies a TM6SF2 variant that confers susceptibility to nonalcoholic fatty liver disease. *Nat. Genet.* **2014**, *46*, 352–356. [CrossRef] [PubMed]

93.    Pirola, C.J.; Sookoian, S. The dual and opposite role of the TM6SF2-rs58542926 variant in protecting against cardiovascular disease and conferring risk for nonalcoholic fatty liver: A meta-analysis. *Hepatology* **2015**, *62*, 1742–1756. [CrossRef] [PubMed]

94.    Smagris, E.; Gilyard, S.; BasuRay, S.; Cohen, J.C.; Hobbs, H.H. Inactivation of TM6SF2, a gene defective in fatty liver disease, impairs lipidation but not secretion of very low density lipoproteins. *J. Biol. Chem.* **2016**. [CrossRef] [PubMed]

95.    Mahdessian, H.; Taxiarchis, A.; Popov, S.; Silveira, A.; Franco-Cereceda, A.; Hamsten, A.; Eriksson, P.; van't Hooft, F. TM6SF2 is a regulator of liver fat metabolism influencing triglyceride secretion and hepatic lipid droplet content. *Proc. Natl. Acad. Sci. USA* **2014**, *111*, 8913–8918. [CrossRef] [PubMed]

96.    Holmen, O.L.; Zhang, H.; Fan, Y.; Hovelson, D.H.; Schmidt, E.M.; Zhou, W.; Guo, Y.; Zhang, J.; Langhammer, A.; Løchen, M.-L.; et al. Systematic evaluation of coding variation identifies a candidate causal variant in TM6SF2 influencing total cholesterol and myocardial infarction risk. *Nat. Genet.* **2014**, *46*, 345–351. [CrossRef] [PubMed]

97.    Zhou, Y.; Llauradó, G.; Orešič, M.; Hyötyläinen, T.; Orho-Melander, M.; Yki-Järvinen, H. Circulating triacylglycerol signatures and insulin sensitivity in NAFLD associated with the E167K variant in TM6SF2. *J. Hepatol.* **2015**, *62*, 657–663. [CrossRef] [PubMed]

98.  Eslam, M.; Mangia, A.; Berg, T.; Chan, H.L.-Y.; Irving, W.L.; Dore, G.J.; Abate, M.L.; Bugianesi, E.; Adams, L.A.; Najim, M.A.M.; *et al.* Diverse impacts of the rs58542926 E167K variant in TM6SF2 on viral and metabolic liver disease phenotypes. *Hepatology* **2016**. [CrossRef] [PubMed]
99.  Goffredo, M.; Caprio, S.; Feldstein, A.E.; D'Adamo, E.; Shaw, M.M.; Pierpont, B.; Savoye, M.; Zhao, H.; Bale, A.E.; Santoro, N. Role of TM6SF2 rs58542926 in the pathogenesis of nonalcoholic pediatric fatty liver disease: A multiethnic study. *Hepatology* **2016**, *63*, 117–125. [CrossRef] [PubMed]
100. Grandone, A.; Cozzolino, D.; Marzuillo, P.; Cirillo, G.; di Sessa, A.; Ruggiero, L.; di Palma, M.R.; Perrone, L.; Miraglia del Giudice, E. TM6SF2 Glu167Lys polymorphism is associated with low levels of LDL-cholesterol and increased liver injury in obese children. *Pediatr. Obes.* **2016**, *11*, 115–119. [CrossRef] [PubMed]
101. European Association for the Study of the Liver (EASL); European Association for the Study of Diabetes (EASD); European Association for the Study of Obesity (EASO). EASL-EASD-EASO Clinical Practice Guidelines for the management of non-alcoholic fatty liver disease. *Diabetologia* **2016**, *9*, 65–90.

# 8

# Molecular Pathogenesis of NASH

**Alessandra Caligiuri, Alessandra Gentilini and Fabio Marra ***

Dipartimento di Medicina Sperimentale e Clinica, Università degli Studi di Firenze, Firenze 50121, Italy;
alessandra.caligiuri@unifi.it (A.C.); alessandra.gentilini@unifi.it (A.G.)
* Correspondence: fabio.marra@unifi.it

Academic Editors: Giovanni Targher and Amedeo Lonardo

**Abstract:** Nonalcoholic steatohepatitis (NASH) is the main cause of chronic liver disease in the Western world and a major health problem, owing to its close association with obesity, diabetes, and the metabolic syndrome. NASH progression results from numerous events originating within the liver, as well as from signals derived from the adipose tissue and the gastrointestinal tract. In a fraction of NASH patients, disease may progress, eventually leading to advanced fibrosis, cirrhosis and hepatocellular carcinoma. Understanding the mechanisms leading to NASH and its evolution to cirrhosis is critical to identifying effective approaches for the treatment of this condition. In this review, we focus on some of the most recent data reported on the pathogenesis of NASH and its fibrogenic progression, highlighting potential targets for treatment or identification of biomarkers of disease progression.

**Keywords:** fibrosis; inflammation; chemokines; genetics; microbiota; pattern-recognition receptors; nuclear receptors; hepatic stellate cells; macrophages

---

## 1. Introduction

Nonalcoholic fatty liver disease (NAFLD) is an expanding health problem, which varies in prevalence among ethnic groups, occurring with an estimated global prevalence of 25% [1]. NAFLD associates with obesity, insulin resistance or type 2 diabetes and other metabolic abnormalities, such as dyslipidemia and hypertension, collectively termed metabolic syndrome. In high risk populations, the prevalence of NAFLD may be as high as 70%–90% [2,3]. NAFLD covers a spectrum of pathological abnormalities. Although most patients have simple steatosis, around 7%–30% develop nonalcoholic steatohepatitis (NASH), that in at least a third of cases progresses to advanced fibrosis or cirrhosis. The tendency to develop hepatic steatosis differs among ethnic groups, with African-Americans having a lower (24%) and Hispanics a higher (45%) frequency of the disease than Americans of European descent (33%). The causes for these ethnic differences in prevalence of hepatic steatosis and liver injury are not entirely understood.

NASH is characterized by hepatocellular damage, inflammation and fibrosis [4,5]. In general, simple steatosis is considered a less severe form of NAFLD, although recent data indicate a possible risk of progression [6,7]. In contrast, NASH is a significant risk factor for the development of cirrhosis and hepatocellular carcinoma [8–10]. Although NASH was first documented more than 30 years ago [11], its pathogenesis is still not fully elucidated. Initially, a two-hit hypothesis, based on appearance of steatosis (first hit), followed by a second hit leading to inflammation, hepatocyte damage, and fibrosis, was proposed by Day and James [12]. While accumulation of triglycerides is necessary for the development of NASH, they may actually have a protective role against hepatocytes lipotoxicity, which is mainly induced by fatty acids and derived metabolites such as diacylglycerols, acylcarnitines or ceramides [13,14]. In addition, it is still unclear whether NASH develops sequentially, on the grounds of a fatty liver, or it is rather a de novo response to a lipotoxic environment. The multiparallel hypothesis proposed more recently [15] suggests that NASH is the result of numerous conditions acting in parallel, including genetic predisposition, abnormal lipid metabolism, oxidative stress, lipotoxicity, mitochondrial dysfunction, altered production of cytokines and adipokines, gut dysbiosis and endoplasmic reticulum stress. According to this hypothesis, hepatic inflammation in NASH may even precede steatosis. As more contributing factors are continuously identified, a more complex picture of NASH pathogenesis is emerging [16] (Figure 1).

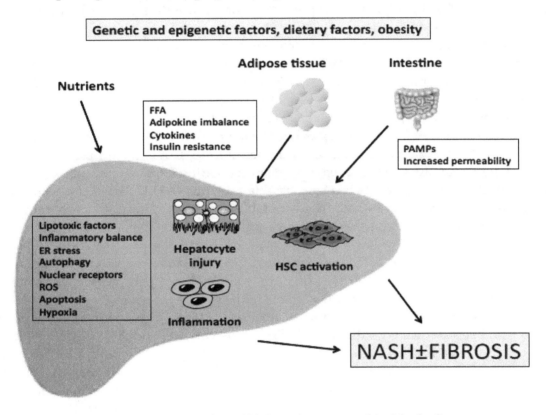

**Figure 1.** Outline of the pathogenesis of NASH. Signals generated inside the liver as a consequence of increased lipid accumulation, together with signals derived from extrahepatic organs cooperate to induce inflammation and fibrosis. FFA, free fatty acids; PAMPs, pathogen-associated molecular patterns; ER, endoplasmic reticulum; ROS, reactive oxygen species; HSC, hepatic stellate cell.

## 2. Genetic Factors

The relevance of genetic factor in the context of NASH has been recently and elegantly outlined by twin studies [17]. A long list of genes potentially implicated in NAFLD appearance and progression has been reported, and these data have been the subject of a recent review [18].

A significant association with a SNP was identified in patatin-like phospholipase domain-containing 3 (*PNPLA3*) on chromosome 22. The variant (rs738409 c.444 C>G, p.I148M), a non-synonymous cytosine to guanine mutation resulting in isoleucine to methionine conversion, correlates with increased hepatic lipid content and predisposes to fatty liver-associated liver disease, from simple steatosis to steatohepatitis, fibrosis and hepatocellular carcinoma [19,20]. *PNPLA3* encodes for a 481 amino acid protein, whose role has not been fully elucidated. It appears to function as acylglycerol hydrolase, acting on triacylglycerol, diacylglycerol, and monoacylglycerol [21,22]. Additional evidence indicates that PNPLA3 also acts as lysophosphatidic acid acetyltransferase [23,24]. Overexpression of the I148M variant in mouse liver promotes accumulation of triacylglycerol, increased synthesis of fatty acids and impaired hydrolysis of triacylglycerol [25]. Moreover, the *PNPLA3* genotype has been reported to influence liver storage of retinol and retinol serum levels in obese subjects [26], suggesting a potential role of PNPLA3 in regulating retinol metabolism and hepatic stellate cell (HSC) biology [27]. Remarkably, PNPLA3 has been recently shown to be expressed in hepatic stellate cells [28]. Interestingly, the prevalence of the *PNPLA3* I148M allele varies considerably among different ethnic groups, with the highest frequency in Hispanics (0.49), and lower frequencies in European Americans (0.23) and African-Americans (0.17) [20]. This is in agreement with the different prevalence of NAFLD in the three ethnic groups.

Carriage of a non-synonymous genetic variant in *TM6SF2* (rs58542926 c.449 C>T, p.E167K) on chromosome 19 (19p13.11) has been reported to correlate with steatosis and increased risk of advanced fibrosis in NAFLD patients [29,30], independently of other factors, including diabetes, obesity, or *PNPLA3* genotype. The minor allele frequency in one of the NAFLD populations tested was 0.12, compared to a frequency of 0.07 in a reference population. TM6SF2, is a transmembrane protein localized in endoplasmic reticulum (ER) and ER–Golgi compartments and functions as a lipid transporter [31]. The amino acid change E167K causes loss of function of TM6SF2 protein. Studies performed in cell lines showed that downregulation of *TM6SF2* reduces lipoproteins and apolipoprotein B (APOB) levels, and increases hepatic deposition of triglycerides and the amount and size of lipid droplets. In contrast, the size and number of lipid droplets diminishes when TM6SF2 is overexpressed, indicating that TM6SF2 plays a role in regulating hepatic lipid efflux [29,31].

A broad spectrum of other genes has been associated with NAFLD. Polymorphism was reported in genes involved in carbohydrate and lipid metabolism, insulin-induced pathways, as well as inflammatory response, oxidative stress and fibrogenesis. A study by Dongiovanni et al. reported that non-synonymous SNPs in ectoenzyme nucleotide pyrophosphate phosphodiesterase 1 (*ENPP1* or *PC1*) (rs1044498, K121Q) and insulin receptor substrate-1 (*IRS1*) (rs1801278, Q972R), are associated with insulin resistance, through impairment of insulin receptor-mediated pathways, such as reduced AKT activation, and promote fibrosis in NAFLD patients [32].

A functional non-synonymous variant (rs1260326, P446L) of glucokinase regulatory protein (GCKR) has also been associated with NAFLD [33]. This variant produces a GCKR with defective inhibitory function, leading to increased glucokinase activity and hepatic glucose uptake [34]. The resultant unimpeded hepatic glycolysis reduces glucose levels, inducing malonyl-CoA synthesis, a substrate for lipogenesis that causes liver fat deposition and impairs mitochondrial β-oxidation. A polymorphism in the solute carrier family 2 member 1 gene (*SLC2A1*), a glucose transporter, has been reported in NAFLD subjects. SLC2A1 downregulation in hepatocytes results in lipid accumulation and oxidative stress [35].

Several genes involved in oxidative stress have been investigated. Two reports correlated the C282Y variant in hemochromatosis gene (HFE) with NASH and higher susceptibility to more severe disease, as fibrosis or cirrhosis [36,37]. However, these findings have not been confirmed by other studies [38–40]. Very recently, the rs641738 genotype at the *MBOAT7-TMC4* locus, encoding for the membrane bound O-acyltransferase domain-containing 7 was associated with more severe liver damage and increased risk of fibrosis in patients with NAFLD. This effect has been ascribed to changes in remodeling of the hepatic phosphatidylinositol acyl-chain [41].

## 3. Epigenetics

Epigenetic changes consist in modifications at the transcriptional level affecting gene expression and phenotype. A number of epigenetic aberrations have been associated with NAFLD pathogenesis, causing alterations in lipid metabolism, insulin resistance (IR), dysfunction of endoplasmic reticulum (ER) and mitochondria, oxidative stress and inflammation [42]. The different epigenetic pathways potentially involved in NAFLD are summarized in Figure 2.

Aberrant DNA methylation is a major epigenetic process in NAFLD development and progression to NASH [43]. It occurs through methyltransferases (DNMTs) that catalyze the conversion of cytosine to 5-methylcytosine [44], leading to gene silencing. It has been reported that mice fed with a methyl-deficient diet show reduced levels of hepatic *S*-adenosylmethionine (SAM), associated with methylation of genes involved in DNA damage and repair, lipid and glucose metabolism and fibrosis progression [45]. In agreement, food-derived methyl donors, such as folate, betaine and choline, responsible for SAM synthesis, counteract DNA methylation [46] whereas folate deficiency correlates with enhanced fatty acid synthesis and hepatic accumulation of triglycerides (TG) via DNA methylation [47]. Methyl donor supplementation reverts liver lipid deposition induced by high fat/high sucrose-diet, lowering global hepatic DNA methylation and methylation levels of the promoter regions of different regulatory factors [48]. Betaine has been demonstrated to diminish the methylation levels of the promoter of microsomal triglyceride transfer protein (MTP), enhancing hepatic TG export and ameliorating liver steatosis in mice administered a high-fat diet (HFD) [43]. In addition, epigenetic changes of peroxisome proliferator-activated receptor gamma (PPARγ) in the liver of NAFLD patients seems to promote IR [49].

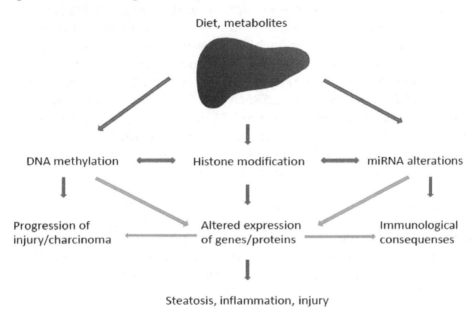

**Figure 2.** Epigenetic pathways implicated in the pathogenesis of NASH. The major pathways and their main effectors are depicted.

Although most epigenetic alterations are transient, DNA methylation can be inherited from parents [50]. It has been reported that maternal Western diet during prenatal time can increase the susceptibility to NAFLD of male progeny [51]. Novel evidence indicates that mitochondrial DNA (mtDNA) methylation may also play a role in NAFLD pathogenesis [52,53]. Liver methylation of *NADH dehydrogenase 6* (*MT-ND6*) correlates with NAFLD severity, resulting in significantly lower expression of MT-ND6 mRNA in NASH than in patients with simple steatosis [54].

Histone acetylation, regulated by histone acetyltransferases (HATs) and histone deacetylases (HDACs), has been extensively associated with NAFLD [55,56]. High-fat maternal diet was shown to lead to depletion of fetal hepatic HDAC1, suggesting that diet-induced maternal obesity can alter fetal chromatin via histone modifications [55]. Carbohydrate-responsive element-binding protein (ChREBP), an activator of lipogenic and glycolytic pathways involved in NAFLD progression, is regulated by the HAT activator p300. Glucose-activated p300 induces ChREBP hyperacetylation, stimulating its transcriptional activity and hepatic lipogenesis in mice, and p300 overexpression is associated with steatosis and IR [56].

NAFLD has been also correlated with histone methylation. Lipid accumulation in the liver of HFD mice has been associated with H3K4 and H3K9 histone trimethylation of peroxisome proliferator-activated receptor alpha (PPARα) and lipolysis-related genes [57]. In addition, trans-generational changes in histone methylation promote lipogenesis and ER stress, acting on endoplasmic reticulum oxidoreductin 1α (ERO1α) and liver X receptor α (LXRα) [58].

Sirtuins (SIRTs) belong to the silent information regulator-2 family. SIRT1 deacetylation has been recognized as a regulatory mechanism for several proteins involved in NAFLD pathogenesis [59] and low SIRT1 expression has been observed in NAFLD models [60]. In addition, SIRT1-mediated regulation of fetal metabolome and epigenome has been reported under maternal HFD [61]. SIRT3 is localized in mitochondria and regulates fatty acid oxidation. SIRT3 knockout mice fed HFD develop hepatic steatosis and IR [62].

MicroRNAs (miRNAs) modulate gene expression via post-transcriptional mechanisms, regulating the main cellular processes, such as lipid metabolism, inflammation, apoptosis, cell growth and differentiation. In the last few years, aberrant miRNA expression has been reported in a number of diseases including metabolic disorders [63,64], whereas an increasing number of dysregulated miRNAs, implicated in fatty acid synthesis, uptake and storage of triglycerides or oxidation, have been recently identified in NAFLD [65] (Table 1). Among these, miR-122, which negatively regulates hepatic lipogenesis, is reduced in NASH patients [66] whereas miR-34a, that induces β-oxidation and inhibits synthesis of fatty acids via a sirtuin1/5′ adenosine monophosphate-activated protein kinase/3-hydroxy-3-methylglutaryl-CoA reductase (SIRT1-AMPK-HMGCR) mechanism, is upregulated in NAFLD patients [67]. miRNA-33a has been recently reported to participate in NASH development, counteracting cholesterol 7alpha-hydroxylase (CYP7A1). Sterol response element-binding protein 2 (SREBP2) binds to its own gene promoter to induce miR-33a, which leads to a decrease in cholesterol efflux to HDL and bile acid synthesis in Cyp7a1-tg mice [68]. In addition, miR-33a inhibits CYP7A1 and bile acid synthesis to inhibit cholesterol catabolism.

**Table 1.** Modulation of miRNA expression relevant to NAFLD/NASH. Δ indicates up- (↑) or downregulation (↓). CYP7A1: cholesterol 7α1-hydroxylase; SREBP2: sterol response element-binding protein 2; SIRT1: sirtuin1; AMPK: 5′ adenosine monophosphate-activated protein kinase; HMGCR: 3-hydroxy-3-methylglutaryl-CoA reductase; FAS: fatty acid synthase; ACC: Acetyl-CoA carboxylase; mTOR: mammalian target of rapamycin; ROS: reactive oxygen species; RAC1: Ras-related C3 botulinum toxin substrate 1; ?: mechanism and/or target unknown.

| miR | Δ | Disease | Model | Role | Validated/ Predicted Target | Reference |
|---|---|---|---|---|---|---|
| 33a | ↑ | NASH | Mouse Liver | Cholesterol and bile acid homeostasis | CYP7A1, SREPB2 | [68] |
| 34a | ↑ | NAFLD/NASH | Human Biopsies | Lipid homeostasis | SIRT1-AMPK-HMGCR | [67,69] |
| 103a2 | ↑ | NAFLD | Human Biopsies | Insulin signaling, metabolism, inflammation | ? | [30,70] |
| 160b | ↑ | NAFLD | Human Biopsies | Insulin signaling | ? | [30] |
| 122 | ↓ | NASH | HFD mice/ Human Biopsies | Lipid and cholesterol metabolism | HMGCR, FAS, SREBP1/2, ACC | [66,71] |
| 301a-3p | ↑ | Steatosis/ NAFLD/NASH | Human Biopsies | ? | ? | [69] |
| 375 | ↓ | NAFLD/NASH/ Cirrhosis | Human Biopsies | ? | ? | [69] |
| 576-5p | ↑ | NAFLD | Human Biopsies | Insulin signaling, metabolic homeostasis, inflammation | mTOR signaling, ephrin B signaling, ROS production, RAC1 | [70] |
| 892a | ↑ | NAFLD | Human Biopsies | Kupffer cell activation ? | ? | [70] |
| I137 | ↑ | NAFLD | Human Biopsies | ? | ? | [70] |
| 1282 | ↓ | NAFLD | Human Biopsies | Insulin signaling, metabolism, inflammation | ? | [70] |
| 3663-5p | ↑ | NAFLD | Human Biopsies | Insulin signaling, metabolism, inflammation | ? | [70] |
| 3924 | ↑ | NAFLD | Human Biopsies | Insulin signaling, metabolism, inflammation | ? | [70] |

More recently, other dysregulated miRNAs have been identified in NAFLD livers [70]. Among these, the most significantly upregulated (miR-103a-2, miR-106b, miR-576-5p, miRPlus-I137, miR-892a, miR-1282, miR-3663-5p, and miR-3924) play critical roles in insulin signaling, metabolism homeostasis, inflammation and cancer. In particular, miR-576-5p influences multiple pathways implied in NAFLD, including mammalian target of rapamycin (mTOR), a kinase modulated by insulin that induces hepatic lipogenesis through a PPARγ-dependent mechanism [72]. miR-576-5p also regulates eukaryotic translation initiation factor 4 (eIF4), p70S6 kinase (p70S6K) and phosphatidylinositol-4,5-bisphosphate 3-kinase (PI3K), pathways associated with insulin action and metabolic control. Moreover, a direct target of miR-576-5p is the small GTPase RAC1, which promotes lipotoxicity via c-Jun N-terminal kinase (JNK) activation. RAC1 is negatively modulated by miR-576-5p, triggering a protective effect against NAFLD progression [72]. Finally, in a study conducted in biopsy-staged NAFLD patients, increased miR-301a-3p and miR-34a-5p and decreased miR-375 significantly correlated with disease progression [69].

## 4. Dietary Factors

Lifestyle changes focusing on weight loss remain the keystone of NAFLD and NASH treatment [73]. Recent reports indicate that lifestyle modifications based on decreased energy intake and/or increased physical activity during 6–12 months cause improvement in biochemical and metabolic parameters and reduce steatosis and inflammation [74]. Conversely, increased consumption of sugar-sweetened food and beverages has been associated with NAFLD development and progression. High intake of fructose, used as food and drink sweetener, is implicated in NAFLD pathogenesis through several mechanisms. In addition, a fructose-enriched diet contributes to induce liver fibrosis in animal models of NASH [75]. Via the portal vein, dietary fructose reaches the liver in high concentrations, exerting a lipogenic action by activation of the transcription factors SREBP1 and ChREBP and subsequent induction of acetyl-CoA carboxylase (ACC) 1, fatty acid synthase (FAS) and stearoyl-CoA desaturase 1 (SCD1) [76]. These effects persist in liver-specific insulin receptor knockout mice, indicating that fructose stimulates lipogenesis independently of insulin signaling [77]. Fructose-induced de novo lipogenesis (DNL), enhancing malonyl-CoA concentration, inhibits mitochondrial β-oxidation and decreases mitochondrial ATP production [78]. In addition, fructose stimulates lipogenesis by inducing ER stress and subsequently activating the transcription factor X-box binding protein 1 (XBP1), which, in turn, upregulates lipogenic enzymes, as demonstrated in mice fed with a 60% fructose diet [79]. In concomitance, phosphorylation of fructose to fructose-1-phosphate leads to depletion of hepatic ATP and increase in ADP and inosine monophosphate (IMP), which is converted to uric acid [80], that promotes steatosis inducing mitochondrial oxidative stress [81]. Generation of reactive oxygen species (ROS) is also induced by fructose metabolism [82], and nutrient-derived ROS have been associated with enhanced steatosis via insulin-independent PI3K pathway [83]. Moreover, upregulating ketohexokinase, fructose potentiates its own metabolism and ketohexokinase inhibition leads to decreased fatty liver and reduced liver inflammation in high-fat/high-sucrose fed mice [84]. Finally, fructose-induced metabolic disorders can be mediated by epigenetic changes, such as alterations in genomic or mitochondrial DNA (mtDNA) methylation [85,86].

Dietary iron overload has been recently implicated in NASH pathogenesis. A study by Handa et al. [87] shows that dietary iron excess leads to a severe NASH phenotype in an obese, diabetogenic mouse model characterized by oxidative stress, inflammation and ballooning. Different molecular mechanisms are involved, including upregulation of cytokines (interleukin 6, IL-6, tumor necrosis factor α, TNFα) and immune mediators (Toll-like receptor 4, TLR4, inducible nitric oxide synthase, NOS, interferon gamma, IFNγ), and induction of inflammasome related factors (NOD like receptor 3, NLRP3, interleukin 18, IL-18) and genes associated with lipid metabolism. Moreover, emerging evidence indicates that hepatic copper (Cu) deficiency is associated with NAFLD development and progression. In an experimental rat model, a Cu deficient diet coupled with high sucrose intake provoked NASH, even in the absence of obesity or severe steatosis. Rats fed low-Cu/high-sucrose diet displayed enhanced liver expression of lipogenic enzymes, such as ATP citrate lyase (ACLY) and FAS, and of inflammatory and pro-fibrogenic factors (TNFα, C–C motif chemokine CCL2, CCL3), together with hepatic stellate cell activation. While low Cu alone promotes lipid peroxidation, as indicated by increased levels of malondialdehyde (MDA), its combination with high sucrose (or fructose), that causes a further reduction of hepatic Cu, causes insulin resistance and liver damage, with hepatocyte ballooning and occurrence of Mallory-Denk bodies. In addition, Cu deficiency influences Fe retention and partitioning in animals as well as in NAFLD patients [88].

Several lines of evidence correlate hepatic free fatty acids (FFAs) and free cholesterol (FC) accumulation to NAFLD pathogenesis. Dysregulation of lipid homeostasis plays an essential role in NAFLD pathogenesis, induced by a surplus of dietary free fatty acids, enhanced DNL and augmented lipolysis [89]. Rather than total hepatic fat content, the role of specific lipid classes in the development and progression of NAFLD is emerging [90]. In particular, accumulation of different lipids as well as upregulation of distinct enzymes mediating DNL was found to be associated with macrovesicular or microvesicular steatosis, the latter correlating with mitochondrial dysfunction and NAFLD [91]. Among toxic lipids, saturated fatty acids have been shown to be elevated in NASH patients [92] and induce inflammation and hepatocyte apoptosis by activating JNK and mitochondrial pathways. Other lipids having a role in NAFLD include ceramide, diacylglycerol (DAG) and sphingosine [90,93–96]. In particular, DAG and ceramide impair insulin capability to stimulate glycogen synthesis and suppress gluconeogenesis, through protein kinase-C epsilon (PKCε) activation [97]. In contrast, unsaturated fatty acids do not affect cell viability and an increase in their content leads to enhanced hepatic synthesis of TG. In turn, TG accumulation is not toxic but may protect the liver from the excessive deposition of toxic TG precursors [98,99]. Omega-3 polyunsaturated fatty acids (PUFAs) plasma levels are reduced in patients with NASH. However, pharmacologic supplementation did not induce an amelioration of the histologic picture of NASH [100], and in an experimental model it was even associated with more severe damage [101].

Emerging evidence underscores the role of cholesterol as a prominent risk factor for the pathogenesis of NAFLD/NASH. In humans a progressive increase in hepatic FC during NAFLD progression to NASH has been observed [102,103]. In experimental models increase in dietary cholesterol has been shown to promote hepatic inflammation and fibrosis [104–106], whereas a cholesterol-free diet ameliorates NASH [107]. The molecular mechanisms underlying FC accumulation during NASH development are multiple and only partially elucidated. Current data indicate that cholesterol homeostasis is dysregulated in NAFLD, due to an increase in cholesterol synthesis and uptake or dysfunction in cholesterol metabolism. Accordingly, the activity of two key regulators of cholesterol synthesis, HMGCR and SREBP2, is elevated in NASH patients [103,108,109]. Similarly, expression analysis of genes involved in cholesterol metabolism reveals a number of altered pathways in individuals with NASH [108].

Cholesterol uptake from lipoproteins is mediated by different proteins, including the low density lipoprotein receptor (LDLR) and the scavenger receptor class B type I (SR-BI) [110]. Hepatic uptake of LDL-cholesterol occurs via the scavenger receptor pathway in unrestrained manner, leading to deposition of cholesterol crystals in hepatocytes and generation of foamy Kupffer cells, two critical features of NASH [111,112]. Intracellular accumulation of free cholesterol represents a key event for inflammasome activation and inflammatory response [112] and sensitizes cells to transforming growth factor beta (TGF-β), TNF-α and Fas, leading to liver damage and disease progression [104,113]. Moreover, LDL cholesterol can be oxidized to oxidized low-density lipoprotein (oxLDL) cholesterol, which has been found in high concentrations in the plasma of NASH patients [114] and induces proinflammatory cytokine secretion accumulating in lysosomes of Kupffer cells [111,112]. Recently, a reduced efflux of FC has been observed in injured (foam) hepatocytes of NAFLD patients, associated with reduced expression of ATP-binding cassette sub-family G member 8 (ABCG8), which regulates cholesterol excretion trough the bile [108]. In addition, decreased expression of CYP7A1 and CYP27A responsible for cholesterol transformation into bile acids (BA) has been found in human NAFLD/NASH [108], as well as in a rat model of NASH induced by dietary cholesterol overload [115].

Oxysterols, the oxidative products of cholesterol generated during bile acid synthesis, have been described to induce liver damage through mitochondrial impairment. A study by Bellanti et al. [116] shows that mice fed high fat/high cholesterol (HF/HC) exhibit high levels of toxic oxysterols, such as triol, and oxidative stress and mitochondrial dysfunction associated with NASH. Accordingly, Huh7 and primary rat hepatocytes co-exposed to triol and palmitic or oleic acid, undergo apoptosis, mediated by impaired mitochondrial respiratory chain [116]. Finally, besides the effects on liver, cholesterol contributes to NASH pathogenesis also by stimulating inflammatory reactions in other tissues, such as adipose tissue and arterial wall, representing a key factor in the multiparallel scenario concurring to NASH [117,118].

## 5. Mitochondrial Dysfunction and Apoptosis

Oxidative stress has been recognized as a major factor in the pathogenesis of NASH. Based on the evidence that a high amount of intracellular ROS are generated in mitochondria and ROS overproduction is elicited in the presence of respiratory chain disruption, mitochondrial impairment has been suggested as a main event in NASH development [83,119,120]. Along these lines, structural and functional defects in mitochondria have been reported in patients with NASH [121,122].

Several mechanisms contribute to mitochondrial impairment and subsequent hepatic cell injury during NASH, mainly associated with lipotoxicity. It has been shown that, following lipid accumulation, water and calcium influx in mitochondria is increased, due to lower phosphorylation of the voltage dependent anion channel (VDAC) in the mitochondrial outer membrane, resulting in cytochrome c release and cell death [123]. Lipotoxic effects in mitochondria are also mediated by JNK; high concentrations of palmitate cause mitochondrial dysfunction and apoptosis through phosphorylation of Sab (SH3BP5), a mitochondrial outer membrane substrate of JNK [124], whereas free cholesterol accumulation in the liver of NASH mice induces mitochondrial permeability, ROS production and apoptosis through JNK1. An emerging role for $NAD^+$ in mitochondrial stress induction during NASH development has been recently shown. Gariani et al. demonstrated that mice fed high-fat/high-sucrose exhibit impaired mitochondrial function associated with lower hepatic $NAD^+$ levels [125]. Conversely, $NAD^+$ repletion displays a protective effect against NAFLD, probably mediated by the induction of mitochondrial unfolded protein response (UPRmt), an adaptive mechanism dependent on the histone deacetylases SIRT1 and SIRT3, aimed to enhance mitochondrial activity and hepatic β-oxidation [126]. Furthermore, recent studies have suggested a role for coenzyme Q (CoQ), which is essential for mitochondrial respiration, in NAFLD development and progression to NASH [127–130]. Abnormal concentrations of CoQ have been found in plasma and liver of NAFLD patients [131] and perturbation in CoQ metabolism was observed in experimental NAFLD during disease progression [132,133].

Other key inducers of mitochondrial dysfunction are lysosomal permeabilization, which is frequently observed in NAFLD patients and associated with caspase activation [134], and ROS generation. CYP2E1 promotes oxidative stress, inflammation and protein modifications, by hydrolyzing molecules such as fatty acids and ethanol into toxic metabolites, including ROS, which cause respiratory chain disruption and mitochondrial damage [135], resulting in hepatocyte injury and progression to NASH [136].

## 6. Necroptosis

Necroptosis is a recently described cell death mechanism, morphologically comparable to necrosis, but consisting in definite biochemical pathways that occur in a programmed mode [137] and are potentially involved in inflammatory disorders, including liver diseases. Necroptosis can be initiated by activation of multiple signals, such as toll-like receptors, death receptors and others, which lead to the assembly of the necrosome, a multiprotein complex consisting in caspase-8,

Fas-Associated protein with Death Domain (FADD), cellular FLICE/caspase 8-like inhibitory protein (cFLIP), and receptor-interacting proteins 1 and 3 (RIP1 and RIP3) [138]. RIP1–RIP3 interaction initiates necroptotic signaling [139]; RIP3 phosphorylates mixed lineage kinase domain-like protein (MLKL), which oligomerizes and translocates to the plasma membrane causing irreversible membrane damage and consequent cell death [140]. In specific cell setting, RIP3 can mediate necroptosis independently of RIP1 [141–143]. In other cell contexts, a RIP3 dependent ROS production may play an additional role [144,145].

Recently, necroptosis has been proposed as a novel mechanism in the pathogenesis of NAFLD both in humans and experimental models. Gautheron et al. found that RIP3 was overexpressed and mediated liver inflammation, activation of hepatic progenitor cells/cholangiocytes and liver fibrosis in NASH patients and in the methionine/choline-deficient (MCD) mouse model of steatohepatitis. They observed that RIP3 induces JNK activation, leading to release of pro-inflammatory mediators, such as CCL2, that further sustain RIP3-dependent signaling, cell death, and liver fibrosis. RIP3-induced pathways were blocked by caspase-8. [146]. A study by Afonso et al. [147] confirmed that hepatic levels of RIP3 are significantly augmented in steatohepatitis and showed that RIP3-dependent MLKL activation is increased in the liver of NAFLD patients as well as in MCD-induced experimental NASH. Moreover, lack of RIP3 ameliorates liver injury, steatosis, inflammation and fibrosis in experimental NASH.

## 7. Endoplasmic Reticulum Stress

ER stress has been implicated in a number of liver diseases, including NASH. ER dysfunction, ATP depletion or other stimuli induce the unfolded protein response (UPR), an adaptive mechanism directed to avoid luminal accumulation of defective proteins and apoptosis initiation. In NAFLD, a cross-talk between insulin signaling and UPR has been reported, involving XBP–1/PI3K interaction and consequent XBP-1 nuclear translocation [148]. Other pathways activated by cellular response to ER stress involve JNK, an activator of inflammation and apoptosis implicated in NAFLD progression to NASH [90] and SREBP-1c, which induces liver fat accumulation, worsening ER stress [149]. In vitro studies show that exposure of hepatic cells to a lipotoxic concentration of palmitate, a saturated fatty acid (SFA), is associated with ER calcium depletion, ROS accumulation and apoptosis [92,150,151]. In fact, increased SFA incorporation in ER membrane, as well as altered phosphatidylcholine/phosphatidylethanolamine ratio, induces disruption of ER membrane and impairment of sarcoendoplasmic reticulum calcium ATPase (SERCA) function, causing a net calcium efflux from ER stores and its subsequent translocation to the mitochondria, with dysregulation of mitochondrial metabolism and oxidative stress. Accordingly SERCA activity is impaired in obese livers [152] and overexpression of SERCA in obese mice improve hepatic ER stress, indicating that SERCA plays a crucial role in lipotoxic-induced ER stress and, indirectly, in mitochondrial dysfunction [152].

## 8. Hypoxia

In experimental NASH, hypoxia causes alterations in lipid homeostasis, upregulating genes involved in lipogenesis, such as SREBP-1c, PPARγ, ACC1 or 2 and downregulating genes implied in lipid metabolism, such as PPARα and carnitine palmitoyltransferase-1 (CPT-1) [153]. Besides lipid metabolism, insulin signaling is also affected and under hypoxic conditions hepatic upregulation of inflammatory cytokines and profibrogenic genes was observed [154]. Moreover, reduced oxygen availability induces secretion of adipokines and inflammatory cytokines in adipose tissue [155], contributing to alter lipid metabolism and glucose homeostasis [156,157]. These effects are mediated by hypoxia-inducible transcription factors (HIF-1α and HIF-2α) that regulate cellular response to oxygen deficiency and can be also activated by other stimuli, including oxidative stress or inflammatory signals [158]. In particular, HIF-1α transcription is induced by nuclear factor kappa-B (NF-κB), and NF-κB activity is crucial for HIF-1α accumulation under oxygen deprivation [159]. Furthermore, hypoxia has been reported to modulate inflammation by regulating TLR expression and function through HIF-1 [160,161]. Along these lines, it is conceivable that the proinflammatory state observed in obese NAFLD patients may be enhanced by hypoxia, due to a positive feedback mechanism involving HIF-1$\alpha$ and NF-$\kappa$B, explaining the exacerbation of liver injury in NAFLD subjects in the presence of obstructive sleep apnea-hypopnea syndrome (OSAHS) [162].

## 9. Inflammation

Inflammation represents a crucial aspect in NASH pathogenesis. Overload of toxic lipids, mainly FFA, causes cellular stress and induces specific signals that trigger hepatocyte apoptosis, the prevailing mechanism of cell death in NASH, correlating with the degree of liver inflammation and fibrosis [163]. Signaling pathways induced by key death receptors, such as TNF-related apoptosis-inducing ligand (TRAIL-R), Fas and tumor necrosis factor receptor (TNFR), are upregulated in NASH, indicating they may have a role in promoting inflammation and chemokine secretion. Although the precise role of Fas and TNFR in NASH in vivo is still controversial, it has been shown that lack of TRAIL-R is protective, as TRAIL-R-deficient mice display reduced steatosis, inflammation and fibrosis in association with lower hepatocyte apoptosis [164]. Moreover, prolonged ER stress and mitochondrial dysfunction, two critical events in NAFLD, have been reported to induce apoptosis through TRAIL-R/caspase 8 [165].

Different types of immune cells are recruited and/or activated to the site of injury, contributing to NAFLD development and progression. Kupffer Cell (KC) activation is critical in NASH and precedes the recruitment of other cells [166]. Lanthier et al. [167] have shown that KC depletion increases insulin sensitivity and ameliorates inflammation and fibrosis. Depending on the settings, different polarization forms have been described for KCs, mainly classified in two phenotypes: M1, pro-inflammatory and M2, considered primarily immunoregulatory [168]. However, markers of both M1 and M2 forms can be expressed at once [169]. Differentiation of KCs towards a M1 phenotype is principally driven by pathogen-associated molecular patterns (PAMPs) that, interacting with TLRs, induce the secretion of various cytokines, such as IL-1$\beta$, IL-12, TNF-$\alpha$, CCL2 and CCL5, concurring to further hepatocyte damage and release of damage-associated molecular patterns (DAMPs). DAMPs, in turn, act on TLRs amplifying KCs activation and inflammation. In addition, some cytokines (i.e., CCL2 and CCL5), induce HSC activation, initiating a fibrogenic response [170]. Activation of KCs in NAFLD is also triggered by toxic lipids, that upregulate TLRs and augment the response to lipopolysaccharide (LPS) [171]. KCs displaying the M2 phenotype produce several factors with anti-inflammatory properties, as IL-4, IL-10, IL-13 and TGF-$\alpha$ [168,169], but different subtypes have been identified with diverse actions. Although it has been reported that induction of peroxisome proliferator-activated receptor delta (PPAR$\delta$) drives KCs toward the M2 form, reducing obesity-induced insulin resistance in mice [172], the role of M2 KCs in NAFLD is still not elucidated [168].

Despite potent antimicrobial and phagocytic properties, neutrophils display scarce specificity. Excess of neutrophil recruitment in NASH crucially contributes to hepatocyte damage, inflammation and fibrosis, through the release of different factors [173,174], including cytotoxic enzymes as myeloperoxidase and elastase. Myeloperoxidase-deficient mice show moderated NASH, associated with lower hepatic secretion of inflammatory cytokines [175]. Similarly, deletion of neutrophil elastase attenuates liver inflammation in experimental NAFLD [176].

Dendritic Cells (DCs) counteract sterile inflammation acting as antigen-presenting cells and eliminating cell debris and apoptotic cells. Studies aimed to establish DCs' function in NASH have shown controversial results [177]. An anti-inflammatory and antifibrotic role of DCs in NASH is suggested by the fact that liver depletion of these cells exacerbates inflammation and fibrosis. According to the study by Henning et al liver infiltrating DCs activate and secrete IL-6, TNF-$\alpha$ and CCL2 [178]. In contrast, other findings report that avoiding the accumulation of DCs subtypes expressing high levels of inflammatory factors limits liver injury in experimental NASH [179].

Natural Killer (NK) cells in the liver are stimulated through several receptors upon interaction with other hepatic cells. In NASH, activation of NK can be achieved by a broad number of ligands and cytokines, but the role of these cells in NAFLD pathogenesis is still controversial [180,181]. Two different phenotypes of NKT cells have been recently associated with liver disease, acting in opposite modes during sterile inflammation: proinflammatory type I and protective type II cells [182]. Although NKT type I cells can be activated by lipids, suggesting their possible involvement in NAFLD, NKT-deficient mice fed HFD are more prone to steatosis and weight gain than wild type mice [183]. In addition, adoptive transfer of NKT cells in leptin-deficient mice ameliorates glucose metabolism and diminishes fatty liver [184]. Furthermore, depletion of NKT can result in activation of KC and secretion of IL-12 [184]. Conversely, clinical studies performed in patients with different stages of NAFLD demonstrate that NKT cells tend to increase in the liver during disease progression [185]. According to these data, NKT cells seem to be depleted in early NAFLD to enhance in the later phases, participating in inflammation and fibrosis [186].

## 10. Hedgehog

Hedgehog (Hh) is a well-characterized factor implied in the fibrogenic process of several organs, including the liver. Hh pathway activation is proportional to the severity and persistence of injury [187], induces a cascade of events concurring to wound healing response and involves various cell types, including damaged ballooned hepatocytes, inflammatory cells (mainly NKT cells and macrophages), ductular/progenitor cells and HSCs [188].

The Hh pathway was associated with severe NASH in a gene profiling study where patients with different severity of the disease were included [189]. In experimental NASH, the Hh pathway leads to proliferation and activation of ductular progenitor cells and HSC, that, in turn, produce Hh ligands and, consequently, soluble mediators such as osteopontin and CXCL-16, responsible for immune cells recruitment and damage progression [190,191]. Moreover, Patched-heterozygous deficient mice, characterized by hyperactivation of the Hh pathway, show exacerbation of the disease following a NASH-inducing diet, whereas liver-specific inhibition of Smo prevents diet-induced liver damage and fibrosis, despite hepatic lipid accumulation [190].

Caspase-2 has been recently identified as a critical factor in NASH pathogenesis, mediating hepatocyte lipoapoptosis. Hepatic caspase-2 was found to be increased both in human and experimental NASH, in association with profibrogenic factors, such as Hh-related genes. When challenged with a HF diet or fed a MCD diet, caspase-2 knockout mice showed lipid-induced hepatic apoptosis, together with decreased activation of Hh signaling and fibrosis [192].

In NAFLD patients, Hh activity and Hh ligands' expression correlates with the degree of fibrosis [193] and elevated Hh activation is associated with hepatocyte ballooning, high presence of progenitor cells and myofibroblasts and portal inflammation [187]. In agreement with these findings, the Pioglitazone vs. Vitamin E vs. Placebo for treatment of NASH (PIVENS) trial demonstrated that amelioration of NASH in response to treatment was associated with a marked decrease of Sonic Hh ligand (Shh) expressing hepatocytes [194].

## 11. Nuclear Receptors

Nuclear receptors are ligand-dependent transcription factors that regulate glucose and lipid metabolism in the liver. Nuclear receptors are divided into seven subfamilies named as NR0-NR6 [195] and NR1 subfamily is of particular importance in NAFLD. This latter group of nuclear receptors is retained in the nucleus and heterodimerizes with the retinoid X receptor (RXR$\alpha$) [195,196] and includes: NR1C1-3 (the peroxisome proliferator-activated receptors, PPAR$\alpha$, $\beta$, $\gamma$), NR1H2-3 (the liver X receptors, LXR$\alpha$, $\beta$), NR1H4 (the farnesoid X receptor, FXR$\alpha$), NR1I2 (the constitutive androstane receptor, CAR), and NR1I3 (the pregnane X receptor, PXR). PPARs inhibit inflammation in the obese state acting on NF-$\kappa$B and AP1 transcription factor and regulate metabolism by inducing transcription of adiponectin (PPAR$\gamma$) and fibroblast growth factor-21 (FGF21) (PPAR$\alpha$ and FXR) [195].

PPARα regulates β-oxidation and cholesterol removal during the fasting state or when metabolism increases in adipose and/or muscle tissues [195]. Hepatic PPARα expression decreases in NAFLD leading to steatosis, but is enhanced following diet and exercise [197,198].

In animal models of steatosis and steatohepatitis, the use of PPARα activators improves the disease [199,200]. In addition, several studies in mice suggest that induction of both PPARβ/δ and PPARγ ameliorates steatosis [201,202]. Indeed, animals treated with PPARα activators show less weight gain than controls, lower levels of epididymal fat, and are protected from atherosclerosis [203]. PPAR activation may also ameliorate fibrosis, since NASH patients treated with pioglitazone (a PPARγ agonist) had improved fibrosis biomarkers [204]. Recent studies show that PPARγ downregulates adipocyte endothelial nitric oxide synthase (eNOS), a molecule that contributes to IR and development of NASH [205]. Since the use of selective PPARα agonists has proven quite ineffective against NAFLD [197] the use of mixed receptor agonists (PPARα and PPARβ/γ) is underway in the therapy for NASH patients and recent results have been reported [206].

PXR, expressed in many tissues but mainly in the liver [207], is released not only by hepatocytes, but also by Kupffer and stellate cells [208]. Two polymorphisms of this gene have been associated with augmented severity of NAFLD: rs7643645/G and rs2461823 [209], whereas a variant encoding a short dominant negative PXR isoform, which inhibits the full-length isoform activity, has been recently described [210]. PXR regulates various genes involved in xenobiotic and drug metabolism, including enzymes [211] that play a role in the oxidative metabolism of lipophilic compounds such as steroids, fatty acids, bile acids, drugs, retinoids, and xenobiotics. PXR activation has been associated with increased severity of steatosis, obesity, insulin resistance and hypercholesterolemia as it enhances hepatic fatty acid uptake and lipogenesis, while it decreases β-oxidation [212,213]. The role of PXR in experimental NAFLD is more complex. While PXR knockout mice are resistant to obesity, they show impaired glucose tolerance, hyperleptinemia and hypoadiponectinemia, together with elevated fasting glucose levels [212]. Recently, it was shown that PXR activation inhibits the production of many NF-κB target genes and increases the production of secreted interleukin-1 receptor antagonist (IL-1RA), reducing the effects of LPS-induced inflammation [214].

Human CAR1-3, expressed mainly in liver and intestine and to a lower extent in other tissues [215], is implicated in protection against toxic food or contaminants [216]. CAR is also associated with lipid metabolism and inflammation in NAFLD. CAR increases in the liver in the fed state, reducing hepatic steatosis, inflammation, insulin resistance and hypercholesterolemia [217]. In animal models, treatment with an agonist of CAR ameliorates diet-induced obesity, hepatic steatosis and diabetes [218]. Moreover, in knockout mice for the low density lipoprotein receptor (LDLR), activation of CAR reduces triglycerides and cholesterol plasma levels [219]. Recently, it has been reported that activated CAR translocates into the nucleus and functions as an adaptor protein to recruit PGC1α to the Cullin1 E3 ligase complex for ubiquitination. The interaction between CAR and PGC1α also induces the degradation of PGC1α and suppression of gluconeogenesis both in vitro and in vivo [220]. CAR can induce carcinogenesis in mice, although this effect has not observed in humans [221]. Indeed, CAR activation in humans may have antiproliferative effects, as demonstrated by a recent report showing that CAR-deficient HepaRG cells have increased expression of proliferative genes [222].

FXR, highly expressed in liver, kidney, intestine, and adrenals, inhibits the expression of CYP7A1 and sterol 12-α-hydroxylase (CYP8B1), genes involved in bile acid synthesis from cholesterol. Besides its central role in bile acid metabolism, FXR activation also regulates the expression of various genes involved in glucose, lipid, and lipoprotein metabolism, crucial in NAFLD [223]. Hepatic FXR inhibits fatty acid synthesis and uptake and upregulates beta oxidation, regulating lipid homeostasis [224]. In NAFLD patients and in animal models, activation of FXR by obeticholic acid (OCA) decreases both steatosis and obesity [225,226]. In HF/HC diet-treated mice, the FXR agonist GW4064 decreased the expression of the hepatic lipid transporter CD36, reducing hepatic steatosis and weight gain [227]. FXR can regulate insulin resistance as recently demonstrated in

NASH patients treated with OCA, which improves insulin sensitivity [228]. Similarly, OCA treatment in Zucker (fa/fa) rats improves insulin sensitivity, and GW4064 treatment, in HF/HC diet mice, reduces hyperinsulinemia and hyperglycemia [226]. Besides OCA and GW4064, further potential novel therapeutic targets in NASH are currently in phase II clinical development [229].

Intestinal activation of FXR reduces weight gain, liver glucose production and steatosis, stimulating human fibroblast growth factor-19 (FGF19). This factor inhibits CYP7A1 resulting in an inhibition of liver bile acid synthesis. Indeed, administration of FGF19 in mice and rats animal models increases fat oxidation and decreases liver triglycerides and glucose levels [230,231]. Recent studies show that activation of intestinal FXR by feraxamine inhibits weight gain induced by diet, hepatic glucose production and steatosis. These effects are mediated by fibroblast growth factor-15 signaling, without interfering with hepatic FXR activation [232]. Intestinal FXR agonism promotes adipose tissue browning and reduces obesity and insulin resistance, suggesting that tissue-specific activation of FXR may be a novel approach to treat NAFLD. Activation of intestinal FXR affords hepatoprotection by restoring hepatic homeostasis, regulating cellular proliferation and decreasing hepatic fibrosis and inflammation [233].

## 12. Pattern Recognition Receptors and the Inflammasomes

Toll-like receptors are highly conserved receptors that recognize endogenous danger signals, such as molecules released by damaged cells (damage-associated molecular patterns, DAMPs) or exogenous danger signals, as gut-derived pathogen-associated molecules (pathogen-associated molecular patterns, PAMPs) [234,235]. Due to the high liver exposure to danger signals via the portal system, TLR-induced pathways play a central role in activation of hepatic cells, primarily Kupffer cells, but also hepatocytes and HSC. As pattern recognition receptors (PRR), TLRs act as defense mechanism, but are also implicated in the pathogenesis of NASH [236,237]. Among NAFLD-related TLRs, TLR2 interacts with a broad range of PAMPs, including peptidoglycan, a surface component of Gram-positive bacteria [238], which appears to be increased in NAFLD [239]. Importantly, inhibition of TLR2 signaling prevents insulin resistance in HFD mice [240], whereas TLR2-deficient mice fed HFD display reduced levels of inflammatory cytokines and do not develop NASH [241].

The role of TLR5 in NAFLD pathogenesis is still unclear, as only a correlation with dysbiosis and metabolic syndrome has been reported [242,243]. TLR9, an intracellular receptor, is activated by unmethylated DNA, typically express in viruses and bacteria but rare in mammalian cells. TLR9 downstream signaling involves IL-1, and is associated with NASH severity and fibrosis [244]. A study conducted in an experimental model of colitis, with high portal levels of LPS, shows increased TLR9 liver expression, associated with hepatic steatosis, inflammation, and fibrosis [245].

The crucial role of TLR4 in NAFLD pathogenesis has been demonstrated in TLR4-deficient mice, that display lower levels of inflammatory mediators and fail to develop NAFLD or insulin resistance [246]. TLR4 plays a major role in linking innate immunity with inflammatory response and the function of TLR4 in Kupffer cells is well characterized [247]. TLR4 is primarily activated by Gram-negative bacterial lipopolysaccharides (LPS), leading to overexpression of cytokines, chemokines and antimicrobial molecules [248,249]. LPS/TLR4 interaction, that requires LPS-binding protein and two co-receptors (CD14 and myeloid differentiation protein 2, MD2), activates downstream pathways in a myeloid differentiation factor (MyD)88-dependent or independent fashion [250]. The MyD88-dependent pathway signals through IκB kinase (IKK)/NF-κB and mitogen activated protein kinase (MAPK)/AP-1, inducing the expression of pro-inflammatory cytokines (TNF-α, IL-1β, IL-6 and IL-12) and genes implicated in the immune response [250]. The MyD88-independent cascade involves IFNs [250]. ROS production and subsequent activation of the unfolded protein response are also induced in TLR4-activated Kupffer cells, representing an additional mechanism triggered by TLRs in NAFLD progression [251].

Besides Kupffer cells, TLR4 is expressed by other hepatic cells, including HSCs, hepatocytes and cholangiocytes and LPS/TLR4 axis plays a critical role in the pathogenesis and progression of fatty liver diseases, as demonstrated by increased levels of portal endotoxins and TLR4 hepatic expression in experimental NASH [252,253]. Based on its expression in HSC, a direct role of TLR4 in liver fibrogenesis has been suggested. According to this hypothesis, the expression of chemokines and adhesion molecules, as well as TGF-β-mediated signaling, are positively modulated by TLR4 [254], while two TLR4 polymorphisms, protective against fibrosis, are associated with a lower apoptotic threshold for HSC [255].

TLR4-mediated inflammatory response can also be elicited by DAMPs released by necrotic cells, such as high mobility group box 1 (HMGB1) or phospholipids. These molecules stimulate monocyte and Kupffer cells to secrete inflammatory mediators (Figure 3). It is noteworthy that, in the presence of high glucose, TLR4 activation and downstream signaling can be triggered by FFA [256], clarifying, at least in part, the mechanism by which saturated fatty acids, frequently enhanced in plasma of obese patients, have toxic effects [257].

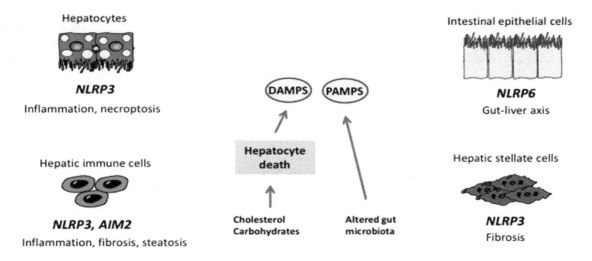

**Figure 3.** Inflammasomes and the liver. In steatosis, hepatic damage leads to generation of damage-associated molecular pattern (DAMPs), while alterations in microbiota lead to increased availability of pathogen-associated molecular patterns (PAMPs). DAMPs and PAMPs act on receptors localized on liver cells leading to activation of different inflammasomes and release of cytokines implicated in NASH. NLRP3: NOD-like receptor family, pyrin domain containing 3; AIM2: Abscent in melanoma 2.

An important role in NASH pathogenesis has been recently ascribed to the nucleotide oligomerization domain (NOD)-like receptors (NLRs). NLR activation in response to DAMPs or PAMPs leads to the assembly of inflammasome, a multiprotein complex required for caspase-1 activity and initiation of inflammatory signals. Full activation of inflammasome, mediated by PRRs via NF-κB, can be induced by a broad spectrum of signals, such as uric acid, ROS, ATP [258] and mitochondrial DNA [259], and results in secretion of mature IL-1 and IL-18 [260,261]. These cytokines, acting on different cell types, elicit inflammatory signals in liver as well as in the adipose tissue and intestine, triggering steatosis, insulin resistance, inflammation and cell death [262]. A role for inflammasomes in NAFLD development and progression to NASH has been shown both in humans and animal models [263,264]. Activation of NLRP3 inflammasome has been reported in MCD diet-induced steatohepatitis [265], as well following protracted HF/HC/HS feeding [266]. Moreover, NLRP3 gain of function correlates with liver fibrosis. Conversely, absence of this receptor appears to improve metabolic activity [267] and diet-induced steatohepatitis [268], although a study by Henao-Mejia et al. [269] demonstrated that lack of NLP3 promotes gut dysbiosis and chronic inflammation. Activation of NLRP3 inflammasome has been associated with hepatocyte pyroptosis, a recently described, inflammasome-mediated cell death mechanism [268,270].

Hepatocyte damage leads to secretion of intracellular molecules, DAMPs, acting as danger signals capable to recruit and/or activate immune cells and initiate an inflammatory response in the absence of pathogens, a mechanism referred as sterile inflammation [271,272]. Several DAMPs have been identified, including nuclear and mitochondrial DNA, purine nucleotides (ATP, UTP), nuclear factors as HMGB1 and uric acid [180,273]. Besides mitochondrial DNA, which activates TLR9, a number of mitochondrial components have been shown to play a part in sterile inflammation [274,275], including formyl-peptides, ATP and ROS, that act by inducing inflammasome activation [276–278]. High concentrations of extracellular ATP, as a consequence of cell death, result in inflammasome activation and IL-1β production, via P2X7 receptor [279]. As binding of ATP to P2X7 provokes pore formation in the plasma membrane, allowing bacterial products to enter the cells, ATP plays a role also in pathogen-associated molecular pattern-induced inflammation [280].

HMGB1 is a constitutively expressed nuclear protein that induces transcriptional activation [281], and is released in response to different stimuli, such as PAMPs and DAMPs [282,283]. HMGB1 interacts with a broad spectrum of receptors (TLR4, TLR2, TLR9, and RAGE) exerting proinflammatory actions in complex with other factors, as single stranded DNA, LPS and IL-1β [284].

In its crystal form, uric acid induce inflammatory response by inflammasome activation in a receptor-independent manner, causing phagosome burst and spill of cytosolic proteases [285]. In some settings, DAMPs can be also secreted independently of apoptosis. HMGB1 production can occur by activated macrophages in response to LPS, TNF, and TGFβ [286]. Moreover, secondary necrosis, due to impaired efferocytosis, may contribute to release of intracellular components amplifying the inflammatory response.

## 13. Adipokines

Adipose tissue is recognized as an endocrine organ that secretes adipokines, which are peptides with autocrine, paracrine and endocrine functions, controlling systemic metabolism and energy homeostasis [287]. Among these, leptin and adiponectin are involved in the pathogenesis of NAFLD and progression to NASH, leptin being identified as a profibrogenic adipokine [285,288]. Adipose tissue also produces other molecules (including classical cytokines), mostly released by endothelial or immune cells, such as TNF-α and IL-6 [289]. Adiponectin has in general a beneficial impact on NAFLD [290], while others, as resistin, TNF-α and IL-6 possibly have an adverse impact. In particular, adiponectin reduces IR and shows anti-steatotic and anti-inflammatory properties, while TNF-α increases IR and displays pro-inflammatory effects [291,292]. In physiologic conditions, cytokine-adipokine interplay is finely regulated, but in some setting, such as increased adipose tissue mass, the critical balance between cytokines and adipokines is compromised, leading to chronic inflammation, IR and NAFLD [292]. Leptin, an adipokine which plays a major role in energy homeostasis, is mainly produced by adipose tissue, but it is also synthesized in other organs [293]. Consequent to an increase in adipose tissue mass, leptin is upregulated, acting as compensatory factor in preserving insulin sensitivity and exerting anti-steatotic effects. Nevertheless, if adipose tissue continues to augment, the compensatory mechanism fails, with a sustained rise in IR and hepatic steatosis [294]. Leptin-mediated dual action has been demonstrated in experimental NAFLD, as in early disease leptin exerts a protective effect by inhibiting hepatic glucose production and de novo lipogenesis through stimulation of fatty acid oxidation, while as NAFLD proceeds, it acts as a pro-fibrogenic and inflammatory factor [294]. Novel evidence indicates that leptin-mediated nicotinamide adenine dinucleotide phosphate (NADPH) oxidase increases the levels of miR21, which is a key regulator of TGF-β signaling. The rise in miR21 increases TGF-β and SMAD2/3-SMAD4 nuclear colocalizations, whilst repressing SMAD7 [295]. In addition, leptin reduces PPAR-γ expression in HSCs, promoting hepatic fibrosis [296]. A recent study, conducted by Heinrich et al., shows that leptin resistance contributes to obesity in null mice mutated for carcinoembryonic antigen cell adhesion molecule 1 (CEACAM1) [297]. CEACAM1 is a molecule that induces insulin clearance [298] and reduces fatty acid synthesis in liver in the presence of insulin resistance, hepatic steatosis and visceral obesity [299]. Furthermore, $(Cc1^{-/-})$ mice develop hyperleptinemia, firstly related to the augmented visceral obesity, followed by hyperphagia and reduced physical activity. These effects are possibly due to leptin resistance and elevated hypothalamic fatty acid synthase activity, that could, in turn, be mediated by both central and peripheral factors [297].

Adiponectin is one of the most abundant adipokines, and is also produced by hepatocytes in response to liver injury [300]. It exhibits anti-steatotic and antiapoptotic actions on hepatocytes and exerts anti-inflammatory and anti-fibrotic effects acting on HSC, Kupffer and sinusoidal cells [301]. Adiponectin amounts drop when adipose mass increases, but the underlying mechanism is not completely elucidated. It may involve adipose tissue hypoxia, oxidative stress [155,302] and increased inflammatory mediator levels [303]. Another potential factor linking adipocyte hypertrophy to reduced adiponectin synthesis is mitochondrial dysfunction [304]. Recent reports show that 11β-hydroxysteroid dehydrogenase type1 (11β-HSD1) expression increases in hypertrophic adipocytes and this could be responsible for mitochondrial dysfunction and reduced adiponectin synthesis.

After NASH progression towards cirrhosis, circulating adiponectin seems to increase [305], probably due to two main mechanisms: a decrease in hepatic clearance of adiponectin and/or a compensatory mechanism aimed to buffer the hyper-secretion of inflammatory cytokines. Recent studies show that in the compensated late stage of NASH, circulating adiponectin is associated with hepatic lipid loss [306]. These data reinforce the theory that adiponectin may be involved in the "burnt-out NASH", characterized by the loss of hepatic lipids, often observed in advanced fibrosis and cirrhosis.

Adipose tissue (mainly visceral) and liver (mainly hepatocytes) are the principal producers of chemerin [307]. Chemerin concentrations, which are generally higher in obesity and IR and drop after weight loss, may modulate insulin resistance and inflammatory responses [308]. Animal models of obesity and IR (*ob/ob* and *db/db* mice) display increased chemerin expression [309,310]. A recent study conducted in NAFLD subjects show that circulating levels of chemerin positively correlate with body mass index (BMI) and are also higher in individuals with impaired glucose tolerance (IGT) or type 2 diabetes. In MCD-induced NASH, hepatic levels of chemerin tend to increase. In human NASH, liver chemerin mRNA is upregulated in respect to healthy controls, but similar levels have been found also in steatosis [311].

## 14. Microbiota

Accumulating evidence indicates that dysregulation of microbiota components are involved in various liver diseases, including NAFLD and NASH, through obesity predisposition, metabolic alterations and liver inflammation. Gut microbiota produces extra energy for the host, processing polysaccharides to short-chain fatty acids (mainly acetate, propionate, and butyrate) [312] and stimulating lipogenesis. A potential role of specific gut microbiome has been suggested in the pathogenesis of NAFLD, as obese mouse models host 50% less *Bacteroides* and more *Firmicutes* compared to lean control [313], and germ-free mice show significantly greater increase in body fat following colonization with an "obese microbiome" [313]. Conversely, a recently described bacterium, *Akkermansia muciniphila*, has been associated with a non-obese phenotype both in humans and animal models, and HFD mice administered with *Akkermansia* show reduced adipose tissue inflammation and increased glucose tolerance [314,315]. The intestinal microflora produces enzymes that metabolize dietary choline, a cell membrane component regulating lipid transport in liver, into methylamines, toxic compounds responsible for inflammation and liver injury [316]. Aberrant microbiota could induce triglyceride accumulation and promote NASH both reducing choline and increasing methylamines [317].

Alterations in bile acid metabolism have been reported during NAFLD development. Intestinal bacteria can modify bile acid pool through the conversion of cholic and chenodeoxycholic acid into secondary bile acids, influencing lipid and glucose homeostasis. In addition, abnormal microbiota can impair bile acid receptor signaling, such as FXR and the G-protein-coupled bile acid-activated receptor TGR5 [318,319], affecting hepatic de novo lipogenesis and very low-density lipoprotein VLDL export [320] as well as glucose metabolism [321,322].

Endogenous ethanol is produced by several microbiome species. Ethanol induces hepatotoxicity stimulating Kupffer cells to produce nitric acid and cytokines, whereas ethanol metabolites promote triglyceride accumulation and oxidative stress in the liver. In addition, ethanol impairs gut mucosal permeability inducing endotoxemia. Enhanced breath ethanol content was found in *ob/ob* mice and it was abolished by antibiotic treatment [323]. Increased ethanol levels were also detected in obese individuals and in children with NASH [324].

The gut microflora plays an important role in the development and function of the host immune system [325]. Through the portal circulation, liver is directly exposed to gut-derived products, being the first line of defense against bacterial toxins. Enhanced levels of circulating LPS and endotoxins have been detected in rodents with diet-induced NAFLD and in NASH patients, respectively. LPS, the active component of endotoxins, interacts with LPS-binding protein and the CD14 receptor, activating TLRs and, consequently, the inflammatory cascade that involves stress-activated protein kinases, JNK, p38, interferon regulatory factor-3 (IRF-3) and NF-κB, pathways implicated in insulin resistance and triglycerides synthesis [252,325].

Finally, a correlation between small intestinal bacterial overgrowth (SIBO) and NAFLD has been observed in clinical and experimental studies [237,326,327]. Bacterial overgrowth in the small intestine, as well as qualitative microbiome abnormalities can impair the barrier functions of the intestinal mucosa, leading to enhanced mucosa permeability and subsequent translocation of endotoxin to the bloodstream [328,329]. Therefore, increased gut permeability represents an additional mechanism in NASH pathogenesis, acting through the accumulation of endotoxin and bacterial metabolites in liver and subsequent induction of inflammatory responses, via activation of pattern recognition receptors.

## 15. Perspectives

Extensive information has accumulated in the past few years on the molecular mechanisms underlying the development of steatohepatitis. This has been paralleled by a number of clinical trials exploring novel approaches, in part derived from preclinical data. Continuing research in this field will be instrumental in providing new targets and biomarkers for the management of this very prevalent condition.

**Acknowledgments:** Work on steatohepatitis in Marra's laboratory is supported by grants from the Italian Ministry for Research (Projects PRIN and FIRB), the European Community (projects FLIP and EPoS), and the CARIPLO Foundation.

**Author Contributions:** Alessandra Caligiuri and Alessandra Gentilini searched the literature, contributed to manuscript organization and wrote the text. Fabio Marra defined manuscript organization and reviewed the final version of the manuscript.

## References

1.    Satapathy, S.K.; Sanyal, A.J. Epidemiology and natural history of nonalcoholic fatty liver disease. *Semin. Liver Dis.* **2015**, *35*, 221–235. [CrossRef] [PubMed]

2.    Vernon, G.; Baranova, A.; Younossi, Z.M. Systematic review: The epidemiology and natural history of non-alcoholic fatty liver disease and non-alcoholic steatohepatitis in adults. *Aliment. Pharmacol. Ther.* **2011**, *34*, 274–285. [CrossRef] [PubMed]

3.    Williams, C.D.; Stengel, J.; Asike, M.I.; Torres, D.M.; Shaw, J.; Contreras, M.; Landt, C.L.; Harrison, S.A. Prevalence of nonalcoholic fatty liver disease and nonalcoholic steatohepatitis among a largely middle-aged population utilizing ultrasound and liver biopsy: A prospective study. *Gastroenterology* **2011**, *140*, 124–131. [CrossRef] [PubMed]

4.    Browning, J.D.; Horton, J.D. Molecular mediators of hepatic steatosis and liver injury. *J. Clin. Investig.* **2004**, *114*, 147–152. [CrossRef] [PubMed]

5.  Brunt, E.M.; Kleiner, D.E.; Wilson, L.A.; Belt, P.; Neuschwander-Tetri, B.A.; Network, N.C.R. Nonalcoholic fatty liver disease (NAFLD) activity score and the histopathologic diagnosis in NAFLD: Distinct clinicopathologic meanings. *Hepatology* **2011**, *53*, 810–820. [CrossRef] [PubMed]

6.  Pais, R.; Charlotte, F.; Fedchuk, L.; Bedossa, P.; Lebray, P.; Poynard, T.; Ratziu, V. A systematic review of follow-up biopsies reveals disease progression in patients with non-alcoholic fatty liver. *J. Hepatol.* **2013**, *59*, 550–556. [CrossRef] [PubMed]

7.  McPherson, S.; Hardy, T.; Henderson, E.; Burt, A.D.; Day, C.P.; Anstee, Q.M. Evidence of NAFLD progression from steatosis to fibrosing-steatohepatitis using paired biopsies: Implications for prognosis and clinical management. *J. Hepatol.* **2015**, *62*, 1148–1155. [CrossRef] [PubMed]

8.  Angulo, P. Long-term mortality in nonalcoholic fatty liver disease: Is liver histology of any prognostic significance? *Hepatology* **2010**, *51*, 373–375. [CrossRef] [PubMed]

9.  Ekstedt, M.; Franzen, L.E.; Mathiesen, U.L.; Thorelius, L.; Holmqvist, M.; Bodemar, G.; Kechagias, S. Long-term follow-up of patients with NAFLD and elevated liver enzymes. *Hepatology* **2006**, *44*, 865–873. [CrossRef] [PubMed]

10.  Adams, L.A.; Lymp, J.F.; St Sauver, J.; Sanderson, S.O.; Lindor, K.D.; Feldstein, A.; Angulo, P. The natural history of nonalcoholic fatty liver disease: A population-based cohort study. *Gastroenterology* **2005**, *129*, 113–121. [CrossRef] [PubMed]

11.  Ludwig, J.; Viggiano, T.R.; McGill, D.B.; Oh, B.J. Nonalcoholic steatohepatitis: Mayo clinic experiences with a hitherto unnamed disease. *Mayo Clin. Proc.* **1980**, *55*, 434–438. [PubMed]

12.  Day, C.P.; James, O.F. Steatohepatitis: A tale of two "hits"? *Gastroenterology* **1998**, *114*, 842–845. [CrossRef]

13.  Cusi, K. Role of obesity and lipotoxicity in the development of nonalcoholic steatohepatitis: Pathophysiology and clinical implications. *Gastroenterology* **2012**, *142*, 711–725. [CrossRef] [PubMed]

14.  Neuschwander-Tetri, B.A. Hepatic lipotoxicity and the pathogenesis of nonalcoholic steatohepatitis: The central role of nontriglyceride fatty acid metabolites. *Hepatology* **2010**, *52*, 774–788. [CrossRef] [PubMed]

15.  Tilg, H.; Moschen, A.R. Evolution of inflammation in nonalcoholic fatty liver disease: The multiple parallel hits hypothesis. *Hepatology* **2010**, *52*, 1836–1846. [CrossRef] [PubMed]

16.  Marra, F.; Lotersztajn, S. Pathophysiology of NASH: Perspectives for a targeted treatment. *Curr. Pharm. Des.* **2013**, *19*, 5250–5269. [CrossRef] [PubMed]

17.  Loomba, R.; Schork, N.; Chen, C.H.; Bettencourt, R.; Bhatt, A.; Ang, B.; Nguyen, P.; Hernandez, C.; Richards, L.; Salotti, J.; et al. Heritability of hepatic fibrosis and steatosis based on a prospective twin study. *Gastroenterology* **2015**, *149*, 1784–1793. [CrossRef] [PubMed]

18.  Anstee, Q.M.; Seth, D.; Day, C.P. Genetic factors that affect risk of alcoholic and nonalcoholic fatty liver disease. *Gastroenterology* **2016**, *150*, 1728–1744. [CrossRef] [PubMed]

19.  Dongiovanni, P.; Donati, B.; Fares, R.; Lombardi, R.; Mancina, R.M.; Romeo, S.; Valenti, L. PNPLA3 I148M polymorphism and progressive liver disease. *World J. Gastroenterol.* **2013**, *19*, 6969–6978. [CrossRef] [PubMed]

20.  Romeo, S.; Kozlitina, J.; Xing, C.; Pertsemlidis, A.; Cox, D.; Pennacchio, L.A.; Boerwinkle, E.; Cohen, J.C.; Hobbs, H.H. Genetic variation in PNPLA3 confers susceptibility to nonalcoholic fatty liver disease. *Nat. Genet.* **2008**, *40*, 1461–1465. [CrossRef] [PubMed]

21.  Speliotes, E.K.; Butler, J.L.; Palmer, C.D.; Voight, B.F.; Consortium, G.; Consortium, M.I.; Nash, C.R.N.; Hirschhorn, J.N. PNPLA3 variants specifically confer increased risk for histologic nonalcoholic fatty liver disease but not metabolic disease. *Hepatology* **2010**, *52*, 904–912. [CrossRef] [PubMed]

22.  Pirazzi, C.; Adiels, M.; Burza, M.A.; Mancina, R.M.; Levin, M.; Stahlman, M.; Taskinen, M.R.; Orho-Melander, M.; Perman, J.; Pujia, A.; et al. Patatin-like phospholipase domain-containing 3 (PNPLA3) I148M (RS738409) affects hepatic VLDL secretion in humans and in vitro. *J. Hepatol.* **2012**, *57*, 1276–1282. [CrossRef] [PubMed]

23.  Kumari, M.; Schoiswohl, G.; Chitraju, C.; Paar, M.; Cornaciu, I.; Rangrez, A.Y.; Wongsiriroj, N.; Nagy, H.M.; Ivanova, P.T.; Scott, S.A.; et al. Adiponutrin functions as a nutritionally regulated lysophosphatidic acid acyltransferase. *Cell Metab.* **2012**, *15*, 691–702. [CrossRef] [PubMed]

24.  Chen, W.; Chang, B.; Li, L.; Chan, L. Patatin-like phospholipase domain-containing 3/adiponutrin deficiency in mice is not associated with fatty liver disease. *Hepatology* **2010**, *52*, 1134–1142. [CrossRef] [PubMed]

25.  Smagris, E.; BasuRay, S.; Li, J.; Huang, Y.; Lai, K.M.; Gromada, J.; Cohen, J.C.; Hobbs, H.H. PNPLA3 I148M knockin mice accumulate PNPLA3 on lipid droplets and develop hepatic steatosis. *Hepatology* **2015**, *61*, 108–118. [CrossRef] [PubMed]

26. Mondul, A.; Mancina, R.M.; Merlo, A.; Dongiovanni, P.; Rametta, R.; Montalcini, T.; Valenti, L.; Albanes, D.; Romeo, S. PNPLA3 I148M variant influences circulating retinol in adults with nonalcoholic fatty liver disease or obesity. *J. Nutr.* **2015**, *145*, 1687–1691. [CrossRef] [PubMed]

27. Kovarova, M.; Konigsrainer, I.; Konigsrainer, A.; Machicao, F.; Haring, H.U.; Schleicher, E.; Peter, A. The genetic variant I148M in *PNPLA3* is associated with increased hepatic retinyl-palmitate storage in humans. *J. Clin. Endocrinol. Metab.* **2015**, *100*, E1568–E1574. [CrossRef] [PubMed]

28. Pirazzi, C.; Valenti, L.; Motta, B.M.; Pingitore, P.; Hedfalk, K.; Mancina, R.M.; Burza, M.A.; Indiveri, C.; Ferro, Y.; Montalcini, T.; et al. PNPLA3 has retinyl-palmitate lipase activity in human hepatic stellate cells. *Hum. Mol. Genet.* **2014**, *23*, 4077–4085. [CrossRef] [PubMed]

29. Kozlitina, J.; Smagris, E.; Stender, S.; Nordestgaard, B.G.; Zhou, H.H.; Tybjaerg-Hansen, A.; Vogt, T.F.; Hobbs, H.H.; Cohen, J.C. Exome-wide association study identifies a *TM6SF2* variant that confers susceptibility to nonalcoholic fatty liver disease. *Nat. Genet.* **2014**, *46*, 352–356. [CrossRef] [PubMed]

30. Liu, Y.L.; Reeves, H.L.; Burt, A.D.; Tiniakos, D.; McPherson, S.; Leathart, J.B.; Allison, M.E.; Alexander, G.J.; Piguet, A.C.; Anty, R.; et al. TM6SF2 RS58542926 influences hepatic fibrosis progression in patients with non-alcoholic fatty liver disease. *Nat. Commun.* **2014**, *5*. [CrossRef] [PubMed]

31. Mahdessian, H.; Taxiarchis, A.; Popov, S.; Silveira, A.; Franco-Cereceda, A.; Hamsten, A.; Eriksson, P.; van't Hooft, F. TM6SF2 is a regulator of liver fat metabolism influencing triglyceride secretion and hepatic lipid droplet content. *Proc. Natl. Acad. Sci. USA* **2014**, *111*, 8913–8918. [CrossRef] [PubMed]

32. Dongiovanni, P.; Valenti, L.; Rametta, R.; Daly, A.K.; Nobili, V.; Mozzi, E.; Leathart, J.B.; Pietrobattista, A.; Burt, A.D.; Maggioni, M.; et al. Genetic variants regulating insulin receptor signalling are associated with the severity of liver damage in patients with non-alcoholic fatty liver disease. *Gut* **2010**, *59*, 267–273. [CrossRef] [PubMed]

33. Beer, N.L.; Tribble, N.D.; McCulloch, L.J.; Roos, C.; Johnson, P.R.; Orho-Melander, M.; Gloyn, A.L. The P446L variant in *GCKR* associated with fasting plasma glucose and triglyceride levels exerts its effect through increased glucokinase activity in liver. *Hum. Mol. Genet.* **2009**, *18*, 4081–4088. [CrossRef] [PubMed]

34. Santoro, N.; Zhang, C.K.; Zhao, H.; Pakstis, A.J.; Kim, G.; Kursawe, R.; Dykas, D.J.; Bale, A.E.; Giannini, C.; Pierpont, B.; et al. Variant in the glucokinase regulatory protein (GCKR) gene is associated with fatty liver in obese children and adolescents. *Hepatology* **2012**, *55*, 781–789. [CrossRef] [PubMed]

35. Tonjes, A.; Scholz, M.; Loeffler, M.; Stumvoll, M. Association of Pro12Ala polymorphism in peroxisome proliferator-activated receptor $\gamma$ with pre-diabetic phenotypes: Meta-analysis of 57 studies on nondiabetic individuals. *Diabetes Care* **2006**, *29*, 2489–2497. [CrossRef] [PubMed]

36. Nelson, J.E.; Bhattacharya, R.; Lindor, K.D.; Chalasani, N.; Raaka, S.; Heathcote, E.J.; Miskovsky, E.; Shaffer, E.; Rulyak, S.J.; Kowdley, K.V. HFE C282Y mutations are associated with advanced hepatic fibrosis in caucasians with nonalcoholic steatohepatitis. *Hepatology* **2007**, *46*, 723–729. [CrossRef] [PubMed]

37. Bugianesi, E.; Manzini, P.; D'Antico, S.; Vanni, E.; Longo, F.; Leone, N.; Massarenti, P.; Piga, A.; Marchesini, G.; Rizzetto, M. Relative contribution of iron burden, HFE mutations, and insulin resistance to fibrosis in nonalcoholic fatty liver. *Hepatology* **2004**, *39*, 179–187. [CrossRef] [PubMed]

38. Valenti, L.; Fracanzani, A.L.; Bugianesi, E.; Dongiovanni, P.; Galmozzi, E.; Vanni, E.; Canavesi, E.; Lattuada, E.; Roviaro, G.; Marchesini, G.; et al. HFE genotype, parenchymal iron accumulation, and liver fibrosis in patients with nonalcoholic fatty liver disease. *Gastroenterology* **2010**, *138*, 905–912. [CrossRef] [PubMed]

39. Raszeja-Wyszomirska, J.; Kurzawski, G.; Lawniczak, M.; Miezynska-Kurtycz, J.; Lubinski, J. Nonalcoholic fatty liver disease and *HFE* gene mutations: A polish study. *World J. Gastroenterol.* **2010**, *16*, 2531–2536. [CrossRef] [PubMed]

40. Al-Serri, A.; Anstee, Q.M.; Valenti, L.; Nobili, V.; Leathart, J.B.; Dongiovanni, P.; Patch, J.; Fracanzani, A.; Fargion, S.; Day, C.P.; et al. The *SOD2* C47T polymorphism influences NAFLD fibrosis severity: Evidence from case-control and intra-familial allele association studies. *J. Hepatol.* **2012**, *56*, 448–454. [CrossRef] [PubMed]

41. Mancina, R.M.; Dongiovanni, P.; Petta, S.; Pingitore, P.; Meroni, M.; Rametta, R.; Boren, J.; Montalcini, T.; Pujia, A.; Wiklund, O.; et al. The *MBOAT7-TMC4* variant rs641738 increases risk of nonalcoholic fatty liver disease in individuals of European descent. *Gastroenterology* **2016**, *150*, 1219–1230. [CrossRef] [PubMed]

42. Sun, C.; Fan, J.G.; Qiao, L. Potential epigenetic mechanism in non-alcoholic fatty liver disease. *Int. J. Mol. Sci.* **2015**, *16*, 5161–5179. [CrossRef] [PubMed]

43.  Wang, L.J.; Zhang, H.W.; Zhou, J.Y.; Liu, Y.; Yang, Y.; Chen, X.L.; Zhu, C.H.; Zheng, R.D.; Ling, W.H.; Zhu, H.L. Betaine attenuates hepatic steatosis by reducing methylation of the *MTTP* promoter and elevating genomic methylation in mice fed a high-fat diet. *J. Nutr. Biochem.* **2014**, *25*, 329–336. [CrossRef] [PubMed]

44.  Iacobazzi, V.; Castegna, A.; Infantino, V.; Andria, G. Mitochondrial DNA methylation as a next-generation biomarker and diagnostic tool. *Mol. Genet. Metab.* **2013**, *110*, 25–34. [CrossRef] [PubMed]

45.  Tryndyak, V.P.; Han, T.; Muskhelishvili, L.; Fuscoe, J.C.; Ross, S.A.; Beland, F.A.; Pogribny, I.P. Coupling global methylation and gene expression profiles reveal key pathophysiological events in liver injury induced by a methyl-deficient diet. *Mol. Nutr. Food Res.* **2011**, *55*, 411–418. [CrossRef] [PubMed]

46.  Kalhan, S.C.; Edmison, J.; Marczewski, S.; Dasarathy, S.; Gruca, L.L.; Bennett, C.; Duenas, C.; Lopez, R. Methionine and protein metabolism in non-alcoholic steatohepatitis: Evidence for lower rate of transmethylation of methionine. *Clin. Sci.* **2011**, *121*, 179–189. [CrossRef] [PubMed]

47.  Zivkovic, A.M.; Bruce German, J.; Esfandiari, F.; Halsted, C.H. Quantitative lipid metabolomic changes in alcoholic micropigs with fatty liver disease. *Alcohol. Clin. Exp. Res.* **2009**, *33*, 751–758. [CrossRef] [PubMed]

48.  Cordero, P.; Campion, J.; Milagro, F.I.; Martinez, J.A. Transcriptomic and epigenetic changes in early liver steatosis associated to obesity: Effect of dietary methyl donor supplementation. *Mol. Genet. Metab.* **2013**, *110*, 388–395. [CrossRef] [PubMed]

49.  Sookoian, S.; Rosselli, M.S.; Gemma, C.; Burgueno, A.L.; Fernandez Gianotti, T.; Castano, G.O.; Pirola, C.J. Epigenetic regulation of insulin resistance in nonalcoholic fatty liver disease: Impact of liver methylation of the peroxisome proliferator-activated receptor γ coactivator 1α promoter. *Hepatology* **2010**, *52*, 1992–2000. [CrossRef] [PubMed]

50.  Wolff, G.L.; Kodell, R.L.; Moore, S.R.; Cooney, C.A. Maternal epigenetics and methyl supplements affect *agouti* gene expression in A$^{vy}$/a mice. *FASEB J.* **1998**, *12*, 949–957. [PubMed]

51.  Pruis, M.G.; Lendvai, A.; Bloks, V.W.; Zwier, M.V.; Baller, J.F.; de Bruin, A.; Groen, A.K.; Plosch, T. Maternal western diet primes non-alcoholic fatty liver disease in adult mouse offspring. *Acta Physiol.* **2014**, *210*, 215–227. [CrossRef] [PubMed]

52.  Chen, G.; Broseus, J.; Hergalant, S.; Donnart, A.; Chevalier, C.; Bolanos-Jimenez, F.; Gueant, J.L.; Houlgatte, R. Identification of master genes involved in liver key functions through transcriptomics and epigenomics of methyl donor deficiency in rat: Relevance to nonalcoholic liver disease. *Mol. Nutr. Food Res.* **2015**, *59*, 293–302. [CrossRef] [PubMed]

53.  Carabelli, J.; Burgueno, A.L.; Rosselli, M.S.; Gianotti, T.F.; Lago, N.R.; Pirola, C.J.; Sookoian, S. High fat diet-induced liver steatosis promotes an increase in liver mitochondrial biogenesis in response to hypoxia. *J. Cell. Mol. Med.* **2011**, *15*, 1329–1338. [CrossRef] [PubMed]

54.  Pirola, C.J.; Gianotti, T.F.; Burgueno, A.L.; Rey-Funes, M.; Loidl, C.F.; Mallardi, P.; Martino, J.S.; Castano, G.O.; Sookoian, S. Epigenetic modification of liver mitochondrial DNA is associated with histological severity of nonalcoholic fatty liver disease. *Gut* **2013**, *62*, 1356–1363. [CrossRef] [PubMed]

55.  Aagaard-Tillery, K.M.; Grove, K.; Bishop, J.; Ke, X.; Fu, Q.; McKnight, R.; Lane, R.H. Developmental origins of disease and determinants of chromatin structure: Maternal diet modifies the primate fetal epigenome. *J. Mol. Endocrinol.* **2008**, *41*, 91–102. [CrossRef] [PubMed]

56.  Bricambert, J.; Miranda, J.; Benhamed, F.; Girard, J.; Postic, C.; Dentin, R. Salt-inducible kinase 2 links transcriptional coactivator p300 phosphorylation to the prevention of ChREBP-dependent hepatic steatosis in mice. *J. Clin. Investig.* **2010**, *120*, 4316–4331. [CrossRef] [PubMed]

57.  Jun, H.J.; Kim, J.; Hoang, M.H.; Lee, S.J. Hepatic lipid accumulation alters global histone H3 Lysine 9 and 4 trimethylation in the peroxisome proliferator-activated receptor α network. *PLoS ONE* **2012**, *7*, e44345. [CrossRef]

58.  Li, J.; Huang, J.; Li, J.S.; Chen, H.; Huang, K.; Zheng, L. Accumulation of endoplasmic reticulum stress and lipogenesis in the liver through generational effects of high fat diets. *J. Hepatol.* **2012**, *56*, 900–907. [CrossRef] [PubMed]

59.  Colak, Y.; Yesil, A.; Mutlu, H.H.; Caklili, O.T.; Ulasoglu, C.; Senates, E.; Takir, M.; Kostek, O.; Yilmaz, Y.; Yilmaz Enc, F.; et al. A potential treatment of non-alcoholic fatty liver disease with SIRT1 activators. *J. Gastrointest. Liver Dis.* **2014**, *23*, 311–319.

60.  Colak, Y.; Ozturk, O.; Senates, E.; Tuncer, I.; Yorulmaz, E.; Adali, G.; Doganay, L.; Enc, F.Y. SIRT1 as a potential therapeutic target for treatment of nonalcoholic fatty liver disease. *Med. Sci. Monit.* **2011**, *17*, HY5–HY9. [CrossRef] [PubMed]

61. Suter, M.A.; Chen, A.; Burdine, M.S.; Choudhury, M.; Harris, R.A.; Lane, R.H.; Friedman, J.E.; Grove, K.L.; Tackett, A.J.; Aagaard, K.M. A maternal high-fat diet modulates fetal SIRT1 histone and protein deacetylase activity in nonhuman primates. *FASEB J.* **2012**, *26*, 5106–5114. [CrossRef] [PubMed]

62. Hirschey, M.D.; Shimazu, T.; Jing, E.; Grueter, C.A.; Collins, A.M.; Aouizerat, B.; Stancakova, A.; Goetzman, E.; Lam, M.M.; Schwer, B.; et al. SIRT3 deficiency and mitochondrial protein hyperacetylation accelerate the development of the metabolic syndrome. *Mol. Cell* **2011**, *44*, 177–190. [CrossRef] [PubMed]

63. Rottiers, V.; Naar, A.M. MicroRNAs in metabolism and metabolic disorders. *Nat. Rev. Mol. Cell Biol.* **2012**, *13*, 239–250. [CrossRef] [PubMed]

64. Williams, M.D.; Mitchell, G.M. MicroRNAs in insulin resistance and obesity. *Exp. Diabetes Res.* **2012**, *2012*. [CrossRef] [PubMed]

65. Ferreira, D.M.; Simao, A.L.; Rodrigues, C.M.; Castro, R.E. Revisiting the metabolic syndrome and paving the way for microRNAs in non-alcoholic fatty liver disease. *FEBS J.* **2014**, *281*, 2503–2524. [CrossRef] [PubMed]

66. Cheung, O.; Puri, P.; Eicken, C.; Contos, M.J.; Mirshahi, F.; Maher, J.W.; Kellum, J.M.; Min, H.; Luketic, V.A.; Sanyal, A.J. Nonalcoholic steatohepatitis is associated with altered hepatic MicroRNA expression. *Hepatology* **2008**, *48*, 1810–1820. [CrossRef] [PubMed]

67. Castro, R.E.; Ferreira, D.M.; Afonso, M.B.; Borralho, P.M.; Machado, M.V.; Cortez-Pinto, H.; Rodrigues, C.M. miR-34a/SIRT1/p53 is suppressed by ursodeoxycholic acid in the rat liver and activated by disease severity in human non-alcoholic fatty liver disease. *J. Hepatol.* **2013**, *58*, 119–125. [CrossRef] [PubMed]

68. Li, T.; Francl, J.M.; Boehme, S.; Chiang, J.Y. Regulation of cholesterol and bile acid homeostasis by the cholesterol 7α-hydroxylase/steroid response element-binding protein 2/microRNA-33a axis in mice. *Hepatology* **2013**, *58*, 1111–1121. [CrossRef] [PubMed]

69. Guo, Y.; Xiong, Y.; Sheng, Q.; Zhao, S.; Wattacheril, J.; Flynn, C.R. A micro-RNA expression signature for human NAFLD progression. *J. Gastroenterol.* **2016**. [CrossRef] [PubMed]

70. Soronen, J.; Yki-Jarvinen, H.; Zhou, Y.; Sadevirta, S.; Sarin, A.P.; Leivonen, M.; Sevastianova, K.; Perttila, J.; Laurila, P.P.; Sigruener, A.; et al. Novel hepatic microRNAs upregulated in human nonalcoholic fatty liver disease. *Physiol. Rep.* **2016**, *4*. [CrossRef] [PubMed]

71. Esau, C.; Davis, S.; Murray, S.F.; Yu, X.X.; Pandey, S.K.; Pear, M.; Watts, L.; Booten, S.L.; Graham, M.; McKay, R.; et al. miR-122 regulation of lipid metabolism revealed by in vivo antisense targeting. *Cell Metab.* **2006**, *3*, 87–98. [CrossRef] [PubMed]

72. Li, Z.; Xu, G.; Qin, Y.; Zhang, C.; Tang, H.; Yin, Y.; Xiang, X.; Li, Y.; Zhao, J.; Mulholland, M.; et al. Ghrelin promotes hepatic lipogenesis by activation of mtor-PPARγ signaling pathway. *Proc. Natl. Acad. Sci. USA* **2014**, *111*, 13163–13168. [CrossRef] [PubMed]

73. Promrat, K.; Kleiner, D.E.; Niemeier, H.M.; Jackvony, E.; Kearns, M.; Wands, J.R.; Fava, J.L.; Wing, R.R. Randomized controlled trial testing the effects of weight loss on nonalcoholic steatohepatitis. *Hepatology* **2010**, *51*, 121–129. [CrossRef] [PubMed]

74. Wong, V.W.; Chan, R.S.; Wong, G.L.; Cheung, B.H.; Chu, W.C.; Yeung, D.K.; Chim, A.M.; Lai, J.W.; Li, L.S.; Sea, M.M.; et al. Community-based lifestyle modification programme for non-alcoholic fatty liver disease: A randomized controlled trial. *J. Hepatol.* **2013**, *59*, 536–542. [CrossRef] [PubMed]

75. Charlton, M.; Krishnan, A.; Viker, K.; Sanderson, S.; Cazanave, S.; McConico, A.; Masuoko, H.; Gores, G. Fast food diet mouse: Novel small animal model of nash with ballooning, progressive fibrosis, and high physiological fidelity to the human condition. *Am. J. Physiol. Gastrointest. Liver Physiol.* **2011**, *301*, G825–G834. [CrossRef] [PubMed]

76. Garbow, J.R.; Doherty, J.M.; Schugar, R.C.; Travers, S.; Weber, M.L.; Wentz, A.E.; Ezenwajiaku, N.; Cotter, D.G.; Brunt, E.M.; Crawford, P.A. Hepatic steatosis, inflammation, and ER stress in mice maintained long term on a very low-carbohydrate ketogenic diet. *Am. J. Physiol. Gastrointest. Liver Physiol.* **2011**, *300*, G956–G967. [CrossRef] [PubMed]

77. Haas, J.T.; Miao, J.; Chanda, D.; Wang, Y.; Zhao, E.; Haas, M.E.; Hirschey, M.; Vaitheesvaran, B.; Farese, R.V., Jr.; Kurland, I.J.; et al. Hepatic insulin signaling is required for obesity-dependent expression of SREBP-1c mRNA but not for feeding-dependent expression. *Cell Metab.* **2012**, *15*, 873–884. [CrossRef] [PubMed]

78. Schmid, A.I.; Szendroedi, J.; Chmelik, M.; Krssak, M.; Moser, E.; Roden, M. Liver ATP synthesis is lower and relates to insulin sensitivity in patients with type 2 diabetes. *Diabetes Care* **2011**, *34*, 448–453. [CrossRef] [PubMed]

79.  Lee, A.H.; Scapa, E.F.; Cohen, D.E.; Glimcher, L.H. Regulation of hepatic lipogenesis by the transcription factor XBP1. *Science* **2008**, *320*, 1492–1496. [CrossRef] [PubMed]

80.  Nakagawa, T.; Hu, H.; Zharikov, S.; Tuttle, K.R.; Short, R.A.; Glushakova, O.; Ouyang, X.; Feig, D.I.; Block, E.R.; Herrera-Acosta, J.; et al. A causal role for uric acid in fructose-induced metabolic syndrome. *Am. J. Physiol. Ren. Physiol.* **2006**, *290*, F625–F631. [CrossRef] [PubMed]

81.  Lanaspa, M.A.; Sanchez-Lozada, L.G.; Choi, Y.J.; Cicerchi, C.; Kanbay, M.; Roncal-Jimenez, C.A.; Ishimoto, T.; Li, N.; Marek, G.; Duranay, M.; et al. Uric acid induces hepatic steatosis by generation of mitochondrial oxidative stress: Potential role in fructose-dependent and -independent fatty liver. *J. Biol. Chem.* **2012**, *287*, 40732–40744. [CrossRef] [PubMed]

82.  Lim, J.S.; Mietus-Snyder, M.; Valente, A.; Schwarz, J.M.; Lustig, R.H. The role of fructose in the pathogenesis of NAFLD and the metabolic syndrome. *Nat. Rev. Gastroenterol. Hepatol.* **2010**, *7*, 251–264. [CrossRef] [PubMed]

83.  Kohli, R.; Pan, X.; Malladi, P.; Wainwright, M.S.; Whitington, P.F. Mitochondrial reactive oxygen species signal hepatocyte steatosis by regulating the phosphatidylinositol 3-kinase cell survival pathway. *J. Biol. Chem.* **2007**, *282*, 21327–21336. [CrossRef] [PubMed]

84.  Ishimoto, T.; Lanaspa, M.A.; Rivard, C.J.; Roncal-Jimenez, C.A.; Orlicky, D.J.; Cicerchi, C.; McMahan, R.H.; Abdelmalek, M.F.; Rosen, H.R.; Jackman, M.R.; et al. High-fat and high-sucrose (western) diet induces steatohepatitis that is dependent on fructokinase. *Hepatology* **2013**, *58*, 1632–1643. [CrossRef] [PubMed]

85.  Ohashi, K.; Munetsuna, E.; Yamada, H.; Ando, Y.; Yamazaki, M.; Taromaru, N.; Nagura, A.; Ishikawa, H.; Suzuki, K.; Teradaira, R.; et al. High fructose consumption induces DNA methylation at PPARα and CPT1A promoter regions in the rat liver. *Biochem. Biophys. Res. Commun.* **2015**, *468*, 185–189. [CrossRef] [PubMed]

86.  Yamazaki, M.; Munetsuna, E.; Yamada, H.; Ando, Y.; Mizuno, G.; Murase, Y.; Kondo, K.; Ishikawa, H.; Teradaira, R.; Suzuki, K.; et al. Fructose consumption induces hypomethylation of hepatic mitochondrial DNA in rats. *Life Sci.* **2016**, *149*, 146–152. [CrossRef] [PubMed]

87.  Handa, P.; Morgan-Stevenson, V.; Maliken, B.D.; Nelson, J.E.; Washington, S.; Westerman, M.; Yeh, M.M.; Kowdley, K.V. Iron overload results in hepatic oxidative stress, immune cell activation, and hepatocellular ballooning injury, leading to nonalcoholic steatohepatitis in genetically obese mice. *Am. J. Physiol. Gastrointest. Liver Physiol.* **2016**, *310*, G117–G127. [CrossRef] [PubMed]

88.  Tallino, S.; Duffy, M.; Ralle, M.; Cortes, M.P.; Latorre, M.; Burkhead, J.L. Nutrigenomics analysis reveals that copper deficiency and dietary sucrose up-regulate inflammation, fibrosis and lipogenic pathways in a mature rat model of nonalcoholic fatty liver disease. *J. Nutr. Biochem.* **2015**, *26*, 996–1006. [CrossRef] [PubMed]

89.  Peverill, W.; Powell, L.W.; Skoien, R. Evolving concepts in the pathogenesis of nash: Beyond steatosis and inflammation. *Int. J. Mol. Sci.* **2014**, *15*, 8591–8638. [CrossRef] [PubMed]

90.  Puri, P.; Mirshahi, F.; Cheung, O.; Natarajan, R.; Maher, J.W.; Kellum, J.M.; Sanyal, A.J. Activation and dysregulation of the unfolded protein response in nonalcoholic fatty liver disease. *Gastroenterology* **2008**, *134*, 568–576. [CrossRef] [PubMed]

91.  Tandra, S.; Yeh, M.M.; Brunt, E.M.; Vuppalanchi, R.; Cummings, O.W.; Unalp-Arida, A.; Wilson, L.A.; Chalasani, N.; Network, N.C.R. Presence and significance of microvesicular steatosis in nonalcoholic fatty liver disease. *J. Hepatol.* **2011**, *55*, 654–659. [CrossRef] [PubMed]

92.  Leamy, A.K.; Egnatchik, R.A.; Young, J.D. Molecular mechanisms and the role of saturated fatty acids in the progression of non-alcoholic fatty liver disease. *Prog. Lipid Res.* **2013**, *52*, 165–174. [CrossRef] [PubMed]

93.  Cheung, O.; Sanyal, A.J. Abnormalities of lipid metabolism in nonalcoholic fatty liver disease. *Semin. Liver Dis.* **2008**, *28*, 351–359. [CrossRef] [PubMed]

94.  Alkhouri, N.; Dixon, L.J.; Feldstein, A.E. Lipotoxicity in nonalcoholic fatty liver disease: Not all lipids are created equal. *Expert Rev. Gastroenterol. Hepatol.* **2009**, *3*, 445–451. [CrossRef] [PubMed]

95.  Pagadala, M.; Kasumov, T.; McCullough, A.J.; Zein, N.N.; Kirwan, J.P. Role of ceramides in nonalcoholic fatty liver disease. *Trends Endocrinol. Metab.* **2012**, *23*, 365–371. [CrossRef] [PubMed]

96.  Brenner, C.; Galluzzi, L.; Kepp, O.; Kroemer, G. Decoding cell death signals in liver inflammation. *J. Hepatol.* **2013**, *59*, 583–594. [CrossRef] [PubMed]

97.  Chaurasia, B.; Summers, S.A. Ceramides—Lipotoxic inducers of metabolic disorders. *Trends Endocrinol. Metab.* **2015**, *26*, 538–550. [CrossRef] [PubMed]

98.　Yamaguchi, K.; Yang, L.; McCall, S.; Huang, J.; Yu, X.X.; Pandey, S.K.; Bhanot, S.; Monia, B.P.; Li, Y.X.; Diehl, A.M. Inhibiting triglyceride synthesis improves hepatic steatosis but exacerbates liver damage and fibrosis in obese mice with nonalcoholic steatohepatitis. *Hepatology* **2007**, *45*, 1366–1374. [CrossRef] [PubMed]

99.　McClain, C.J.; Barve, S.; Deaciuc, I. Good fat/bad fat. *Hepatology* **2007**, *45*, 1343–1346. [CrossRef] [PubMed]

100.　Sanyal, A.J. Reply: To PMID 24818764. *Gastroenterology* **2015**, *148*, 262–263. [CrossRef] [PubMed]

101.　Provenzano, A.; Milani, S.; Vizzutti, F.; Delogu, W.; Navari, N.; Novo, E.; Maggiora, M.; Maurino, V.; Laffi, G.; Parola, M.; et al. N-3 polyunsaturated fatty acids worsen inflammation and fibrosis in experimental nonalcoholic steatohepatitis. *Liver Int.* **2014**, *34*, 918–930. [CrossRef] [PubMed]

102.　Puri, P.; Baillie, R.A.; Wiest, M.M.; Mirshahi, F.; Choudhury, J.; Cheung, O.; Sargeant, C.; Contos, M.J.; Sanyal, A.J. A lipidomic analysis of nonalcoholic fatty liver disease. *Hepatology* **2007**, *46*, 1081–1090. [CrossRef] [PubMed]

103.　Caballero, F.; Fernandez, A.; De Lacy, A.M.; Fernandez-Checa, J.C.; Caballeria, J.; Garcia-Ruiz, C. Enhanced free cholesterol, SREBP-2 and star expression in human nash. *J. Hepatol.* **2009**, *50*, 789–796. [CrossRef] [PubMed]

104.　Mari, M.; Caballero, F.; Colell, A.; Morales, A.; Caballeria, J.; Fernandez, A.; Enrich, C.; Fernandez-Checa, J.C.; Garcia-Ruiz, C. Mitochondrial free cholesterol loading sensitizes to TNF- and FAS-mediated steatohepatitis. *Cell Metab.* **2006**, *4*, 185–198. [CrossRef] [PubMed]

105.　Savard, C.; Tartaglione, E.V.; Kuver, R.; Haigh, W.G.; Farrell, G.C.; Subramanian, S.; Chait, A.; Yeh, M.M.; Quinn, L.S.; Ioannou, G.N. Synergistic interaction of dietary cholesterol and dietary fat in inducing experimental steatohepatitis. *Hepatology* **2013**, *57*, 81–92. [CrossRef] [PubMed]

106.　Van Rooyen, D.M.; Larter, C.Z.; Haigh, W.G.; Yeh, M.M.; Ioannou, G.; Kuver, R.; Lee, S.P.; Teoh, N.C.; Farrell, G.C. Hepatic free cholesterol accumulates in obese, diabetic mice and causes nonalcoholic steatohepatitis. *Gastroenterology* **2011**, *141*, 1393–1403. [CrossRef] [PubMed]

107.　Wouters, K.; van Gorp, P.J.; Bieghs, V.; Gijbels, M.J.; Duimel, H.; Lutjohann, D.; Kerksiek, A.; van Kruchten, R.; Maeda, N.; Staels, B.; et al. Dietary cholesterol, rather than liver steatosis, leads to hepatic inflammation in hyperlipidemic mouse models of nonalcoholic steatohepatitis. *Hepatology* **2008**, *48*, 474–486. [CrossRef] [PubMed]

108.　Min, H.K.; Kapoor, A.; Fuchs, M.; Mirshahi, F.; Zhou, H.; Maher, J.; Kellum, J.; Warnick, R.; Contos, M.J.; Sanyal, A.J. Increased hepatic synthesis and dysregulation of cholesterol metabolism is associated with the severity of nonalcoholic fatty liver disease. *Cell Metab.* **2012**, *15*, 665–674. [CrossRef] [PubMed]

109.　Simonen, P.; Kotronen, A.; Hallikainen, M.; Sevastianova, K.; Makkonen, J.; Hakkarainen, A.; Lundbom, N.; Miettinen, T.A.; Gylling, H.; Yki-Jarvinen, H. Cholesterol synthesis is increased and absorption decreased in non-alcoholic fatty liver disease independent of obesity. *J. Hepatol.* **2011**, *54*, 153–159. [CrossRef] [PubMed]

110.　Cortes, V.A.; Busso, D.; Maiz, A.; Arteaga, A.; Nervi, F.; Rigotti, A. Physiological and pathological implications of cholesterol. *Front. Biosci.* **2014**, *19*, 416–428. [CrossRef]

111.　Walenbergh, S.M.; Koek, G.H.; Bieghs, V.; Shiri-Sverdlov, R. Non-alcoholic steatohepatitis: The role of oxidized low-density lipoproteins. *J. Hepatol.* **2013**, *58*, 801–810. [CrossRef] [PubMed]

112.　Hendrikx, T.; Walenbergh, S.M.; Hofker, M.H.; Shiri-Sverdlov, R. Lysosomal cholesterol accumulation: Driver on the road to inflammation during atherosclerosis and non-alcoholic steatohepatitis. *Obes. Rev.* **2014**, *15*, 424–433. [CrossRef] [PubMed]

113.　Tomita, K.; Teratani, T.; Suzuki, T.; Shimizu, M.; Sato, H.; Narimatsu, K.; Okada, Y.; Kurihara, C.; Irie, R.; Yokoyama, H.; et al. Free cholesterol accumulation in hepatic stellate cells: Mechanism of liver fibrosis aggravation in nonalcoholic steatohepatitis in mice. *Hepatology* **2014**, *59*, 154–169. [CrossRef] [PubMed]

114.　Chalasani, N.; Younossi, Z.; Lavine, J.E.; Diehl, A.M.; Brunt, E.M.; Cusi, K.; Charlton, M.; Sanyal, A.J. The diagnosis and management of non-alcoholic fatty liver disease: Practice guideline by the American association for the study of liver diseases, American college of gastroenterology, and the American gastroenterological association. *Hepatology* **2012**, *55*, 2005–2023. [CrossRef] [PubMed]

115.　Spolding, B.; Connor, T.; Wittmer, C.; Abreu, L.L.; Kaspi, A.; Ziemann, M.; Kaur, G.; Cooper, A.; Morrison, S.; Lee, S.; et al. Rapid development of non-alcoholic steatohepatitis in psammomys obesus (Israeli Sand Rat). *PLoS ONE* **2014**, *9*, e92656. [CrossRef] [PubMed]

116.　Bellanti, F.; Mitarotonda, D.; Tamborra, R.; Blonda, M.; Iannelli, G.; Petrella, A.; Sanginario, V.; Iuliano, L.; Vendemiale, G.; Serviddio, G. Oxysterols induce mitochondrial impairment and hepatocellular toxicity in non-alcoholic fatty liver disease. *Free Radic. Biol. Med.* **2014**, *75*, S16–S17. [CrossRef] [PubMed]

117. Tall, A.R.; Yvan-Charvet, L. Cholesterol, inflammation and innate immunity. *Nat. Rev. Immunol.* **2015**, *15*, 104–116. [CrossRef] [PubMed]

118. Chung, S.; Cuffe, H.; Marshall, S.M.; McDaniel, A.L.; Ha, J.H.; Kavanagh, K.; Hong, C.; Tontonoz, P.; Temel, R.E.; Parks, J.S. Dietary cholesterol promotes adipocyte hypertrophy and adipose tissue inflammation in visceral, but not in subcutaneous, fat in monkeys. *Arterioscler. Thromb. Vasc. Biol.* **2014**, *34*, 1880–1887. [CrossRef] [PubMed]

119. Serviddio, G.; Bellanti, F.; Vendemiale, G.; Altomare, E. Mitochondrial dysfunction in nonalcoholic steatohepatitis. *Expert Rev. Gastroenterol. Hepatol.* **2011**, *5*, 233–244. [CrossRef] [PubMed]

120. Tessari, P.; Coracina, A.; Cosma, A.; Tiengo, A. Hepatic lipid metabolism and non-alcoholic fatty liver disease. *Nutr. Metab. Cardiovasc. Dis.* **2009**, *19*, 291–302. [CrossRef] [PubMed]

121. Nassir, F.; Ibdah, J.A. Role of mitochondria in nonalcoholic fatty liver disease. *Int. J. Mol. Sci.* **2014**, *15*, 8713–8742. [CrossRef] [PubMed]

122. Mailloux, R.J.; Florian, M.; Chen, Q.; Yan, J.; Petrov, I.; Coughlan, M.C.; Laziyan, M.; Caldwell, D.; Lalande, M.; Patry, D.; et al. Exposure to a northern contaminant mixture (NCM) alters hepatic energy and lipid metabolism exacerbating hepatic steatosis in obese JCR rats. *PLoS ONE* **2014**, *9*, e106832. [CrossRef] [PubMed]

123. Martel, C.; Allouche, M.; Esposti, D.D.; Fanelli, E.; Boursier, C.; Henry, C.; Chopineau, J.; Calamita, G.; Kroemer, G.; Lemoine, A.; et al. Glycogen synthase kinase 3-mediated voltage-dependent anion channel phosphorylation controls outer mitochondrial membrane permeability during lipid accumulation. *Hepatology* **2013**, *57*, 93–102. [CrossRef] [PubMed]

124. Win, S.; Than, T.A.; Le, B.H.; Garcia-Ruiz, C.; Fernandez-Checa, J.C.; Kaplowitz, N. Sab (Sh3bp5) dependence of JNK mediated inhibition of mitochondrial respiration in palmitic acid induced hepatocyte lipotoxicity. *J. Hepatol.* **2015**, *62*, 1367–1374. [CrossRef] [PubMed]

125. Penke, M.; Larsen, P.S.; Schuster, S.; Dall, M.; Jensen, B.A.; Gorski, T.; Meusel, A.; Richter, S.; Vienberg, S.G.; Treebak, J.T.; et al. Hepatic nad salvage pathway is enhanced in mice on a high-fat diet. *Mol. Cell. Endocrinol.* **2015**, *412*, 65–72. [CrossRef] [PubMed]

126. Gariani, K.; Menzies, K.J.; Ryu, D.; Wegner, C.J.; Wang, X.; Ropelle, E.R.; Moullan, N.; Zhang, H.; Perino, A.; Lemos, V.; et al. Eliciting the mitochondrial unfolded protein response by nicotinamide adenine dinucleotide repletion reverses fatty liver disease in mice. *Hepatology* **2016**, *63*, 1190–1204. [CrossRef] [PubMed]

127. Bentinger, M.; Brismar, K.; Dallner, G. The antioxidant role of coenzyme Q. *Mitochondrion* **2007**, *7*, S41–S50. [CrossRef] [PubMed]

128. Nowicka, B.; Kruk, J. Occurrence, biosynthesis and function of isoprenoid quinones. *Biochim. Biophys. Acta* **2010**, *1797*, 1587–1605. [CrossRef] [PubMed]

129. Laredj, L.N.; Licitra, F.; Puccio, H.M. The molecular genetics of coenzyme Q biosynthesis in health and disease. *Biochimie* **2014**, *100*, 78–87. [CrossRef] [PubMed]

130. Bentinger, M.; Tekle, M.; Dallner, G. Coenzyme Q—Biosynthesis and functions. *Biochem. Biophys. Res. Commun.* **2010**, *396*, 74–79. [CrossRef] [PubMed]

131. Yesilova, Z.; Yaman, H.; Oktenli, C.; Ozcan, A.; Uygun, A.; Cakir, E.; Sanisoglu, S.Y.; Erdil, A.; Ates, Y.; Aslan, M.; et al. Systemic markers of lipid peroxidation and antioxidants in patients with nonalcoholic fatty liver disease. *Am. J. Gastroenterol.* **2005**, *100*, 850–855. [CrossRef] [PubMed]

132. Huertas, J.R.; Battino, M.; Lenaz, G.; Mataix, F.J. Changes in mitochondrial and microsomal rat liver coenzyme Q9 and Q10 content induced by dietary fat and endogenous lipid peroxidation. *FEBS Lett.* **1991**, *287*, 89–92. [CrossRef]

133. Bravo, E.; Palleschi, S.; Rossi, B.; Napolitano, M.; Tiano, L.; D'Amore, E.; Botham, K.M. Coenzyme Q metabolism is disturbed in high fat diet-induced non-alcoholic fatty liver disease in rats. *Int. J. Mol. Sci.* **2012**, *13*, 1644–1657. [CrossRef] [PubMed]

134. Feldstein, A.E.; Werneburg, N.W.; Canbay, A.; Guicciardi, M.E.; Bronk, S.F.; Rydzewski, R.; Burgart, L.J.; Gores, G.J. Free fatty acids promote hepatic lipotoxicity by stimulating TNF-α expression via a lysosomal pathway. *Hepatology* **2004**, *40*, 185–194. [CrossRef] [PubMed]

135. Aubert, J.; Begriche, K.; Knockaert, L.; Robin, M.A.; Fromenty, B. Increased expression of cytochrome P450 2E1 in nonalcoholic fatty liver disease: Mechanisms and pathophysiological role. *Clin. Res. Hepatol. Gastroenterol.* **2011**, *35*, 630–637. [CrossRef] [PubMed]

136. Abdelmegeed, M.A.; Banerjee, A.; Yoo, S.H.; Jang, S.; Gonzalez, F.J.; Song, B.J. Critical role of cytochrome P450 2E1 (CYP2E1) in the development of high fat-induced non-alcoholic steatohepatitis. *J. Hepatol.* **2012**, *57*, 860–866. [CrossRef] [PubMed]

137. Guicciardi, M.E.; Malhi, H.; Mott, J.L.; Gores, G.J. Apoptosis and necrosis in the liver. *Compr. Physiol.* **2013**, *3*, 977–1010. [PubMed]

138. Hirsova, P.; Gores, G.J. Death receptor-mediated cell death and proinflammatory signaling in nonalcoholic steatohepatitis. *Cell. Mol. Gastroenterol. Hepatol.* **2015**, *1*, 17–27. [CrossRef] [PubMed]

139. Li, J.; McQuade, T.; Siemer, A.B.; Napetschnig, J.; Moriwaki, K.; Hsiao, Y.S.; Damko, E.; Moquin, D.; Walz, T.; McDermott, A.; et al. The RIP1/RIP3 necrosome forms a functional amyloid signaling complex required for programmed necrosis. *Cell* **2012**, *150*, 339–350. [CrossRef] [PubMed]

140. Wang, H.; Sun, L.; Su, L.; Rizo, J.; Liu, L.; Wang, L.F.; Wang, F.S.; Wang, X. Mixed lineage kinase domain-like protein MLKL causes necrotic membrane disruption upon phosphorylation by RIP3. *Mol. Cell* **2014**, *54*, 133–146. [CrossRef] [PubMed]

141. Zhang, D.W.; Shao, J.; Lin, J.; Zhang, N.; Lu, B.J.; Lin, S.C.; Dong, M.Q.; Han, J. RIP3, an energy metabolism regulator that switches TNF-induced cell death from apoptosis to necrosis. *Science* **2009**, *325*, 332–336. [CrossRef] [PubMed]

142. Upton, J.W.; Kaiser, W.J.; Mocarski, E.S. Virus inhibition of RIP3-dependent necrosis. *Cell Host Microbe* **2010**, *7*, 302–313. [CrossRef] [PubMed]

143. Moujalled, D.M.; Cook, W.D.; Okamoto, T.; Murphy, J.; Lawlor, K.E.; Vince, J.E.; Vaux, D.L. TNF can activate RIPK3 and cause programmed necrosis in the absence of RIPK1. *Cell Death Dis.* **2013**, *4*. [CrossRef] [PubMed]

144. Degterev, A.; Huang, Z.; Boyce, M.; Li, Y.; Jagtap, P.; Mizushima, N.; Cuny, G.D.; Mitchison, T.J.; Moskowitz, M.A.; Yuan, J. Chemical inhibitor of nonapoptotic cell death with therapeutic potential for ischemic brain injury. *Nat. Chem. Biol.* **2005**, *1*, 112–119. [CrossRef] [PubMed]

145. Zhao, J.; Jitkaew, S.; Cai, Z.; Choksi, S.; Li, Q.; Luo, J.; Liu, Z.G. Mixed lineage kinase domain-like is a key receptor interacting protein 3 downstream component of TNF-induced necrosis. *Proc. Natl. Acad. Sci. USA* **2012**, *109*, 5322–5327. [CrossRef] [PubMed]

146. Gautheron, J.; Vucur, M.; Reisinger, F.; Cardenas, D.V.; Roderburg, C.; Koppe, C.; Kreggenwinkel, K.; Schneider, A.T.; Bartneck, M.; Neumann, U.P.; et al. A positive feedback loop between RIP3 and JNK controls non-alcoholic steatohepatitis. *EMBO Mol. Med.* **2014**, *6*, 1062–1074. [CrossRef] [PubMed]

147. Afonso, M.B.; Rodrigues, P.M.; Carvalho, T.; Caridade, M.; Borralho, P.; Cortez-Pinto, H.; Castro, R.E.; Rodrigues, C.M. Necroptosis is a key pathogenic event in human and experimental murine models of non-alcoholic steatohepatitis. *Clin. Sci.* **2015**, *129*, 721–739. [CrossRef] [PubMed]

148. Park, S.W.; Zhou, Y.; Lee, J.; Lu, A.; Sun, C.; Chung, J.; Ueki, K.; Ozcan, U. The regulatory subunits of PI3K, p85α and p85β, interact with XBP-1 and increase its nuclear translocation. *Nat. Med.* **2010**, *16*, 429–437. [CrossRef] [PubMed]

149. Kapoor, A.; Sanyal, A.J. Endoplasmic reticulum stress and the unfolded protein response. *Clin. Liver Dis.* **2009**, *13*, 581–590. [CrossRef] [PubMed]

150. Padilla, A.; Descorbeth, M.; Almeyda, A.L.; Payne, K.; de Leon, M. Hyperglycemia magnifies Schwann cell dysfunction and cell death triggered by PA-induced lipotoxicity. *Brain Res.* **2011**, *1370*, 64–79. [CrossRef] [PubMed]

151. Wei, Y.; Wang, D.; Topczewski, F.; Pagliassotti, M.J. Saturated fatty acids induce endoplasmic reticulum stress and apoptosis independently of ceramide in liver cells. *Am. J. Physiol. Endocrinol. Metab.* **2006**, *291*, E275–E281. [CrossRef] [PubMed]

152. Fu, S.; Yang, L.; Li, P.; Hofmann, O.; Dicker, L.; Hide, W.; Lin, X.; Watkins, S.M.; Ivanov, A.R.; Hotamisligil, G.S. Aberrant lipid metabolism disrupts calcium homeostasis causing liver endoplasmic reticulum stress in obesity. *Nature* **2011**, *473*, 528–531. [CrossRef] [PubMed]

153. Arias-Loste, M.T.; Fabrega, E.; Lopez-Hoyos, M.; Crespo, J. The crosstalk between hypoxia and innate immunity in the development of obesity-related nonalcoholic fatty liver disease. *BioMed Res. Int.* **2015**, *2015*. [CrossRef] [PubMed]

154. Qu, A.; Taylor, M.; Xue, X.; Matsubara, T.; Metzger, D.; Chambon, P.; Gonzalez, F.J.; Shah, Y.M. Hypoxia-inducible transcription factor 2α promotes steatohepatitis through augmenting lipid accumulation, inflammation, and fibrosis. *Hepatology* **2011**, *54*, 472–483. [CrossRef] [PubMed]

155. Ye, J.; Gao, Z.; Yin, J.; He, Q. Hypoxia is a potential risk factor for chronic inflammation and adiponectin reduction in adipose tissue of *ob/ob* and dietary obese mice. *Am. J. Physiol. Endocrinol. Metab.* **2007**, *293*, E1118–E1128. [CrossRef] [PubMed]
156. Hodson, L. Adipose tissue oxygenation: Effects on metabolic function. *Adipocyte* **2014**, *3*, 75–80. [CrossRef] [PubMed]
157. Hodson, L.; Humphreys, S.M.; Karpe, F.; Frayn, K.N. Metabolic signatures of human adipose tissue hypoxia in obesity. *Diabetes* **2013**, *62*, 1417–1425. [CrossRef] [PubMed]
158. Eltzschig, H.K.; Carmeliet, P. Hypoxia and inflammation. *N. Engl. J. Med.* **2011**, *364*, 656–665. [PubMed]
159. Rius, J.; Guma, M.; Schachtrup, C.; Akassoglou, K.; Zinkernagel, A.S.; Nizet, V.; Johnson, R.S.; Haddad, G.G.; Karin, M. NF-κB links innate immunity to the hypoxic response through transcriptional regulation of HIF-1α. *Nature* **2008**, *453*, 807–811. [CrossRef] [PubMed]
160. Kuhlicke, J.; Frick, J.S.; Morote-Garcia, J.C.; Rosenberger, P.; Eltzschig, H.K. Hypoxia inducible factor (HIF)-1 coordinates induction of toll-like receptors TLR2 and TLR6 during hypoxia. *PLoS ONE* **2007**, *2*, e1364. [CrossRef] [PubMed]
161. Kim, S.Y.; Choi, Y.J.; Joung, S.M.; Lee, B.H.; Jung, Y.S.; Lee, J.Y. Hypoxic stress up-regulates the expression of toll-like receptor 4 in macrophages via hypoxia-inducible factor. *Immunology* **2010**, *129*, 516–524. [CrossRef] [PubMed]
162. Aron-Wisnewsky, J.; Minville, C.; Tordjman, J.; Levy, P.; Bouillot, J.L.; Basdevant, A.; Bedossa, P.; Clement, K.; Pepin, J.L. Chronic intermittent hypoxia is a major trigger for non-alcoholic fatty liver disease in morbid obese. *J. Hepatol.* **2012**, *56*, 225–233. [CrossRef] [PubMed]
163. Feldstein, A.E.; Canbay, A.; Angulo, P.; Taniai, M.; Burgart, L.J.; Lindor, K.D.; Gores, G.J. Hepatocyte apoptosis and FAS expression are prominent features of human nonalcoholic steatohepatitis. *Gastroenterology* **2003**, *125*, 437–443. [CrossRef]
164. Idrissova, L.; Malhi, H.; Werneburg, N.W.; LeBrasseur, N.K.; Bronk, S.F.; Fingas, C.; Tchkonia, T.; Pirtskhalava, T.; White, T.A.; Stout, M.B.; et al. Trail receptor deletion in mice suppresses the inflammation of nutrient excess. *J. Hepatol.* **2015**, *62*, 1156–1163. [CrossRef] [PubMed]
165. Lu, M.; Lawrence, D.A.; Marsters, S.; Acosta-Alvear, D.; Kimmig, P.; Mendez, A.S.; Paton, A.W.; Paton, J.C.; Walter, P.; Ashkenazi, A. Opposing unfolded-protein-response signals converge on death receptor 5 to control apoptosis. *Science* **2014**, *345*, 98–101. [CrossRef] [PubMed]
166. Gadd, V.L.; Skoien, R.; Powell, E.E.; Fagan, K.J.; Winterford, C.; Horsfall, L.; Irvine, K.; Clouston, A.D. The portal inflammatory infiltrate and ductular reaction in human nonalcoholic fatty liver disease. *Hepatology* **2014**, *59*, 1393–1405. [CrossRef] [PubMed]
167. Lanthier, N. Targeting Kupffer cells in non-alcoholic fatty liver disease/non-alcoholic steatohepatitis: Why and how? *World J. Hepatol.* **2015**, *7*, 2184–2188. [CrossRef] [PubMed]
168. Dixon, L.J.; Barnes, M.; Tang, H.; Pritchard, M.T.; Nagy, L.E. Kupffer cells in the liver. *Compr. Physiol.* **2013**, *3*, 785–797. [PubMed]
169. Tacke, F.; Zimmermann, H.W. Macrophage heterogeneity in liver injury and fibrosis. *J. Hepatol.* **2014**, *60*, 1090–1096. [CrossRef] [PubMed]
170. Marra, F.; Tacke, F. Roles for chemokines in liver disease. *Gastroenterology* **2014**, *147*, 577–594. [CrossRef] [PubMed]
171. Leroux, A.; Ferrere, G.; Godie, V.; Cailleux, F.; Renoud, M.L.; Gaudin, F.; Naveau, S.; Prevot, S.; Makhzami, S.; Perlemuter, G.; et al. Toxic lipids stored by Kupffer cells correlates with their pro-inflammatory phenotype at an early stage of steatohepatitis. *J. Hepatol.* **2012**, *57*, 141–149. [CrossRef] [PubMed]
172. Chinetti-Gbaguidi, G.; Staels, B. Macrophage polarization in metabolic disorders: Functions and regulation. *Curr. Opin. Lipidol.* **2011**, *22*, 365–372. [CrossRef] [PubMed]
173. Xu, R.; Huang, H.; Zhang, Z.; Wang, F.S. The role of neutrophils in the development of liver diseases. *Cell. Mol. Immunol.* **2014**, *11*, 224–231. [CrossRef] [PubMed]
174. Ibusuki, R.; Uto, H.; Arima, S.; Mawatari, S.; Setoguchi, Y.; Iwashita, Y.; Hashimoto, S.; Maeda, T.; Tanoue, S.; Kanmura, S.; et al. Transgenic expression of human neutrophil peptide-1 enhances hepatic fibrosis in mice fed a choline-deficient, l-amino acid-defined diet. *Liver Int.* **2013**, *33*, 1549–1556. [CrossRef] [PubMed]
175. Rensen, S.S.; Bieghs, V.; Xanthoulea, S.; Arfianti, E.; Bakker, J.A.; Shiri-Sverdlov, R.; Hofker, M.H.; Greve, J.W.; Buurman, W.A. Neutrophil-derived myeloperoxidase aggravates non-alcoholic steatohepatitis in low-density lipoprotein receptor-deficient mice. *PLoS ONE* **2012**, *7*, e52411. [CrossRef] [PubMed]

176. Talukdar, S.; Oh da, Y.; Bandyopadhyay, G.; Li, D.; Xu, J.; McNelis, J.; Lu, M.; Li, P.; Yan, Q.; Zhu, Y.; et al. Neutrophils mediate insulin resistance in mice fed a high-fat diet through secreted elastase. *Nat. Med.* **2012**, *18*, 1407–1412. [CrossRef] [PubMed]

177. Tacke, F.; Yoneyama, H. From NAFLD to NASH to fibrosis to HCC: Role of dendritic cell populations in the liver. *Hepatology* **2013**, *58*, 494–496. [CrossRef] [PubMed]

178. Henning, J.R.; Graffeo, C.S.; Rehman, A.; Fallon, N.C.; Zambirinis, C.P.; Ochi, A.; Barilla, R.; Jamal, M.; Deutsch, M.; Greco, S.; et al. Dendritic cells limit fibroinflammatory injury in nonalcoholic steatohepatitis in mice. *Hepatology* **2013**, *58*, 589–602. [CrossRef] [PubMed]

179. Sutti, S.; Locatelli, I.; Bruzzi, S.; Jindal, A.; Vacchiano, M.; Bozzola, C.; Albano, E. CX3CR1-expressing inflammatory dendritic cells contribute to the progression of steatohepatitis. *Clin. Sci.* **2015**, *129*, 797–808. [CrossRef] [PubMed]

180. Ganz, M.; Szabo, G. Immune and inflammatory pathways in NASH. *Hepatol. Int.* **2013**, *7*, 771–781. [CrossRef] [PubMed]

181. Tian, Z.; Chen, Y.; Gao, B. Natural killer cells in liver disease. *Hepatology* **2013**, *57*, 1654–1662. [CrossRef] [PubMed]

182. Kumar, V. NKT-cell subsets: Promoters and protectors in inflammatory liver disease. *J. Hepatol.* **2013**, *59*, 618–620. [CrossRef] [PubMed]

183. Martin-Murphy, B.V.; You, Q.; Wang, H.; De La Houssaye, B.A.; Reilly, T.P.; Friedman, J.E.; Ju, C. Mice lacking natural killer T cell are more susceptible to metabolic alterations following high fat diet feeding. *PLoS ONE* **2014**, *9*, e80949. [CrossRef] [PubMed]

184. Kremer, M.; Thomas, E.; Milton, R.J.; Perry, A.W.; van Rooijen, N.; Wheeler, M.D.; Zacks, S.; Fried, M.; Rippe, R.A.; Hines, I.N. Kupffer cell and interleukin-12-dependent loss of natural killer T cell in hepatosteatosis. *Hepatology* **2010**, *51*, 130–141. [CrossRef] [PubMed]

185. Syn, W.K.; Oo, Y.H.; Pereira, T.A.; Karaca, G.F.; Jung, Y.; Omenetti, A.; Witek, R.P.; Choi, S.S.; Guy, C.D.; Fearing, C.M.; et al. Accumulation of natural killer T cells in progressive nonalcoholic fatty liver disease. *Hepatology* **2010**, *51*, 1998–2007. [CrossRef] [PubMed]

186. Tajiri, K.; Shimizu, Y. Role of NKT cells in the pathogenesis of NAFLD. *Int. J. Hepatol.* **2012**, *2012*. [CrossRef] [PubMed]

187. Guy, C.D.; Suzuki, A.; Zdanowicz, M.; Abdelmalek, M.F.; Burchette, J.; Unalp, A.; Diehl, A.M.; Nash, C.R.N. Hedgehog pathway activation parallels histologic severity of injury and fibrosis in human nonalcoholic fatty liver disease. *Hepatology* **2012**, *55*, 1711–1721. [CrossRef] [PubMed]

188. Verdelho Machado, M.; Diehl, A.M. Role of Hedgehog Signaling Pathway in NASH. *Int. J. Mol. Sci.* **2016**, *17*. [CrossRef] [PubMed]

189. Moylan, C.A.; Pang, H.; Dellinger, A.; Suzuki, A.; Garrett, M.E.; Guy, C.D.; Murphy, S.K.; Ashley-Koch, A.E.; Choi, S.S.; Michelotti, G.A.; et al. Hepatic gene expression profiles differentiate presymptomatic patients with mild versus severe nonalcoholic fatty liver disease. *Hepatology* **2014**, *59*, 471–482. [CrossRef] [PubMed]

190. Kwon, H.; Song, K.; Han, C.; Chen, W.; Wang, Y.; Dash, S.; Lim, K.; Wu, T. Inhibition of hedgehog signaling ameliorates hepatic inflammation in mice with nonalcoholic fatty liver disease. *Hepatology* **2015**, *63*, 1155–1169. [CrossRef] [PubMed]

191. Syn, W.K.; Choi, S.S.; Liaskou, E.; Karaca, G.F.; Agboola, K.M.; Oo, Y.H.; Mi, Z.; Pereira, T.A.; Zdanowicz, M.; Malladi, P.; et al. Osteopontin is induced by hedgehog pathway activation and promotes fibrosis progression in nonalcoholic steatohepatitis. *Hepatology* **2011**, *53*, 106–115. [CrossRef] [PubMed]

192. Machado, M.V.; Michelotti, G.A.; Pereira, T.; Boursier, J.; Swiderska-Syn, M.; Karaca, G.; Xie, G.; Guy, C.D.; Bohinc, B.; Lindblom, K.R.; et al. Reduced lipoapoptosis, hedgehog pathway activation and fibrosis in caspase-2 deficient mice with non-alcoholic steatohepatitis. *Gut* **2015**, *64*, 1148–1157. [CrossRef] [PubMed]

193. Machado, M.V.; Michelotti, G.A.; Pereira, T.A.; Xie, G.; Premont, R.; Cortez-Pinto, H.; Diehl, A.M. Accumulation of duct cell with activated YAP parallels fibrosis progression in non-alcoholic fatty liver disease. *J. Hepatol.* **2015**, *63*, 962–970. [CrossRef] [PubMed]

194. Guy, C.D.; Suzuki, A.; Abdelmalek, M.F.; Burchette, J.L.; Diehl, A.M. Treatment response in the PIVENS trial is associated with decreased hedgehog pathway activity. *Hepatology* **2015**, *61*, 98–107. [CrossRef] [PubMed]

195. Evans, R.M.; Mangelsdorf, D.J. Nuclear receptors, RXR, and the big bang. *Cell* **2014**, *157*, 255–266. [CrossRef] [PubMed]

196. Fuchs, C.D.; Traussnigg, S.A.; Trauner, M. Nuclear receptor modulation for the treatment of nonalcoholic fatty liver disease. *Semin. Liver Dis.* **2016**, *36*, 69–86. [CrossRef] [PubMed]

197. Tailleux, A.; Wouters, K.; Staels, B. Roles of PPARs in NAFLD: Potential therapeutic targets. *Biochim. Biophys. Acta* **2012**, *1821*, 809–818. [CrossRef] [PubMed]

198. Francque, S.; Verrijken, A.; Caron, S.; Prawitt, J.; Paumelle, R.; Derudas, B.; Lefebvre, P.; Taskinen, M.R.; Van Hul, W.; Mertens, I.; et al. PPARα gene expression correlates with severity and histological treatment response in patients with non-alcoholic steatohepatitis. *J. Hepatol.* **2015**, *63*, 164–173. [CrossRef] [PubMed]

199. Reddy, J.K.; Rao, M.S. Lipid metabolism and liver inflammation. II. Fatty liver disease and fatty acid oxidation. *Am. J. Physiol. Gastrointest. Liver Physiol.* **2006**, *290*, G852–G858. [CrossRef] [PubMed]

200. Ip, E.; Farrell, G.; Hall, P.; Robertson, G.; Leclercq, I. Administration of the potent PPARα agonist, Wy-14,643, reverses nutritional fibrosis and steatohepatitis in mice. *Hepatology* **2004**, *39*, 1286–1296. [CrossRef] [PubMed]

201. Shan, W.; Nicol, C.J.; Ito, S.; Bility, M.T.; Kennett, M.J.; Ward, J.M.; Gonzalez, F.J.; Peters, J.M. Peroxisome proliferator-activated receptor-β/δ protects against chemically induced liver toxicity in mice. *Hepatology* **2008**, *47*, 225–235. [CrossRef] [PubMed]

202. Kawaguchi, K.; Sakaida, I.; Tsuchiya, M.; Omori, K.; Takami, T.; Okita, K. Pioglitazone prevents hepatic steatosis, fibrosis, and enzyme-altered lesions in rat liver cirrhosis induced by a choline-deficient L-amino acid-defined diet. *Biochem. Biophys. Res. Commun.* **2004**, *315*, 187–195. [CrossRef] [PubMed]

203. Stienstra, R.; Duval, C.; Muller, M.; Kersten, S. PPARs, obesity, and inflammation. *PPAR Res.* **2007**, *2007*. [CrossRef] [PubMed]

204. Lutchman, G.; Modi, A.; Kleiner, D.E.; Promrat, K.; Heller, T.; Ghany, M.; Borg, B.; Loomba, R.; Liang, T.J.; Premkumar, A.; et al. The effects of discontinuing pioglitazone in patients with nonalcoholic steatohepatitis. *Hepatology* **2007**, *46*, 424–429. [CrossRef] [PubMed]

205. Yamada, Y.; Eto, M.; Ito, Y.; Mochizuki, S.; Son, B.K.; Ogawa, S.; Iijima, K.; Kaneki, M.; Kozaki, K.; Toba, K.; et al. Suppressive role of PPARγ-regulated endothelial nitric oxide synthase in adipocyte lipolysis. *PLoS ONE* **2015**, *10*, e0136597. [CrossRef] [PubMed]

206. Ratziu, V.; Harrison, S.A.; Francque, S.; Bedossa, P.; Lehert, P.; Serfaty, L.; Romero-Gomez, M.; Boursier, J.; Abdelmalek, M.; Caldwell, S.; et al. Elafibranor, an agonist of the peroxisome proliferator-activated receptor-α and -β, induces resolution of nonalcoholic steatohepatitis without fibrosis worsening. *Gastroenterology* **2016**, *150*, 1147–1159. [CrossRef] [PubMed]

207. Lamba, V.; Yasuda, K.; Lamba, J.K.; Assem, M.; Davila, J.; Strom, S.; Schuetz, E.G. PXR (NR1I2): Splice variants in human tissues, including brain, and identification of neurosteroids and nicotine as PXR activators. *Toxicol. Appl. Pharmacol.* **2004**, *199*, 251–265. [CrossRef] [PubMed]

208. Haughton, E.L.; Tucker, S.J.; Marek, C.J.; Durward, E.; Leel, V.; Bascal, Z.; Monaghan, T.; Koruth, M.; Collie-Duguid, E.; Mann, D.A.; et al. Pregnane X receptor activators inhibit human hepatic stellate cell transdifferentiation in vitro. *Gastroenterology* **2006**, *131*, 194–209. [CrossRef] [PubMed]

209. Sookoian, S.; Castano, G.O.; Burgueno, A.L.; Gianotti, T.F.; Rosselli, M.S.; Pirola, C.J. The nuclear receptor PXR gene variants are associated with liver injury in nonalcoholic fatty liver disease. *Pharmacogenet. Genom.* **2010**, *20*, 1–8. [CrossRef] [PubMed]

210. Breuker, C.; Planque, C.; Rajabi, F.; Nault, J.C.; Couchy, G.; Zucman-Rossi, J.; Evrard, A.; Kantar, J.; Chevet, E.; Bioulac-Sage, P.; et al. Characterization of a novel PXR isoform with potential dominant-negative properties. *J. Hepatol.* **2014**, *61*, 609–616. [CrossRef] [PubMed]

211. Monostory, K.; Dvorak, Z. Steroid regulation of drug-metabolizing cytochromes P450. *Curr. Drug Metab.* **2011**, *12*, 154–172. [CrossRef] [PubMed]

212. Spruiell, K.; Richardson, R.M.; Cullen, J.M.; Awumey, E.M.; Gonzalez, F.J.; Gyamfi, M.A. Role of pregnane X receptor in obesity and glucose homeostasis in male mice. *J. Biol. Chem.* **2014**, *289*, 3244–3261. [CrossRef] [PubMed]

213. Li, L.; Li, H.; Garzel, B.; Yang, H.; Sueyoshi, T.; Li, Q.; Shu, Y.; Zhang, J.; Hu, B.; Heyward, S.; et al. SLC13A5 is a novel transcriptional target of the pregnane X receptor and sensitizes drug-induced steatosis in human liver. *Mol. Pharmacol.* **2015**, *87*, 674–682. [CrossRef] [PubMed]

214. Sun, M.; Cui, W.; Woody, S.K.; Staudinger, J.L. Pregnane X receptor modulates the inflammatory response in primary cultures of hepatocytes. *Drug Metab. Dispos.* **2015**, *43*, 335–343. [CrossRef] [PubMed]

215. Nishimura, M.; Naito, S.; Yokoi, T. Tissue-specific mRNA expression profiles of human nuclear receptor subfamilies. *Drug Metab. Pharmacokinet.* **2004**, *19*, 135–149. [CrossRef] [PubMed]

216. Beilke, L.D.; Aleksunes, L.M.; Holland, R.D.; Besselsen, D.G.; Beger, R.D.; Klaassen, C.D.; Cherrington, N.J. Constitutive androstane receptor-mediated changes in bile acid composition contributes to hepatoprotection from lithocholic acid-induced liver injury in mice. *Drug Metab. Dispos.* **2009**, *37*, 1035–1045. [CrossRef] [PubMed]
217. Fisher, C.D.; Lickteig, A.J.; Augustine, L.M.; Ranger-Moore, J.; Jackson, J.P.; Ferguson, S.S.; Cherrington, N.J. Hepatic cytochrome P450 enzyme alterations in humans with progressive stages of nonalcoholic fatty liver disease. *Drug Metab. Dispos.* **2009**, *37*, 2087–2094. [CrossRef] [PubMed]
218. Gao, J.; He, J.; Zhai, Y.; Wada, T.; Xie, W. The constitutive androstane receptor is an anti-obesity nuclear receptor that improves insulin sensitivity. *J. Biol. Chem.* **2009**, *284*, 25984–25992. [CrossRef] [PubMed]
219. Sberna, A.L.; Assem, M.; Xiao, R.; Ayers, S.; Gautier, T.; Guiu, B.; Deckert, V.; Chevriaux, A.; Grober, J.; Le Guern, N.; et al. Constitutive androstane receptor activation decreases plasma apolipoprotein B-containing lipoproteins and atherosclerosis in low-density lipoprotein receptor-deficient mice. *Arterioscler. Thromb. Vasc. Biol.* **2011**, *31*, 2232–2239. [CrossRef] [PubMed]
220. Gao, J.; Yan, J.; Xu, M.; Ren, S.; Xie, W. CAR suppresses hepatic gluconeogenesis by facilitating the ubiquitination and degradation of PGC1α. *Mol. Endocrinol.* **2015**, *29*, 1558–1570. [CrossRef] [PubMed]
221. Dong, B.; Lee, J.S.; Park, Y.Y.; Yang, F.; Xu, G.; Huang, W.; Finegold, M.J.; Moore, D.D. Activating CAR and β-catenin induces uncontrolled liver growth and tumorigenesis. *Nat. Commun.* **2015**, *6*. [CrossRef] [PubMed]
222. Li, D.; Mackowiak, B.; Brayman, T.G.; Mitchell, M.; Zhang, L.; Huang, S.M.; Wang, H. Genome-wide analysis of human constitutive androstane receptor (CAR) transcriptome in wild-type and CAR-knockout HepaRG cells. *Biochem. Pharmacol.* **2015**, *98*, 190–202. [CrossRef] [PubMed]
223. Kunne, C.; Acco, A.; Duijst, S.; de Waart, D.R.; Paulusma, C.C.; Gaemers, I.; Oude Elferink, R.P. FXR-dependent reduction of hepatic steatosis in a bile salt deficient mouse model. *Biochim. Biophys. Acta* **2014**, *1842*, 739–746. [CrossRef] [PubMed]
224. Pineda Torra, I.; Claudel, T.; Duval, C.; Kosykh, V.; Fruchart, J.C.; Staels, B. Bile acids induce the expression of the human peroxisome proliferator-activated receptor α gene via activation of the farnesoid X receptor. *Mol. Endocrinol.* **2003**, *17*, 259–272. [CrossRef] [PubMed]
225. Neuschwander-Tetri, B.A.; Loomba, R.; Sanyal, A.J.; Lavine, J.E.; van Natta, M.L.; Abdelmalek, M.F.; Chalasani, N.; Dasarathy, S.; Diehl, A.M.; Hameed, B.; et al. Farnesoid X nuclear receptor ligand obeticholic acid for non-cirrhotic, non-alcoholic steatohepatitis (FLINT): A multicentre, randomised, placebo-controlled trial. *Lancet* **2015**, *385*, 956–965. [CrossRef]
226. Cipriani, S.; Mencarelli, A.; Palladino, G.; Fiorucci, S. FXR activation reverses insulin resistance and lipid abnormalities and protects against liver steatosis in zucker (FA/FA) obese rats. *J. Lipid Res.* **2010**, *51*, 771–784. [CrossRef] [PubMed]
227. Ma, Y.; Huang, Y.; Yan, L.; Gao, M.; Liu, D. Synthetic FXR agonist GW4064 prevents diet-induced hepatic steatosis and insulin resistance. *Pharm. Res.* **2013**, *30*, 1447–1457. [CrossRef] [PubMed]
228. Mudaliar, S.; Henry, R.R.; Sanyal, A.J.; Morrow, L.; Marschall, H.U.; Kipnes, M.; Adorini, L.; Sciacca, C.I.; Clopton, P.; Castelloe, E.; et al. Efficacy and safety of the farnesoid x receptor agonist obeticholic acid in patients with type 2 diabetes and nonalcoholic fatty liver disease. *Gastroenterology* **2013**, *145*, 574–582. [CrossRef] [PubMed]
229. Jahn, D.; Rau, M.; Wohlfahrt, J.; Hermanns, H.M.; Geier, A. Non-alcoholic steatohepatitis: From pathophysiology to novel therapies. *Dig. Dis.* **2016**, *34*, 356–363. [CrossRef] [PubMed]
230. Tomlinson, E.; Fu, L.; John, L.; Hultgren, B.; Huang, X.; Renz, M.; Stephan, J.P.; Tsai, S.P.; Powell-Braxton, L.; French, D.; et al. Transgenic mice expressing human fibroblast growth factor-19 display increased metabolic rate and decreased adiposity. *Endocrinology* **2002**, *143*, 1741–1747. [CrossRef] [PubMed]
231. Fu, L.; John, L.M.; Adams, S.H.; Yu, X.X.; Tomlinson, E.; Renz, M.; Williams, P.M.; Soriano, R.; Corpuz, R.; Moffat, B.; et al. Fibroblast growth factor 19 increases metabolic rate and reverses dietary and leptin-deficient diabetes. *Endocrinology* **2004**, *145*, 2594–2603. [CrossRef] [PubMed]
232. Fang, S.; Suh, J.M.; Reilly, S.M.; Yu, E.; Osborn, O.; Lackey, D.; Yoshihara, E.; Perino, A.; Jacinto, S.; Lukasheva, Y.; et al. Intestinal FXR agonism promotes adipose tissue browning and reduces obesity and insulin resistance. *Nat. Med.* **2015**, *21*, 159–165. [CrossRef] [PubMed]
233. Degirolamo, C.; Modica, S.; Vacca, M.; Di Tullio, G.; Morgano, A.; D'Orazio, A.; Kannisto, K.; Parini, P.; Moschetta, A. Prevention of spontaneous hepatocarcinogenesis in farnesoid X receptor-null mice by intestinal-specific farnesoid x receptor reactivation. *Hepatology* **2015**, *61*, 161–170. [CrossRef] [PubMed]

234. Seki, E.; Brenner, D.A. Toll-like receptors and adaptor molecules in liver disease: Update. *Hepatology* **2008**, *48*, 322–335. [CrossRef] [PubMed]

235. Strowig, T.; Henao-Mejia, J.; Elinav, E.; Flavell, R. Inflammasomes in health and disease. *Nature* **2012**, *481*, 278–286. [CrossRef] [PubMed]

236. Vanni, E.; Bugianesi, E. The gut-liver axis in nonalcoholic fatty liver disease: Another pathway to insulin resistance? *Hepatology* **2009**, *49*, 1790–1792. [CrossRef] [PubMed]

237. Miele, L.; Valenza, V.; La Torre, G.; Montalto, M.; Cammarota, G.; Ricci, R.; Masciana, R.; Forgione, A.; Gabrieli, M.L.; Perotti, G.; et al. Increased intestinal permeability and tight junction alterations in nonalcoholic fatty liver disease. *Hepatology* **2009**, *49*, 1877–1887. [CrossRef] [PubMed]

238. Akira, S.; Uematsu, S.; Takeuchi, O. Pathogen recognition and innate immunity. *Cell* **2006**, *124*, 783–801. [CrossRef] [PubMed]

239. Raman, M.; Ahmed, I.; Gillevet, P.M.; Probert, C.S.; Ratcliffe, N.M.; Smith, S.; Greenwood, R.; Sikaroodi, M.; Lam, V.; Crotty, P.; et al. Fecal microbiome and volatile organic compound metabolome in obese humans with nonalcoholic fatty liver disease. *Clin. Gastroenterol. Hepatol.* **2013**, *11*, 868–875. [CrossRef] [PubMed]

240. Douhara, A.; Moriya, K.; Yoshiji, H.; Noguchi, R.; Namisaki, T.; Kitade, M.; Kaji, K.; Aihara, Y.; Nishimura, N.; Takeda, K.; et al. Reduction of endotoxin attenuates liver fibrosis through suppression of hepatic stellate cell activation and remission of intestinal permeability in a rat non-alcoholic steatohepatitis model. *Mol. Med. Rep.* **2015**, *11*, 1693–1700. [CrossRef] [PubMed]

241. Ehses, J.A.; Meier, D.T.; Wueest, S.; Rytka, J.; Boller, S.; Wielinga, P.Y.; Schraenen, A.; Lemaire, K.; Debray, S.; van Lommel, L.; et al. Toll-like receptor 2-deficient mice are protected from insulin resistance and β cell dysfunction induced by a high-fat diet. *Diabetologia* **2010**, *53*, 1795–1806. [CrossRef] [PubMed]

242. Vijay-Kumar, M.; Aitken, J.D.; Carvalho, F.A.; Cullender, T.C.; Mwangi, S.; Srinivasan, S.; Sitaraman, S.V.; Knight, R.; Ley, R.E.; Gewirtz, A.T. Metabolic syndrome and altered gut microbiota in mice lacking toll-like receptor 5. *Science* **2010**, *328*, 228–231. [CrossRef] [PubMed]

243. Al-Daghri, N.M.; Clerici, M.; Al-Attas, O.; Forni, D.; Alokail, M.S.; Alkharfy, K.M.; Sabico, S.; Mohammed, A.K.; Cagliani, R.; Sironi, M. A nonsense polymorphism (R392X) in TLR5 protects from obesity but predisposes to diabetes. *J. Immunol.* **2013**, *190*, 3716–3720. [CrossRef] [PubMed]

244. Miura, K.; Kodama, Y.; Inokuchi, S.; Schnabl, B.; Aoyama, T.; Ohnishi, H.; Olefsky, J.M.; Brenner, D.A.; Seki, E. Toll-like receptor 9 promotes steatohepatitis by induction of interleukin-1β in mice. *Gastroenterology* **2010**, *139*, 323–334. [CrossRef] [PubMed]

245. Gabele, E.; Dostert, K.; Hofmann, C.; Wiest, R.; Scholmerich, J.; Hellerbrand, C.; Obermeier, F. DSS induced colitis increases portal LPS levels and enhances hepatic inflammation and fibrogenesis in experimental NASH. *J. Hepatol.* **2011**, *55*, 1391–1399. [CrossRef] [PubMed]

246. Csak, T.; Velayudham, A.; Hritz, I.; Petrasek, J.; Levin, I.; Lippai, D.; Catalano, D.; Mandrekar, P.; Dolganiuc, A.; Kurt-Jones, E.; et al. Deficiency in myeloid differentiation factor-2 and toll-like receptor 4 expression attenuates nonalcoholic steatohepatitis and fibrosis in mice. *Am. J. Physiol. Gastrointest. Liver Physiol.* **2011**, *300*, G433–G441. [CrossRef] [PubMed]

247. Dolganiuc, A.; Norkina, O.; Kodys, K.; Catalano, D.; Bakis, G.; Marshall, C.; Mandrekar, P.; Szabo, G. Viral and host factors induce macrophage activation and loss of toll-like receptor tolerance in chronic HCV infection. *Gastroenterology* **2007**, *133*, 1627–1636. [CrossRef] [PubMed]

248. Beutler, B. Inferences, questions and possibilities in toll-like receptor signalling. *Nature* **2004**, *430*, 257–263. [CrossRef] [PubMed]

249. Kawasaki, T.; Kawai, T. Toll-like receptor signaling pathways. *Front. Immunol.* **2014**, *5*. [CrossRef] [PubMed]

250. Guo, J.; Friedman, S.L. Toll-like receptor 4 signaling in liver injury and hepatic fibrogenesis. *Fibrogenes. Tissue Repair* **2010**, *3*. [CrossRef] [PubMed]

251. Ye, D.; Li, F.Y.; Lam, K.S.; Li, H.; Jia, W.; Wang, Y.; Man, K.; Lo, C.M.; Li, X.; Xu, A. Toll-like receptor-4 mediates obesity-induced non-alcoholic steatohepatitis through activation of X-box binding protein-1 in mice. *Gut* **2012**, *61*, 1058–1067. [CrossRef] [PubMed]

252. Rivera, C.A.; Adegboyega, P.; van Rooijen, N.; Tagalicud, A.; Allman, M.; Wallace, M. Toll-like receptor-4 signaling and Kupffer cells play pivotal roles in the pathogenesis of non-alcoholic steatohepatitis. *J. Hepatol.* **2007**, *47*, 571–579. [CrossRef] [PubMed]

253. Szabo, G.; Bala, S. Alcoholic liver disease and the gut-liver axis. *World J. Gastroenterol.* **2010**, *16*, 1321–1329. [CrossRef] [PubMed]

254. Seki, E.; de Minicis, S.; Osterreicher, C.H.; Kluwe, J.; Osawa, Y.; Brenner, D.A.; Schwabe, R.F. TLR4 enhances TGF-β signaling and hepatic fibrosis. *Nat. Med.* **2007**, *13*, 1324–1332. [CrossRef] [PubMed]

255. Guo, J.; Loke, J.; Zheng, F.; Hong, F.; Yea, S.; Fukata, M.; Tarocchi, M.; Abar, O.T.; Huang, H.; Sninsky, J.J.; et al. Functional linkage of cirrhosis-predictive single nucleotide polymorphisms of toll-like receptor 4 to hepatic stellate cell responses. *Hepatology* **2009**, *49*, 960–968. [CrossRef] [PubMed]

256. Dasu, M.R.; Jialal, I. Free fatty acids in the presence of high glucose amplify monocyte inflammation via toll-like receptors. *Am. J. Physiol. Endocrinol. Metab.* **2011**, *300*, E145–E154. [CrossRef] [PubMed]

257. Shi, H.; Kokoeva, M.V.; Inouye, K.; Tzameli, I.; Yin, H.; Flier, J.S. TLR4 links innate immunity and fatty acid-induced insulin resistance. *J. Clin. Investig.* **2006**, *116*, 3015–3025. [CrossRef] [PubMed]

258. Dostert, C.; Petrilli, V.; van Bruggen, R.; Steele, C.; Mossman, B.T.; Tschopp, J. Innate immune activation through NALP3 inflammasome sensing of asbestos and silica. *Science* **2008**, *320*, 674–677. [CrossRef] [PubMed]

259. Shimada, K.; Crother, T.R.; Karlin, J.; Dagvadorj, J.; Chiba, N.; Chen, S.; Ramanujan, V.K.; Wolf, A.J.; Vergnes, L.; Ojcius, D.M.; et al. Oxidized mitochondrial DNA activates the NLRP3 inflammasome during apoptosis. *Immunity* **2012**, *36*, 401–414. [CrossRef] [PubMed]

260. Martinon, F.; Burns, K.; Tschopp, J. The inflammasome: A molecular platform triggering activation of inflammatory caspases and processing of proIL-β. *Mol. Cell* **2002**, *10*, 417–426. [CrossRef]

261. Szabo, G.; Csak, T. Inflammasomes in liver diseases. *J. Hepatol.* **2012**, *57*, 642–654. [CrossRef] [PubMed]

262. Dixon, L.J.; Flask, C.A.; Papouchado, B.G.; Feldstein, A.E.; Nagy, L.E. Caspase-1 as a central regulator of high fat diet-induced non-alcoholic steatohepatitis. *PLoS ONE* **2013**, *8*, e56100. [CrossRef] [PubMed]

263. Stienstra, R.; Joosten, L.A.; Koenen, T.; van Tits, B.; van Diepen, J.A.; van den Berg, S.A.; Rensen, P.C.; Voshol, P.J.; Fantuzzi, G.; Hijmans, A.; et al. The inflammasome-mediated caspase-1 activation controls adipocyte differentiation and insulin sensitivity. *Cell Metab.* **2010**, *12*, 593–605. [CrossRef] [PubMed]

264. Membrez, M.; Ammon-Zufferey, C.; Philippe, D.; Aprikian, O.; Monnard, I.; Mace, K.; Darimont, C. Interleukin-18 protein level is upregulated in adipose tissue of obese mice. *Obesity* **2009**, *17*, 393–395. [CrossRef] [PubMed]

265. Csak, T.; Pillai, A.; Ganz, M.; Lippai, D.; Petrasek, J.; Park, J.K.; Kodys, K.; Dolganiuc, A.; Kurt-Jones, E.A.; Szabo, G. Both bone marrow-derived and non-bone marrow-derived cells contribute to AIM2 and NLRP3 inflammasome activation in a MyD88-dependent manner in dietary steatohepatitis. *Liver Int.* **2014**, *34*, 1402–1413. [CrossRef] [PubMed]

266. Ganz, M.; Bukong, T.N.; Csak, T.; Saha, B.; Park, J.K.; Ambade, A.; Kodys, K.; Szabo, G. Progression of non-alcoholic steatosis to steatohepatitis and fibrosis parallels cumulative accumulation of danger signals that promote inflammation and liver tumors in a high fat-cholesterol-sugar diet model in mice. *J. Transl. Med.* **2015**, *13*. [CrossRef] [PubMed]

267. Vandanmagsar, B.; Youm, Y.H.; Ravussin, A.; Galgani, J.E.; Stadler, K.; Mynatt, R.L.; Ravussin, E.; Stephens, J.M.; Dixit, V.D. The NLRP3 inflammasome instigates obesity-induced inflammation and insulin resistance. *Nat. Med.* **2011**, *17*, 179–188. [CrossRef] [PubMed]

268. Wree, A.; McGeough, M.D.; Pena, C.A.; Schlattjan, M.; Li, H.; Inzaugarat, M.E.; Messer, K.; Canbay, A.; Hoffman, H.M.; Feldstein, A.E. NLRP3 inflammasome activation is required for fibrosis development in NAFLD. *J. Mol. Med.* **2014**, *92*, 1069–1082. [CrossRef] [PubMed]

269. Henao-Mejia, J.; Elinav, E.; Jin, C.; Hao, L.; Mehal, W.Z.; Strowig, T.; Thaiss, C.A.; Kau, A.L.; Eisenbarth, S.C.; Jurczak, M.J.; et al. Inflammasome-mediated dysbiosis regulates progression of NAFLD and obesity. *Nature* **2012**, *482*, 179–185. [CrossRef] [PubMed]

270. Wree, A.; Eguchi, A.; McGeough, M.D.; Pena, C.A.; Johnson, C.D.; Canbay, A.; Hoffman, H.M.; Feldstein, A.E. NLRP3 inflammasome activation results in hepatocyte pyroptosis, liver inflammation, and fibrosis in mice. *Hepatology* **2014**, *59*, 898–910. [CrossRef] [PubMed]

271. Seki, E.; Schwabe, R.F. Hepatic inflammation and fibrosis: Functional links and key pathways. *Hepatology* **2015**, *61*, 1066–1079. [CrossRef] [PubMed]

272. Luedde, T.; Kaplowitz, N.; Schwabe, R.F. Cell death and cell death responses in liver disease: Mechanisms and clinical relevance. *Gastroenterology* **2014**, *147*, 765–783. [CrossRef] [PubMed]

273. Huebener, P.; Pradere, J.P.; Hernandez, C.; Gwak, G.Y.; Caviglia, J.M.; Mu, X.; Loike, J.D.; Jenkins, R.E.; Antoine, D.J.; Schwabe, R.F. The HMGB1/RAGE axis triggers neutrophil-mediated injury amplification following necrosis. *J. Clin. Investig.* **2015**, *125*, 539–550. [CrossRef] [PubMed]

274. Zhang, Q.; Raoof, M.; Chen, Y.; Sumi, Y.; Sursal, T.; Junger, W.; Brohi, K.; Itagaki, K.; Hauser, C.J. Circulating mitochondrial damps cause inflammatory responses to injury. *Nature* **2010**, *464*, 104–107. [CrossRef] [PubMed]

275. Tschopp, J. Mitochondria: Sovereign of inflammation? *Eur. J. Immunol.* **2011**, *41*, 1196–1202. [CrossRef] [PubMed]

276. Carp, H. Mitochondrial N-formylmethionyl proteins as chemoattractants for neutrophils. *J. Exp. Med.* **1982**, *155*, 264–275. [CrossRef] [PubMed]

277. Iyer, S.S.; Pulskens, W.P.; Sadler, J.J.; Butter, L.M.; Teske, G.J.; Ulland, T.K.; Eisenbarth, S.C.; Florquin, S.; Flavell, R.A.; Leemans, J.C.; et al. Necrotic cells trigger a sterile inflammatory response through the NLRP3 inflammasome. *Proc. Natl. Acad. Sci. USA* **2009**, *106*, 20388–20393. [CrossRef] [PubMed]

278. Nakahira, K.; Haspel, J.A.; Rathinam, V.A.; Lee, S.J.; Dolinay, T.; Lam, H.C.; Englert, J.A.; Rabinovitch, M.; Cernadas, M.; Kim, H.P.; et al. Autophagy proteins regulate innate immune responses by inhibiting the release of mitochondrial DNA mediated by the NALP3 inflammasome. *Nat. Immunol.* **2011**, *12*, 222–230. [CrossRef] [PubMed]

279. Coddou, C.; Yan, Z.; Obsil, T.; Huidobro-Toro, J.P.; Stojilkovic, S.S. Activation and regulation of purinergic P2X receptor channels. *Pharmacol. Rev.* **2011**, *63*, 641–683. [CrossRef] [PubMed]

280. Di Virgilio, F. Liaisons dangereuses: P2X$_7$ and the inflammasome. *Trends Pharmacol. Sci.* **2007**, *28*, 465–472. [CrossRef] [PubMed]

281. Stros, M. HMGB proteins: Interactions with DNA and chromatin. *Biochim. Biophys. Acta* **2010**, *1799*, 101–113. [CrossRef] [PubMed]

282. Scaffidi, P.; Misteli, T.; Bianchi, M.E. Release of chromatin protein HMGB1 by necrotic cells triggers inflammation. *Nature* **2002**, *418*, 191–195. [CrossRef] [PubMed]

283. Tsung, A.; Klune, J.R.; Zhang, X.; Jeyabalan, G.; Cao, Z.; Peng, X.; Stolz, D.B.; Geller, D.A.; Rosengart, M.R.; Billiar, T.R. HMGB1 release induced by liver ischemia involves toll-like receptor 4 dependent reactive oxygen species production and calcium-mediated signaling. *J. Exp. Med.* **2007**, *204*, 2913–2923. [CrossRef] [PubMed]

284. Bianchi, M.E. HMGB1 loves company. *J. Leukoc. Biol.* **2009**, *86*, 573–576. [CrossRef] [PubMed]

285. Hornung, V.; Bauernfeind, F.; Halle, A.; Samstad, E.O.; Kono, H.; Rock, K.L.; Fitzgerald, K.A.; Latz, E. Silica crystals and aluminum salts activate the NALP3 inflammasome through phagosomal destabilization. *Nat. Immunol.* **2008**, *9*, 847–856. [CrossRef] [PubMed]

286. Lotze, M.T.; Tracey, K.J. High-mobility group box 1 protein (HMGB1): Nuclear weapon in the immune arsenal. *Nat. Rev. Immunol.* **2005**, *5*, 331–342. [CrossRef] [PubMed]

287. Bluher, M. Clinical relevance of adipokines. *Diabetes Metab. J.* **2012**, *36*, 317–327. [CrossRef] [PubMed]

288. Marra, F.; Bertolani, C. Adipokines in liver diseases. *Hepatology* **2009**, *50*, 957–969. [CrossRef] [PubMed]

289. Polyzos, S.A.; Kountouras, J.; Zavos, C. Nonalcoholic fatty liver disease: The pathogenetic roles of insulin resistance and adipocytokines. *Curr. Mol. Med.* **2009**, *9*, 299–314. [CrossRef] [PubMed]

290. Polyzos, S.A.; Kountouras, J.; Zavos, C.; Tsiaousi, E. The role of adiponectin in the pathogenesis and treatment of non-alcoholic fatty liver disease. *Diabetes Obes. Metab.* **2010**, *12*, 365–383. [CrossRef] [PubMed]

291. Polyzos, S.A.; Kountouras, J.; Zavos, C. The multi-hit process and the antagonistic roles of tumor necrosis factor-α and adiponectin in non alcoholic fatty liver disease. *Hippokratia* **2009**, *13*, 127. [PubMed]

292. Tilg, H.; Hotamisligil, G.S. Nonalcoholic fatty liver disease: Cytokine-adipokine interplay and regulation of insulin resistance. *Gastroenterology* **2006**, *131*, 934–945. [CrossRef] [PubMed]

293. Moon, H.S.; Dalamaga, M.; Kim, S.Y.; Polyzos, S.A.; Hamnvik, O.P.; Magkos, F.; Paruthi, J.; Mantzoros, C.S. Leptin's role in lipodystrophic and nonlipodystrophic insulin-resistant and diabetic individuals. *Endocr. Rev.* **2013**, *34*, 377–412. [CrossRef] [PubMed]

294. Polyzos, S.A.; Kountouras, J.; Mantzoros, C.S. Leptin in nonalcoholic fatty liver disease: A narrative review. *Metabolism* **2015**, *64*, 60–78. [CrossRef] [PubMed]

295. Dattaroy, D.; Pourhoseini, S.; Das, S.; Alhasson, F.; Seth, R.K.; Nagarkatti, M.; Michelotti, G.A.; Diehl, A.M.; Chatterjee, S. Micro-RNA 21 inhibition of SMAD7 enhances fibrogenesis via leptin-mediated NADPH oxidase in experimental and human nonalcoholic steatohepatitis. *Am. J. Physiol. Gastrointest. Liver Physiol.* **2015**, *308*, G298–G312. [CrossRef] [PubMed]

296. Zhou, Q.; Guan, W.; Qiao, H.; Cheng, Y.; Li, Z.; Zhai, X.; Zhou, Y. Gata binding protein 2 mediates leptin inhibition of PPARγ1 expression in hepatic stellate cells and contributes to hepatic stellate cell activation. *Biochim. Biophys. Acta* **2014**, *1842*, 2367–2377. [CrossRef] [PubMed]

297. Heinrich, G.; Russo, L.; Castaneda, T.R.; Pfeiffer, V.; Ghadieh, H.E.; Ghanem, S.S.; Wu, J.; Faulkner, L.D.; Ergun, S.; McInerney, M.F.; et al. Leptin resistance contributes to obesity in mice with null mutation of carcinoembryonic antigen-related cell adhesion molecule 1. *J. Biol. Chem.* **2016**, *291*, 11124–11132. [CrossRef] [PubMed]

298. Poy, M.N.; Yang, Y.; Rezaei, K.; Fernstrom, M.A.; Lee, A.D.; Kido, Y.; Erickson, S.K.; Najjar, S.M. CEACAM1 regulates insulin clearance in liver. *Nat. Genet.* **2002**, *30*, 270–276. [CrossRef] [PubMed]

299. DeAngelis, A.M.; Heinrich, G.; Dai, T.; Bowman, T.A.; Patel, P.R.; Lee, S.J.; Hong, E.G.; Jung, D.Y.; Assmann, A.; Kulkarni, R.N.; et al. Carcinoembryonic antigen-related cell adhesion molecule 1: A link between insulin and lipid metabolism. *Diabetes* **2008**, *57*, 2296–2303. [CrossRef] [PubMed]

300. Yoda-Murakami, M.; Taniguchi, M.; Takahashi, K.; Kawamata, S.; Saito, K.; Choi-Miura, N.H.; Tomita, M. Change in expression of GBP28/adiponectin in carbon tetrachloride-administrated mouse liver. *Biochem. Biophys. Res. Commun.* **2001**, *285*, 372–377. [CrossRef] [PubMed]

301. Heiker, J.T.; Kosel, D.; Beck-Sickinger, A.G. Molecular mechanisms of signal transduction via adiponectin and adiponectin receptors. *Biol. Chem.* **2010**, *391*, 1005–1018. [CrossRef] [PubMed]

302. Jiang, C.; Qu, A.; Matsubara, T.; Chanturiya, T.; Jou, W.; Gavrilova, O.; Shah, Y.M.; Gonzalez, F.J. Disruption of hypoxia-inducible factor 1 in adipocytes improves insulin sensitivity and decreases adiposity in high-fat diet-fed mice. *Diabetes* **2011**, *60*, 2484–2495. [CrossRef] [PubMed]

303. Otani, H. Oxidative stress as pathogenesis of cardiovascular risk associated with metabolic syndrome. *Antioxid. Redox Signal.* **2011**, *15*, 1911–1926. [CrossRef] [PubMed]

304. Kusminski, C.M.; Scherer, P.E. Mitochondrial dysfunction in white adipose tissue. *Trends Endocrinol. Metab.* **2012**, *23*, 435–443. [CrossRef] [PubMed]

305. Polyzos, S.A.; Kountouras, J.; Zavos, C. Nonlinear distribution of adiponectin in patients with nonalcoholic fatty liver disease limits its use in linear regression analysis. *J. Clin. Gastroenterol.* **2010**, *44*, 229–230. [CrossRef] [PubMed]

306. Van der Poorten, D.; Samer, C.F.; Ramezani-Moghadam, M.; Coulter, S.; Kacevska, M.; Schrijnders, D.; Wu, L.E.; McLeod, D.; Bugianesi, E.; Komuta, M.; et al. Hepatic fat loss in advanced nonalcoholic steatohepatitis: Are alterations in serum adiponectin the cause? *Hepatology* **2013**, *57*, 2180–2188. [CrossRef] [PubMed]

307. Bozaoglu, K.; Bolton, K.; McMillan, J.; Zimmet, P.; Jowett, J.; Collier, G.; Walder, K.; Segal, D. Chemerin is a novel adipokine associated with obesity and metabolic syndrome. *Endocrinology* **2007**, *148*, 4687–4694. [CrossRef] [PubMed]

308. Sell, H.; Divoux, A.; Poitou, C.; Basdevant, A.; Bouillot, J.L.; Bedossa, P.; Tordjman, J.; Eckel, J.; Clement, K. Chemerin correlates with markers for fatty liver in morbidly obese patients and strongly decreases after weight loss induced by bariatric surgery. *J. Clin. Endocrinol. Metab.* **2010**, *95*, 2892–2896. [CrossRef] [PubMed]

309. Ernst, M.C.; Issa, M.; Goralski, K.B.; Sinal, C.J. Chemerin exacerbates glucose intolerance in mouse models of obesity and diabetes. *Endocrinology* **2010**, *151*, 1998–2007. [CrossRef] [PubMed]

310. Yoshimura, T.; Oppenheim, J.J. Chemerin reveals its chimeric nature. *J. Exp. Med.* **2008**, *205*, 2187–2190. [CrossRef] [PubMed]

311. Krautbauer, S.; Wanninger, J.; Eisinger, K.; Hader, Y.; Beck, M.; Kopp, A.; Schmid, A.; Weiss, T.S.; Dorn, C.; Buechler, C. Chemerin is highly expressed in hepatocytes and is induced in non-alcoholic steatohepatitis liver. *Exp. Mol. Pathol.* **2013**, *95*, 199–205. [CrossRef] [PubMed]

312. Topping, D.L.; Clifton, P.M. Short-chain fatty acids and human colonic function: Roles of resistant starch and nonstarch polysaccharides. *Physiol. Rev.* **2001**, *81*, 1031–1064. [PubMed]

313. Turnbaugh, P.J.; Ley, R.E.; Mahowald, M.A.; Magrini, V.; Mardis, E.R.; Gordon, J.I. An obesity-associated gut microbiome with increased capacity for energy harvest. *Nature* **2006**, *444*, 1027–1031. [CrossRef] [PubMed]

314. Shin, N.R.; Lee, J.C.; Lee, H.Y.; Kim, M.S.; Whon, T.W.; Lee, M.S.; Bae, J.W. An increase in the *Akkermansia* spp. population induced by metformin treatment improves glucose homeostasis in diet-induced obese mice. *Gut* **2014**, *63*, 727–735. [CrossRef] [PubMed]

315. Karlsson, C.L.; Onnerfalt, J.; Xu, J.; Molin, G.; Ahrne, S.; Thorngren-Jerneck, K. The microbiota of the gut in preschool children with normal and excessive body weight. *Obesity* **2012**, *20*, 2257–2261. [CrossRef] [PubMed]

316. Zeisel, S.H.; Wishnok, J.S.; Blusztajn, J.K. Formation of methylamines from ingested choline and lecithin. *J. Pharmacol. Exp. Ther.* **1983**, *225*, 320–324. [PubMed]

317. Spencer, M.D.; Hamp, T.J.; Reid, R.W.; Fischer, L.M.; Zeisel, S.H.; Fodor, A.A. Association between composition of the human gastrointestinal microbiome and development of fatty liver with choline deficiency. *Gastroenterology* **2011**, *140*, 976–986. [CrossRef] [PubMed]

318. Sinal, C.J.; Tohkin, M.; Miyata, M.; Ward, J.M.; Lambert, G.; Gonzalez, F.J. Targeted disruption of the nuclear receptor FXR/BAR impairs bile acid and lipid homeostasis. *Cell* **2000**, *102*, 731–744. [CrossRef]

319. Hylemon, P.B.; Zhou, H.; Pandak, W.M.; Ren, S.; Gil, G.; Dent, P. Bile acids as regulatory molecules. *J. Lipid Res.* **2009**, *50*, 1509–1520. [CrossRef] [PubMed]

320. Tremaroli, V.; Backhed, F. Functional interactions between the gut microbiota and host metabolism. *Nature* **2012**, *489*, 242–249. [CrossRef] [PubMed]

321. Prawitt, J.; Abdelkarim, M.; Stroeve, J.H.; Popescu, I.; Duez, H.; Velagapudi, V.R.; Dumont, J.; Bouchaert, E.; van Dijk, T.H.; Lucas, A.; et al. Farnesoid X receptor deficiency improves glucose homeostasis in mouse models of obesity. *Diabetes* **2011**, *60*, 1861–1871. [CrossRef] [PubMed]

322. Thomas, C.; Gioiello, A.; Noriega, L.; Strehle, A.; Oury, J.; Rizzo, G.; Macchiarulo, A.; Yamamoto, H.; Mataki, C.; Pruzanski, M.; et al. TGR5-mediated bile acid sensing controls glucose homeostasis. *Cell Metab.* **2009**, *10*, 167–177. [CrossRef] [PubMed]

323. Cope, K.; Risby, T.; Diehl, A.M. Increased gastrointestinal ethanol production in obese mice: Implications for fatty liver disease pathogenesis. *Gastroenterology* **2000**, *119*, 1340–1347. [CrossRef] [PubMed]

324. Zhu, L.; Baker, S.S.; Gill, C.; Liu, W.; Alkhouri, R.; Baker, R.D.; Gill, S.R. Characterization of gut microbiomes in nonalcoholic steatohepatitis (NASH) patients: A connection between endogenous alcohol and NASH. *Hepatology* **2013**, *57*, 601–609. [CrossRef] [PubMed]

325. Noverr, M.C.; Huffnagle, G.B. Does the microbiota regulate immune responses outside the gut? *Trends Microbiol.* **2004**, *12*, 562–568. [CrossRef] [PubMed]

326. Sabate, J.M.; Jouet, P.; Harnois, F.; Mechler, C.; Msika, S.; Grossin, M.; Coffin, B. High prevalence of small intestinal bacterial overgrowth in patients with morbid obesity: A contributor to severe hepatic steatosis. *Obes. Surg.* **2008**, *18*, 371–377. [CrossRef] [PubMed]

327. Wigg, A.J.; Roberts-Thomson, I.C.; Dymock, R.B.; McCarthy, P.J.; Grose, R.H.; Cummins, A.G. The role of small intestinal bacterial overgrowth, intestinal permeability, endotoxaemia, and tumour necrosis factor $\alpha$ in the pathogenesis of non-alcoholic steatohepatitis. *Gut* **2001**, *48*, 206–211. [CrossRef] [PubMed]

328. Minemura, M.; Shimizu, Y. Gut microbiota and liver diseases. *World J. Gastroenterol.* **2015**, *21*, 1691–1702. [CrossRef] [PubMed]

329. Fukui, H. Gut-liver axis in liver cirrhosis: How to manage leaky gut and endotoxemia. *World J. Hepatol.* **2015**, *7*, 425–442. [CrossRef] [PubMed]

# 9

# Relationship between Non-Alcoholic Fatty Liver Disease and Psoriasis: A Novel Hepato-Dermal Axis?

Alessandro Mantovani [1], Paolo Gisondi [2], Amedeo Lonardo [3] and Giovanni Targher [1,*]

[1]  Section of Endocrinology, Diabetes and Metabolism, Department of Medicine,
    University and Azienda Ospedaliera Universitaria Integrata of Verona, Piazzale Stefani, 1,
    Verona 37126, Italy; alessandro.mantovani24@gmail.com

[2]  Section of Dermatology, Department of Medicine, University and Azienda Ospedaliera Universitaria
    Integrata of Verona, Piazzale Stefani, 1, Verona 37126, Italy; paolo.gisondi@univr.it

[3]  Outpatient Liver Clinic and Division of Internal Medicine—Department of Biomedical,
    Metabolic and Neural Sciences, NOCSAE, University of Modena and Reggio Emilia and
    Azienda USL Modena, Baggiovara, Modena 41126, Italy; a.lonardo@libero.it

*   Correspondence: giovanni.targher@univr.it

Academic Editor: Johannes Haybaeck

**Abstract:** Over the past 10 years, it has become increasingly evident that nonalcoholic fatty liver disease (NAFLD) is a multisystem disease that affects multiple extra-hepatic organ systems and interacts with the regulation of several metabolic and immunological pathways. In this review we discuss the rapidly expanding body of clinical and epidemiological evidence supporting a strong association between NAFLD and chronic plaque psoriasis. We also briefly discuss the possible biological mechanisms underlying this association, and discuss treatment options for psoriasis that may influence NAFLD development and progression. Recent observational studies have shown that the prevalence of NAFLD (as diagnosed either by imaging or by histology) is remarkably higher in psoriatic patients (occurring in up to 50% of these patients) than in matched control subjects. Notably, psoriasis is associated with NAFLD even after adjusting for metabolic syndrome traits and other potential confounding factors. Some studies have also suggested that psoriatic patients are more likely to have the more advanced forms of NAFLD than non-psoriatic controls, and that psoriatic patients with NAFLD have more severe psoriasis than those without NAFLD. In conclusion, the published evidence argues for more careful evaluation and surveillance of NAFLD among patients with psoriasis.

**Keywords:** nonalcoholic fatty liver disease; NAFLD; nonalcoholic steatohepatitis; management; psoriasis

## 1. Introduction

Psoriasis is a chronic, immune-mediated, inflammatory skin disease that affects approximately 2%–3% of the adults in the general population of Western countries [1,2]. This disease is known for its typical cutaneous manifestations; described as well-demarcated, erythematous oval plaques with adherent silvery scales. However, recent studies have also linked psoriasis with multiple comorbid conditions, including arthritis, uveitis, inflammatory bowel diseases, depression, osteoporosis, cardiovascular disease and metabolic syndrome [3].

In parallel, nonalcoholic fatty liver disease (NAFLD) is the most frequent liver disease worldwide, affecting an estimated 30% of the adult population in developed countries [4,5]. NAFLD and the metabolic syndrome are mutually and bi-directionally associated, as these two pathologic conditions share insulin resistance as a common pathophysiological mechanism [6–8]. NAFLD encompasses a spectrum of pathologic conditions ranging from simple steatosis to nonalcoholic steatohepatitis ((NASH) featuring steatosis associated with inflammatory changes, hepatocellular ballooning and pericellular fibrosis), to advanced fibrosis and cirrhosis. NAFLD is projected to become the most common indication for liver transplantation in the United States by 2030 [5,9]. However, over the past 10 years, it has become increasingly clear that NAFLD is not only associated with increased liver-related mortality or morbidity, but also is a multisystem disease affecting a variety of extra-hepatic organ systems, including the heart and the vascular system [9,10]. Cardiovascular disease represents the primary cause of mortality in NAFLD patients [9,10].

In this updated review we will discuss the clinical evidence supporting a link between NAFLD and chronic plaque psoriasis, and the putative mechanisms underlying this association. We will also briefly discuss some of the therapeutic options for psoriasis that may influence NAFLD development and progression. We extensively searched PubMed database to identify original articles published through December 31st 2015, using the following key-words "nonalcoholic fatty liver disease" or "NAFLD" combined with "chronic plaque psoriasis", "psoriasis" or "psoriatic treatment".

## 2. Epidemiology, Clinical Manifestations and Pathogenesis of Psoriasis

Psoriasis is a chronic, recurrent, immune-mediated inflammatory disease of the skin, affecting approximately 2%–3% of the general adult population in many parts of the world [1]. The prevalence of this disease in adults ranges from approximately 1% (United States) to 8.5% (Norway). The incidence estimate varies from approximately 80/100,000 person-years (United States) to 230/100,000 person-years (Italy) [1]. Epidemiological studies suggest that the prevalence of psoriasis varies according to increasing age and is more common in countries more distant from the equator [1]. However, additional studies are needed to better understand the epidemiology of psoriasis and trends in incidence over time.

Psoriasis manifests as raised, irregularly round and well-demarcated erythematous lesions that are usually covered by silver scales (Figure 1).

Psoriatic lesions are distributed symmetrically on the scalp, elbows, knees, lumbo-sacral area and in the body folds. Psoriatic lesions are frequently symptomatic with pruritus by far the most bothersome skin symptom reported by the patients, even for those with limited disease, followed by scaling and flaking. Psoriasis may have a negative impact on the physical, emotional and psychosocial wellbeing of affected patients. About one third of patients have symptoms of arthritis, which might be very disabling in the more severe cases [11]. Psoriasis is also frequently associated with multiple metabolic co-morbidities, including abdominal overweight or obesity, type 2 diabetes, metabolic syndrome and NAFLD [3,12,13].

The exact aetiology of psoriasis is largely unknown. However, strong evidence indicates that psoriasis is a chronic inflammatory skin disease, occurring against a predisposing genetic background. The pathogenesis of psoriasis is complex, with a combination of genetic and environmental factors playing an integrated role [2]. The contribution of genetic factors to the pathogenesis of psoriasis is extensive, with the human leukocyte antigen (HLA)-C*06 showing the most significant association, although genome-wide association studies have identified more than 35 psoriasis risk gene regions primarily involved in innate and adaptive immunity [14]. A deregulated cytokine network occurs in psoriasis, leading to the release of multiple pro-inflammatory mediators from immune cells, which in turn induce increased keratinocyte proliferation [15]. Psoriasis is thought to be a T cell-driven disease, with the Th1 and Th17 cell populations playing a major role. These immune cells produce a variety of pro-inflammatory cytokines, including tumour necrosis factor (TNF)-α, interleukin (IL)-6, IL-17, IL-22 and interferon-gamma, resulting in abnormal differentiation and proliferation of keratinocytes, blood vessels dilatation and inflammatory infiltration of leukocytes into the dermis and epidermis [15,16]. A number of environmental factors have been also identified as possible triggers of psoriasis, including physical traumas (known as Koebner's phenomenon), bacterial infections, stressful life events or use of some drugs, such as interferon α and lithium salts [2,15]. However, more precise identification of genetic and environmental factors that are potentially involved in the development of psoriasis will help to better elucidate the pathogenesis of this disease and identify new targets for a more specific and effective treatment.

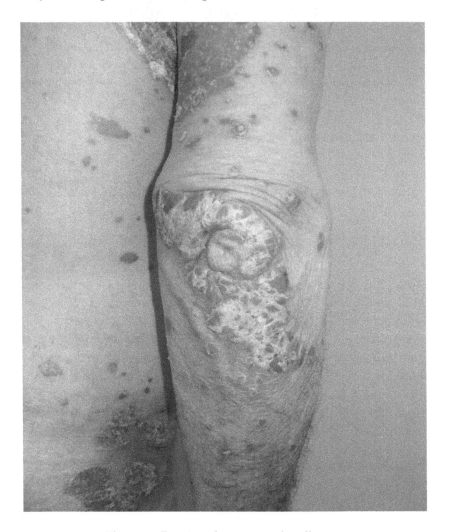

**Figure 1.** Psoriatic lesions on the elbows.

### 3. Epidemiological Evidence Linking Nonalcoholic Fatty Liver Disease (NAFLD) to Psoriasis

Given the strong relationship of the metabolic syndrome with both psoriasis [3,12,13] and NAFLD [4–6], it is perhaps not surprising that these two latter diseases may coexist within the same individual.

In a case report published in 2001 Lonardo *et al.* [17] were the first to describe three cases of concurrent psoriasis vulgaris and NASH, diagnosed on biopsy. All patients were obese and had other features of the metabolic syndrome. Similarly, Matsumoto *et al.* [18] described a case of a young obese psoriatic man with NASH that improved after hypocaloric diet.

As detailed in Table 1, after these pioneering case reports, multiple observational (cross-sectional and case-control) studies have recently assessed whether NAFLD (as diagnosed either by ultrasonography or by histology) is associated with psoriasis [19–27].

**Table 1.** Principal studies examining the relationship between NAFLD and psoriasis (ordered by publication year).

| Authors, Year (Reference) | Study Characteristics | NAFLD Diagnosis | Main Findings |
|---|---|---|---|
| Gisondi et al. 2009 [19] | Cross-sectional: 130 consecutive Italian patients with chronic plaque psoriasis and 260 healthy controls matched for age, sex and BMI | Ultrasonography | Prevalence of NAFLD was remarkably higher in psoriatic patients than in matched controls (47% vs. 28%; p < 0.001). Patients with psoriasis and NAFLD were more likely to have metabolic syndrome and had higher serum C-reactive protein concentrations and greater severity of psoriasis according to PASI score than those with psoriasis alone. At multivariate linear regression analysis, NAFLD was associated with higher PASI score (standardized β coefficient 0.19, p = 0.03), independent of age, sex, BMI, psoriasis duration and alcohol consumption |
| Miele et al. 2009 [20] | Retrospective, case-control: 142 Italian patients with psoriasis and 125 non-psoriatic patients with biopsy-proven NAFLD comparable for age and BMI | Ultrasonography and biopsy | Prevalence of NAFLD was 59.2% in the cohort of psoriatic patients. In these patients NAFLD was significantly associated with metabolic syndrome and psoriatic arthritis. Compared with the non-psoriatic NAFLD cohort, psoriatic patients with NAFLD were likely to have more severe NAFLD reflected by either non-invasive NAFLD Fibrosis score or AST/ALT ratio >1 |
| Madanagobalane et al. 2012 [21] | Cross-sectional: 333 Indian psoriatic patients and 330 controls matched for age, sex and BMI | Ultrasonography and liver enzymes | Prevalence of NAFLD was higher in psoriatic patients than in matched controls (17.4% vs. 7.9%; p < 0.005). Psoriatic patients with NAFLD had more severe psoriasis than those without NAFLD. In a subset of participants, psoriatic patients had more severe forms of NAFLD than non-psoriatic patients with NAFLD (as estimated by non-invasive fibrosis markers) |
| van der Voort et al. 2014 [22] | Cross-sectional: population-based cohort of 2292 Dutch elderly participants (the Rotterdam Study) | Ultrasonography | Prevalence of psoriasis was 5.1% (by a validated algorithm). Prevalence of NAFLD was higher in psoriatic patients than in participants without psoriasis (46.2% vs. 33.3%, p = 0.005). Psoriasis was associated with NAFLD (OR 1.70, 95% CI 1.1–2.6, p = 0.01), independent of age, sex, alcohol consumption, pack-years and smoking status, metabolic syndrome, and serum ALT levels |
| van der Voort et al. 2015 [23] | Cross-sectional: population-based cohort of 1535 elderly participants (the Rotterdam Study) of whom 74 (4.7%) had psoriasis | Ultrasonography and transient elastography (Fibroscan) | Prevalence of NAFLD was higher in subjects with psoriasis than in those without psoriasis (44.3% vs. 34%, p < 0.05). Moreover, prevalence of advanced liver fibrosis was 8.1% in psoriatic patients compared with 3.6% in the control group (p < 0.05). Multivariate logistic regression analysis revealed that the risk of advanced liver fibrosis remained higher in psoriatic patients after adjustment for age, sex, alcohol consumption, serum ALT levels, presence of metabolic syndrome and hepatic steatosis (OR 2.57, 95% CI 1.0–6.6) |
| Gisondi et al. 2015 [24] | Cross-sectional: 124 Italian patients with psoriasis and 79 healthy controls | Ultrasonography | Prevalence of NAFLD was higher in psoriatic patients than in controls (44% vs. 26%, p < 0.001). NAFLD fibrosis score was also higher in psoriatic patients (p < 0.001). Multivariate regression analysis revealed that psoriasis was associated with higher NAFLD fibrosis score, independent of age, sex, BMI, hypertension and pre-existing diabetes |
| Abedini et al. 2015 [25] | Cross-sectional: 123 Iranian patients with psoriasis and 123 healthy controls matched by age, sex and BMI | Ultrasonography | Prevalence of NAFLD was higher in psoriatic patients than in matched controls (65.6% vs. 35%, p < 0.01). Multivariate logistic regression analysis revealed that PASI score, waist circumference, hypertension and serum aminotransferase levels independently predicted the ultrasonographic severity of NAFLD |
| Roberts et al. 2015 [26] | Cross-sectional: 103 United States adult patients with a diagnosis of psoriasis or psoriatic arthritis | Ultrasonography and biopsy (available in a subgroup of 52 patients) | The overall prevalence of NAFLD was 47%. The prevalence of NASH was 22% in those who underwent liver biopsy. Psoriatic patients with NAFLD had higher mean PASI scores than those without NAFLD |
| Candia et al. 2015 [27] | Systematic review and meta-analysis: 7 case-control studies included | Ultrasonography and liver enzymes | Psoriatic patients had an increased risk of prevalent NAFLD compared with control subjects (6 studies, n = 267,761 patients, OR 2.15, 95% CI 1.6–2.9, p < 0.05). The risk of prevalent NAFLD was higher in patients with psoriatic arthritis (3 studies, n = 505 patients, OR 2.25, 95% CI 1.4–3.7, p < 0.05) and in those with moderate-to-severe psoriasis compared with patients with mild psoriasis (2 studies, n = 51,930 patients, OR 2.07, 95% CI 1.6–2.7, p < 0.05) |

Abbreviations: ALT, alanine aminotransferase; AST, aspartate aminotransferase; BMI, body mass index; CI, confidence interval; NAFLD, nonalcoholic fatty liver disease; NASH, nonalcoholic steatohepatitis; PASI, psoriasis area and severity index; OR, odds ratio.

For instance, in a case-control study involving 130 consecutive patients with chronic plaque psoriasis (none of whom treated with methotrexate or other potentially hepato-toxic drugs) and 260 matched healthy controls, Gisondi et al. [19] have documented that NAFLD prevalence was almost two times higher among psoriatic patients than among control individuals (47% vs. 28%, $p < 0.001$). This difference remained significant (37% vs. 21%; $p < 0.01$), even after excluding subjects with mild-moderate alcohol consumption (i.e., those who drank less than 30 grams of alcohol per day). Patients with psoriasis and NAFLD were also more likely to have higher circulating levels of C-reactive protein, IL-6 and lower adiponectin levels than those without NAFLD. Furthermore, NAFLD was associated with a greater clinical severity of psoriasis as estimated by the Psoriasis Area and Severity Index (PASI) score after adjusting for many cardio-metabolic risk factors [19]. This score measures the severity of psoriatic lesions (evaluating the degree of erythema, thickness, and scaling of psoriatic plaques in four separate body areas) based on area coverage and plaque appearance.

In another retrospective study Miele et al. [20] found a NAFLD prevalence of 59.2% in an outpatient cohort of 142 adults with psoriasis. Although there were no differences in PASI score between psoriatic patients with or without NAFLD, those with NAFLD were more likely to have psoriatic arthritis and more severe NAFLD as estimated non-invasively with the NAFLD fibrosis score. Unfortunately, data on liver biopsy were available only for five psoriatic patients, but revealed that three of these patients had histologically proven NASH.

Interestingly, in a large population-based cohort study which included 2292 elderly individuals of whom 5.1% had psoriasis, van der Voort et al. [22] documented that the prevalence of NAFLD on ultrasonography was greater among psoriatic patients than among the reference group without psoriasis (46.2% vs. 33.3%, $p = 0.005$). Notably, multivariate regression analysis revealed that psoriatic participants were 70% more likely to have NAFLD than those without psoriasis (odds ratio (OR) 1.70, 95% confidence interval (CI) 1.1–2.6, $p = 0.01$), independent of metabolic syndrome and other common NAFLD risk factors. In a subsequent analysis of the same cohort, the authors have also reported that the prevalence of advanced hepatic fibrosis, as detected by transient elastography, was greater among those with psoriasis than among those without this disease (8.1% vs. 3.6%, $p < 0.05$), and that psoriatic patients were twice as likely to have advanced hepatic fibrosis, irrespective of common risk factors (adjusted-OR 2.57, 95% CI 1.0–6.6) [23]. Similarly, in a smaller case-control study, Gisondi et al. [24] reported that the NAFLD fibrosis score (i.e., a non-invasive scoring system that identifies advanced hepatic fibrosis) was higher in psoriatic patients than in control subjects, and psoriasis predicted advanced liver fibrosis, independently of coexisting metabolic syndrome features and other potential confounding factors.

Recently, in a cross-sectional study involving 103 United States middle-aged adult patients with psoriasis or psoriatic arthritis recruited over a 24-month period, Roberts et al. [26] found that the prevalence of ultrasound-diagnosed NAFLD was 47%, whereas that of NASH was 22% among those ($n = 52$) who underwent liver biopsy. Moreover, similarly to previous studies, the authors also found that psoriatic patients with NAFLD had significantly higher PASI scores than those without this disease.

Finally, a recent systematic review and meta-analysis of seven case-control studies confirmed that psoriatic patients had a two-fold increased rate of prevalent NAFLD compared with non-psoriatic control individuals, and that this risk was higher among those with either more severe psoriasis or psoriatic arthritis. Interestingly, the significant relationship between psoriasis and NAFLD was consistent in all studies included in this meta-analysis and was maintained even when the studies of lower methodological quality (due to poorly documented diagnosis of NAFLD or insufficient adjustment for potential confounding variables) were excluded from the analysis [27]. However, it is important to note that the cross-sectional nature of the above-mentioned studies does not permit to ascertain the temporality and causality of the association between NAFLD and psoriasis [19–27]. Future follow-up studies are required to improve our understanding of this topic.

That said, the data available to date show that NAFLD prevalence is very high in patients with psoriasis (affecting up to 50% of these patients), independent of coexisting metabolic syndrome components. In addition, the relatively advanced stage of NASH revealed by the biopsies from psoriatic patients suggests the possibility of an increased risk of long-term liver-related complications in this patient population. Thus, the current evidence argues for more careful monitoring and evaluation of the presence of NAFLD in people with chronic plaque psoriasis.

## 4. Potential Biological Mechanisms Linking Psoriasis and NAFLD

To date, the underlying mechanisms linking NAFLD to psoriasis are complex and not fully understood. However, identification of the pathophysiological mechanisms linking these two diseases is of clinical relevance because it may offer the promise for novel pharmacological approaches.

Psoriasis and NAFLD share multiple inflammatory and cytokine-mediated mechanisms and are part of an intriguing network of genetic, clinical and pathophysiological features. Indeed, it is possible to assume that the mechanisms underlying the association between NAFLD and psoriasis are multifactorial (involving both genetic and environmental factors) and often overlap with metabolic abnormalities, which frequently coexist in psoriatic patients.

The schematic Figure 2 shows the possible links between expanded visceral adipose tissue, steatotic liver and psoriatic skin, and the signals passing between these three organs.

Although the liver is a key regulator of glucose metabolism, and is the leading source of multiple inflammatory and coagulation factors [5,9,28], the close inter-relationships of psoriasis and NAFLD with visceral obesity and insulin resistance make it very difficult to distinguish the individual contribution of NAFLD to the inflammatory and metabolic manifestations of psoriasis. Although the studies available in the literature do not allow to clearly determine the directionality of the association between NAFLD and psoriasis, it is conceivable that several pro-inflammatory cytokines (e.g., IL-6, IL-17, TNF-$\alpha$) that are locally over-produced by lymphocytes and keratinocytes into the skin of psoriatic patients may contribute, at least in part, to the pathogenesis of systemic insulin resistance [29,30], and that psoriatic patients with greater insulin resistance are the ones who get NAFLD. Undoubtedly, an expanded and inflamed (dysfunctional) visceral adipose tissue plays a key role in the development of insulin resistance, chronic inflammation and NAFLD, possibly through the secretion of multiple factors, such as increased release of non-esterified fatty acids, increased production of various hormones and pro-inflammatory adipocytokines (including also TNF-$\alpha$, IL-6, leptin, visfatin, and resistin), and decreased production of adiponectin [9,31–34]. In the presence of obesity and insulin resistance, there is an increased influx of non-esterified fatty acids to the liver. There is now substantial evidence that non-esterified fatty acids play a key role in directly promoting liver injury by increasing intra-hepatic oxidative stress and by activating inflammatory pathways [9,31–34]. The central role of hepatocyte cytokine production in NAFLD progression is supported by studies showing that cytokines may replicate all of the histological features associated with NASH, including neutrophil chemotaxis, hepatocyte necrosis and stellate cell activation [9,31–34]. It is possible to assume that the increased release of non-esterified free fatty acids from the expanded and dysfunctional adipose tissue, in presence of insulin resistance, may also exert a deleterious impact on inflammatory skin lesions in psoriasis. However, to our knowledge, there are currently no reliable data regarding a direct pathogenic role of non-esterified fatty acids in the pathogenesis of psoriasis. Further studies are required to better elucidate this topic.

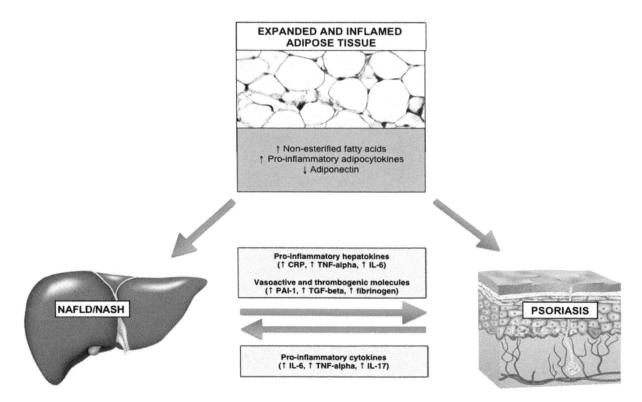

**Figure 2.** Possible mechanisms linking expanded and inflamed (dysfunctional) visceral adipose tissue, psoriasis and nonalcoholic fatty liver disease. Abbreviations: CRP, C-reactive protein; IL-6, interleukin-6; IL-17, interleukin-17; NAFLD, nonalcoholic fatty liver disease; NASH, nonalcoholic steatohepatitis; PAI-1, plasminogen activator inhibitor-1; TGF-β, transforming growth factor-β; TNF-α, tumor necrosis factor-α.

To date, accumulating evidence indicates that NAFLD, especially its necro-inflammatory and progressive form (NASH), may exacerbate insulin resistance, predisposes to atherogenic dyslipidemia and releases a myriad of pro-inflammatory, pro-coagulant, pro-oxidant and pro-fibrogenic mediators (e.g., C-reactive protein, IL-6, fibrinogen, plasminogen activator inhibitor-1, transforming growth factor-β) that may play important roles in the pathophysiology of psoriasis [5,9,31,35]. It is possible to hypothesize that the release of these pro-inflammatory, pro-oxidant and pro-atherogenic mediators from the steatotic and inflamed liver (which is also one of the most important mechanisms by which fatty liver directly contributes to the development of cardiovascular disease and type 2 diabetes [5,9,36]) may adversely influence the severity of psoriasis by increased keratinocyte proliferation, increased inflammation, and up-regulation of various vascular adhesion molecules. Experimentally, it has been also shown that induction of oxazolone-induced skin inflammation is more evident in NAFLD mice than in normal mice; oxazolone challenge significantly increases ear thickness, ear weight, nuclear factor-κB activity, and histological features of skin inflammation in NAFLD mice as compared to normal mice [37]. The oxazolone-induced skin inflammation model is not specifically designed to study the pathogenesis of psoriasis. Nevertheless, this simple mouse model of NAFLD-enhanced skin inflammation might be used to evaluate new therapeutic strategies for treatment of NAFLD with associated skin inflammation and also to understand the nexus between these two co-morbidities.

## 5. Treatment for Psoriasis and Its Potential Implications for NAFLD

Detailed discussion of treatment options for psoriasis is beyond the scope of this review and have been recently discussed elsewhere [38]. There are numerous treatment options against psoriasis and they are classified as topical, systemic or phototherapy. Systemic drugs such as methotrexate, cyclosporine and acitretin are indicated for moderate-to-severe psoriasis, especially when the disease is either widespread or resistant to topical therapy. In the case of intolerance, inefficacy or contraindication to either phototherapy or conventional systemic treatments, patients with psoriasis are eligible for newer biological agents, which include TNF-α antagonists (etanercept, adalimumab and infliximab), the anti-IL-2/23 monoclonal antibody ustekinumab, and the anti-IL-17 monoclonal antibodies secukinumab and ixekizumab [38].

From a clinical perspective, understanding whether psoriatic patients have underlying metabolic comorbidities, including NAFLD, is important to ensure that treatment is safe [38,39]. Indeed, while phototherapy or topical treatments are not expected to cause significant changes in metabolic parameters and liver function tests, some pharmacological treatments may negatively influence metabolic comorbidities (including NAFLD) or exert interactions with drugs that are commonly used to treat them [39].

In particular, methotrexate should be administered with caution in the presence of obesity, type 2 diabetes or NAFLD because of the increased risk of drug-induced hepatic fibrosis [40–42]. Indeed, psoriatic patients with type 2 diabetes or obesity are at higher risk of developing hepatic fibrosis during methotrexate treatment compared with those without such metabolic comorbidities [39]. The liver injury induced by methotrexate appears to mimic NAFLD histologically. So, drug induced liver injury should be always considered in a patient with hepatic steatosis who has been previously treated with methotrexate [40,41]. Similarly, cyclosporine should be used cautiously among psoriatic patients with coexisting metabolic syndrome. This drug may worsen type 2 diabetes, exacerbate arterial hypertension and predispose to atherogenic dyslipidemia and hyperuricemia [38,43]. Moreover, the drug interaction between cyclosporine and statins may also increase the risk of rhabdomyolysis [44]. In some cases, cyclosporine may induce liver injury and cholestasis with increased levels of serum aminotransferases, bilirubin and alkaline phosphatase [38,43]. However, cyclosporine-induced hepatitis is a relatively rare event that is less common than nephrotoxicity and occurs more frequently among liver-transplant patients. Acitretin is a vitamin A derivative that has been used to treat psoriasis since the early 1980s. The use of acitretin is limited by its potential adverse effects (e.g., muco-cutaneous effects, dyslipidemia and hepatotoxicity). These effects may be reduced by using lower doses of acitretin or in combination with other therapies [43,45].

Biologic drugs represent a major advancement in the treatment of psoriasis [38]. Generally, biologic agents do not seem to negatively affect metabolic parameters and serum liver enzyme levels as conventional systemic treatments can. Indeed, the drug survival of biologics is higher than that of conventional treatments because they are better tolerated in the longer term. Although the effects of TNF-α inhibitors on insulin sensitivity are a matter of intense debate [38,43,46], preliminary evidence suggests that treatment with etanercept (i.e., a TNF-α inhibitor) may improve both plasma glucose levels and insulin resistance indices [47], and that patients with psoriasis or rheumatoid arthritis receiving TNF-α inhibitors exhibit a lower risk of new-onset type 2 diabetes compared with those receiving other non-biological disease-modifying anti-rheumatic drugs [48]. Clinically meaningful dyslipidemia has been rarely reported in patients receiving etanercept or other TNF-α antagonists, so that it is not a serious concern in routine clinical practice [49]. A significant body weight gain, mainly due to increased fat mass, has been also documented among psoriatic patients receiving TNF-α antagonists [38,39,43], whereas it is not observed among those receiving the anti-IL-12/23 monoclonal antibody ustekinumab [50]. Mild to moderate elevations in serum transaminases may be observed in some patients receiving TNF-α antagonists (especially infliximab [51]), but they usually return to normal after discontinuation of the drug [38,43,52]. In a small clinical trial, Campanati et al. [53] have recently compared the effect of a 24-week treatment with etanercept versus phototherapy on serum markers of hepatic fibrosis in 89 overweight patients with psoriasis and NAFLD. Notably, they found that there were significant improvements in the aspartate aminotransferase-to-alanine aminotransferase ratio, serum C-reactive protein levels and insulin resistance indices only among psoriatic patients receiving etanercept. This finding suggests that etanercept is more efficacious to reduce the risk of hepatic fibrosis than phototherapy, and that this effect might be mainly dependent on its metabolic and anti-inflammatory properties. However, additional studies with more accurate and direct measures of hepatic fibrosis are needed to further examine this topic. Recently, preliminary evidence has suggested that NAFLD might also be a side effect of TNF-α inhibitor treatment in some cases, and that previous methotrexate exposure and patatin-like phospholipase domain-containing protein-3 (PNPLA3) genotype might be the most important risk factors [54]. Even though only few cases have been reported in the literature, TNF-α inhibitors may induce autoimmune hepatitis, granulomatous hepatitis, and reactivation of viral hepatitis [38,52].

Finally, similarly to patients with NAFLD, lifestyle interventions (hypocaloric diet, exercise and avoiding alcohol consumption) are the mainstay treatment for the majority of psoriatic patients because they may also improve the response to pharmacological treatments for psoriasis [38,39,43]. It is known that the risk of psoriasis and its clinical severity are closely associated with the degree of overweight/obesity of this patient population. Although weight loss alone may be insufficient for maintaining skin disease remission in obese patients with psoriasis [55], some recent intervention trials have demonstrated that treatment with a low-energy diet showed a trend towards significant improvement in PASI scores among overweight or obese patients with psoriasis, and that body weight reduction in psoriatic patients receiving either low-dose cyclosporine or biologics increased the efficacy of these drugs [56–58]. A recent systematic review and meta-analysis including four small randomized clinical trials with either pioglitazone or rosiglitazone that examined the efficacy of glitazones on psoriasis severity has concluded that pioglitazone may exert some positive effect on psoriasis [59]. However, the clinical significance of this effect and role of this drug in management of psoriatic patients deserve further study.

There are as yet few proven therapies available for patients with NAFLD and NASH, and current therapeutic strategies are specifically directed towards improving features of the metabolic syndrome [5,9,36]. Pioglitazone has the best evidence-based data for NASH treatment. To date, however, lifestyle changes are the more effective therapeutic option that is sharable between patients with NAFLD and those with psoriasis. To our knowledge, no randomized clinical trials have specifically examined the effects of chronic treatment with the newer biologic agents on histologic features of NAFLD. Therefore, additional studies are required to evaluate the best approach to management of NAFLD among patients with psoriasis.

## 6. Conclusions

Although the published evidence is restricted to observational (cross-sectional and case-control) studies [17–27], a growing body of clinical evidence suggests a strong relationship between NAFLD and psoriasis. Published studies indicate that NAFLD is a very frequent condition among adult patients with psoriasis (affecting up to 50% of these patients) and that patients with psoriasis and NAFLD are more likely to have metabolic syndrome and a more severe degree of skin disease than their counterparts without NAFLD. In addition, psoriatic patients are at higher risk of developing the more severe forms of NAFLD (i.e., about a quarter of these patients may develop NASH during the course of the disease). However, further research is required to ascertain whether NAFLD is merely an epiphenomen of coexisting metabolic syndrome features, or is an independent risk factor for the development and progression of psoriasis. Additional studies are also needed to better elucidate the putative biological mechanisms linking NAFLD with psoriasis. Specific mediators of this novel "hepato-dermal axis" need to be further investigated in order to discover innovative drugs and treatments.

In the meantime, given the strong association between NAFLD and psoriasis, we believe that health care providers following psoriatic patients should be mindful of this potentially progressive liver disease that is commonly observed among psoriatic patients. The presence of NAFLD should be also taken into consideration when choosing pharmacological treatment, as some conventional drugs for psoriasis are potentially hepatotoxic.

These findings imply that psoriatic patients should be routinely screened for NAFLD and that consideration should be given to referring these patients to a hepatologist for further evaluation. The optimal method of screening is presently unknown. However, given the intrinsic limitations of serum liver enzyme levels as initial screening test for NAFLD, we think liver ultrasound and transient elastography combined with the use of the NAFLD fibrosis score or other non-invasive fibrosis scoring systems are useful as first-line options in identifying patients with suspected NASH to submit to biopsy among those with psoriasis [60–62]. Moreover, all these patients should be followed regularly to monitor the development of liver-related, metabolic and cardiovascular complications [63].

**Acknowledgments: Acknowledgments:** Giovanni Targher is supported in part by grants from the University School of Medicine of Verona.

**Author Contributions: Author Contributions:** Alessandro Mantovani and Giovanni Targher conceived the study and researched the data. Paolo Gisondi and Amedeo Lonardo contributed to discussion and reviewed/edited the manuscript. Giovanni Targher wrote the manuscript.

# References

1. Parisi, R.; Symmons, D.P.; Griffiths, C.E.; Ashcroft, D.M. Global epidemiology of psoriasis: A systematic review of incidence and prevalence. *J. Investig. Dermatol.* **2013**, *133*, 377–385. [CrossRef] [PubMed]
2. Griffiths, C.E.; Barker, J.N. Pathogenesis and clinical features of psoriasis. *Lancet* **2007**, *370*, 263–271. [CrossRef]
3. Gottlieb, A.B.; Chao, C.; Dann, F. Psoriasis comorbidities. *J. Dermatol. Treat.* **2008**, *19*, 5–21. [CrossRef] [PubMed]
4. Non-alcoholic fatty liver disease (NAFLD) Study Group, dedicated to the memory of Prof. Paola Loria; Lonardo, A.; Bellentani, S.; Argo, C.K.; Ballestri, S.; Byrne, C.D.; Caldwell, S.H.; Cortez-Pinto, H.; Grieco, A.; Machado, M.V.; *et al.* Epidemiological modifiers of non-alcoholic fatty liver disease: Focus on high-risk groups. *Dig. Liver Dis.* **2015**, *47*, 997–1006.
5. Anstee, Q.M.; Targher, G.; Day, C.P. Progression of NAFLD to diabetes mellitus, cardiovascular disease or cirrhosis. *Nat. Rev. Gastroenterol. Hepatol.* **2013**, *10*, 330–344. [CrossRef] [PubMed]
6. Lonardo, A.; Ballestri, S.; Marchesini, G.; Angulo, P.; Loria, P. Nonalcoholic fatty liver disease: A precursor of the metabolic syndrome. *Dig. Liver Dis.* **2015**, *47*, 181–190. [CrossRef] [PubMed]
7. Zhang, Y.; Zhang, T.; Zhang, C.; Tang, F.; Zhong, N.; Li, H.; Song, X.; Lin, H.; Liu, Y.; Xue, F. Identification of reciprocal causality between non-alcoholic fatty liver disease and metabolic syndrome by a simplified Bayesian network in a Chinese population. *BMJ Open* **2015**, *5*. [CrossRef] [PubMed]
8. Ballestri, S.; Zona, S.; Targher, G.; Romagnoli, D.; Baldelli, E.; Nascimbeni, F.; Roverato, A.; Guaraldi, G.; Lonardo, A. Nonalcoholic fatty liver disease is associated with an almost two-fold increased risk of incident type 2 diabetes and metabolic syndrome. Evidence from a systematic review and meta-analysis. *J. Gastroenterol. Hepatol.* **2015**. [CrossRef] [PubMed]
9. Byrne, C.D.; Targher, G. NAFLD: A multisystem disease. *J. Hepatol.* **2015**, *62*, S47–S64. [CrossRef] [PubMed]
10. Ballestri, S.; Lonardo, A.; Bonapace, S.; Byrne, C.D.; Loria, P.; Targher, G. Risk of cardiovascular, cardiac and arrhythmic complications in patients with non-alcoholic fatty liver disease. *World J. Gastroenterol.* **2014**, *20*, 1724–1745. [CrossRef] [PubMed]
11. Ogdie, A.; Gelfand, J.M. Clinical risk factors for the development of psoriatic arthritis among patients with psoriasis: A review of available evidence. *Curr. Rheumatol. Rep.* **2015**, *17*. [CrossRef] [PubMed]
12. Sommer, D.M.; Jenisch, S.; Suchan, M.; Christophers, E.; Weichenthal, M. Increased prevalence of the metabolic syndrome in patients with moderate to severe psoriasis. *Arch. Dermatol. Res.* **2006**, *298*, 321–328. [CrossRef] [PubMed]
13. Gisondi, P.; Tessari, G.; Conti, A.; Piaserico, S.; Schianchi, S.; Peserico, A.; Giannetti, A.; Girolomoni, G. Prevalence of metabolic syndrome in patients with psoriasis: A hospital-based case-control study. *Br. J. Dermatol.* **2007**, *157*, 68–73. [CrossRef] [PubMed]
14. Chandra, A.; Ray, A.; Senapati, S.; Chatterjee, R. Genetic and epigenetic basis of psoriasis pathogenesis. *Mol. Immunol.* **2015**, *64*, 313–323. [CrossRef] [PubMed]

15. Lowes, M.A.; Suarez-Farinas, M.; Krueger, J.G. Immunology of psoriasis. *Annu. Rev. Immunol.* **2014**, *32*, 227–255. [CrossRef] [PubMed]

16. Durham, L.E.; Kirkham, B.W.; Taams, L.S. Contribution of the IL-17 pathway to psoriasis and psoriatic arthritis. *Curr. Rheumatol. Rep.* **2015**, *17*. [CrossRef] [PubMed]

17. Lonardo, A.; Loria, P.; Carulli, N. Concurrent non-alcoholic steatohepatitis and psoriasis. Report of three cases from the POLI.ST.E.N.A. Study. *Dig. Liver Dis.* **2001**, *33*, 86–87. [CrossRef]

18. Matsumoto, T.; Suziki, N.; Watanabe, H.; Irie, M.; Iwata, K.; Anan, A.; Nakane, H.; Yoshikane, M.; Nishizawa, S.; Sohda, T.; *et al.* Nonalcoholic steatohepatitis associated with psoriasis vulgaris. *J. Gastroenterol.* **2004**, *39*, 1102–1110. [CrossRef] [PubMed]

19. Gisondi, P.; Targher, G.; Zoppini, G.; Girolomoni, G. Non-alcoholic fatty liver disease in patients with chronic plaque psoriasis. *J. Hepatol.* **2009**, *51*, 758–764. [CrossRef] [PubMed]

20. Miele, L.; Vallone, S.; Cefalo, C.; la Torre, G.; di Stasi, C.; Vecchio, F.M.; D'Agostino, M.; Gabrieli, M.L.; Vero, V.; Biolato, M.; *et al.* Prevalence, characteristics and severity of non-alcoholic fatty liver disease in patients with chronic plaque psoriasis. *J. Hepatol.* **2009**, *51*, 778–786. [CrossRef] [PubMed]

21. Madanagobalane, S.; Anandan, S. The increased prevalence of non-alcoholic fatty liver disease in psoriatic patients: A study from South India. *Australas. J. Dermatol.* **2012**, *53*, 190–197. [CrossRef] [PubMed]

22. Van der Voort, E.A.; Koehler, E.M.; Dowlatshahi, E.A.; Hofman, A.; Stricker, B.H.; Janssen, H.L.; Schouten, J.N.; Nijsten, T. Psoriasis is independently associated with nonalcoholic fatty liver disease in patients 55 years old or older: Results from a population-based study. *J. Am. Acad. Dermatol.* **2014**, *70*, 517–524. [CrossRef] [PubMed]

23. Van der Voort, E.A.; Koehler, E.M.; Nijsten, T.; Stricker, B.H.; Hofman, A.; Janssen, H.L.; Schouten, J.N.; Wakkee, M. Increased prevalence of advanced liver fibrosis in patients with psoriasis: A cross-sectional analysis from the Rotterdam study. *Acta Derm. Venereol.* **2015**. [CrossRef] [PubMed]

24. Gisondi, P.; Barba, E.; Girolomoni, G. Non-alcoholic fatty liver disease fibrosis score in patients with psoriasis. *J. Eur. Acad. Dermatol. Venereol.* **2015**, *30*, 282–287. [CrossRef] [PubMed]

25. Abedini, R.; Salehi, M.; Lajevardi, V.; Beygi, S. Patients with psoriasis are at a higher risk of developing nonalcoholic fatty liver disease. *Clin. Exp. Dermatol.* **2015**, *40*, 722–727. [CrossRef] [PubMed]

26. Roberts, K.K.; Cochet, A.E.; Lamb, P.B.; Brown, P.J.; Battafarano, D.F.; Brunt, E.M.; Harrison, S.A. The prevalence of NAFLD and NASH among patients with psoriasis in a tertiary care dermatology and rheumatology clinic. *Aliment. Pharmacol. Ther.* **2015**, *41*, 293–300. [CrossRef] [PubMed]

27. Candia, R.; Ruiz, A.; Torres-Robles, R.; Chávez-Tapia, N.; Méndez-Sánchez, N.; Arrese, M. Risk of non-alcoholic fatty liver disease in patients with psoriasis: A systematic review and meta-analysis. *J. Eur. Acad. Dermatol. Venereol.* **2015**, *29*, 656–662. [CrossRef] [PubMed]

28. Birkenfeld, A.L.; Shulman, G.I. Nonalcoholic fatty liver disease, hepatic insulin resistance, and type 2 diabetes. *Hepatology* **2014**, *59*, 713–723. [CrossRef] [PubMed]

29. Shoelson, S.E.; Lee, J.; Goldfine, A.B. Inflammation and insulin resistance. *J. Clin. Investig.* **2006**, *116*, 1793–1801. [CrossRef] [PubMed]

30. Ucak, S.; Ekmekci, T.; Basat, O. Comparison of various insulin sensitivity indices in psoriatic patients and their relationship with types of psoriasis. *J. Eur. Acad. Dermatol. Venereol.* **2006**, *20*, 517–522. [CrossRef] [PubMed]

31. Byrne, C.D.; Targher, G. Ectopic fat, insulin resistance, and nonalcoholic fatty liver disease: Implications for cardiovascular disease. *Arterioscler. Thromb. Vasc. Biol.* **2014**, *34*, 1155–1161. [CrossRef] [PubMed]

32. Loria, P.; Carulli, L.; Bertolotti, M.; Lonardo, A. Endocrine and liver interaction: The role of endocrine pathways in NASH. *Nat. Rev. Gastroenterol. Hepatol.* **2009**, *6*, 236–247. [CrossRef] [PubMed]

33. Shulmann, G.I. Ectopic fat in insulin resistance, dyslipidemia, and cardiometabolic disease. *N. Engl. J. Med.* **2014**, *371*, 1131–1141. [CrossRef] [PubMed]

34. Hunter, C.A.; Jones, S.A. IL-6 as a keystone cytokine in health and disease. *Nat. Immunol.* **2015**, *16*, 448–457. [CrossRef] [PubMed]

35. Stefan, N.; Häring, H.U. The role of hepatokines in metabolism. *Nat. Rev. Endocrinol.* **2013**, *9*, 144–152. [CrossRef] [PubMed]

36. Targher, G.; Day, C.P.; Bonora, E. Risk of cardiovascular disease in patients with nonalcoholic fatty liver disease. *N. Engl. J. Med.* **2010**, *363*, 1341–1350.

37.  Kulkarni, N.M.; Jaji, M.S.; Shetty, P.; Kurhe, Y.V.; Chaudhary, S.; Vijaykant, G.; Raghul, J.; Vishwakarma, S.L.; Rajesh, B.N.; Mookkan, J.; *et al.* A novel animal model of metabolic syndrome with non-alcoholic fatty liver disease and skin inflammation. *Pharm. Biol.* **2015**, *53*, 1110–1117. [CrossRef] [PubMed]

38.  Nast, A.; Gisondi, P.; Ormerod, A.D.; Saiag, P.; Smith, C.; Spuls, P.I.; Arenberger, P.; Bachelez, H.; Barker, J.; Dauden, E.; *et al.* European S3-Guidelines on the systemic treatment of psoriasis vulgaris—Update 2015—Short version—EDF in cooperation with EADV and IPC. *J. Eur. Acad. Dermatol. Venereol.* **2015**, *29*, 2277–2294. [CrossRef] [PubMed]

39.  Gisondi, P.; Galvan, A.; Idolazzi, L.; Girolomoni, G. Management of moderate to severe psoriasis in patients with metabolic comorbidities. *Front. Med.* **2015**, *2*. [CrossRef] [PubMed]

40.  Kalb, R.E.; Strober, B.; Weinstein, G.; Lebwohl, M. Methotrexate and psoriasis: 2009 National psoriasis foundation consensus conference. *J. Am. Acad. Dermatol.* **2009**, *60*, 824–837. [CrossRef] [PubMed]

41.  Hardwick, R.N.; Clarke, J.D.; Lake, A.D.; Canet, M.J.; Anumol, T.; Street, S.M.; Merrell, M.D.; Goedken, M.J.; Snyder, S.A.; Cherrington, N.J. Increased susceptibility to methotrexate-induced toxicity in nonalcoholic steatohepatitis. *Toxicol. Sci.* **2014**, *142*, 45–55. [CrossRef] [PubMed]

42.  Rosenberg, P.; Urwitz, H.; Johannesson, A.; Ros, A.M.; Lindholm, J.; Kinnman, N.; Hultcrantz, R. Psoriasis patients with diabetes type 2 are at high risk of developing liver fibrosis during methotrexate treatment. *J. Hepatol.* **2007**, *46*, 1111–1118. [CrossRef] [PubMed]

43.  Gisondi, P.; Cazzaniga, S.; Chimenti, S.; Giannetti, A.; Maccarone, M.; Picardo, M.; Girolomoni, G.; Naldi, L. Psocare Study Group. Metabolic abnormalities associated with initiation of systemic treatment for psoriasis: Evidence from the Italian Psocare Registry. *J. Eur. Acad. Dermatol. Venereol.* **2013**, *27*, e30–e41. [CrossRef] [PubMed]

44.  Neuvonen, P.J.; Niemi, M.; Backman, J.T. Drug interactions with lipid-lowering drugs: Mechanisms and clinical relevance. *Clin. Pharmacol. Ther.* **2006**, *80*, 565–581. [CrossRef] [PubMed]

45.  Dunn, L.K.; Gaar, L.R.; Yentzer, B.A.; O'Neill, J.L.; Feldman, S.R. Acitretin in dermatology: A review. *J. Drugs Dermatol.* **2011**, *10*, 772–782. [PubMed]

46.  Martinez Abundis, E.; Reynoso-von, D.C.; Hernandez-Salazar, E.; Gonzalez-Ortiz, M. Effect of etanercept on insulin secretion and insulin sensitivity in a randomized trial with psoriatic patients at risk for developing type 2 diabetes mellitus. *Arch. Dermatol. Res.* **2007**, *299*, 461–465. [CrossRef] [PubMed]

47.  Stanley, T.L.; Zanni, M.V.; Johnsen, S.; Rasheed, S.; Makimura, H.; Lee, H.; Khor, V.K.; Ahima, R.S.; Grinspoon, S.K. TNF-α antagonism with etanercept decreases glucose and increases the proportion of high molecular weight adiponectin in obese subjects with features of the metabolic syndrome. *J. Clin. Endocrinol. Metab.* **2011**, *96*, E146–E150. [CrossRef] [PubMed]

48.  Solomon, D.H.; Massarotti, E.; Garg, R.; Liu, J.; Canning, C.; Schneeweiss, S. Association between disease-modifying anti-rheumatic drugs and diabetes risk in patients with rheumatoid arthritis and psoriasis. *JAMA* **2011**, *305*, 2525–2531. [CrossRef] [PubMed]

49.  Lestre, S.; Diamantino, F.; Veloso, L.; Fidalgo, A.; Ferreira, A. Effects of etanercept treatment on lipid profile in patients with moderate-to-severe chronic plaque psoriasis: A retrospective cohort study. *Eur. J. Dermatol.* **2011**, *21*, 916–920. [PubMed]

50.  Gisondi, P.; Conti, A.; Galdo, G.; Piaserico, S.; de Simone, C.; Girolomoni, G. Ustekinumab does not increase body mass index in patients with chronic plaque psoriasis: A prospective cohort study. *Br. J. Dermatol.* **2013**, *168*, 1124–1127. [CrossRef] [PubMed]

51.  Tobon, G.J.; Cañas, C.; Jaller, J.J.; Restrepo, J.C.; Anaya, J.M. Serious liver disease induced by infliximab. *Clin. Rheumatol.* **2007**, *26*, 578–581. [CrossRef] [PubMed]

52.  Tan, K.W.; Griffiths, C.E. Novel systemic therapies for the treatment of psoriasis. *Expert. Opin. Pharmacother.* **2016**, *17*, 79–92. [CrossRef] [PubMed]

53.  Campanati, A.; Ganzetti, G.; di Sario, A.; Damiani, A.; Sandroni, L.; Rosa, L.; Benedetti, A.; Offidani, A. The effect of etanercept on hepatic fibrosis risk in patients with non-alcoholic fatty liver disease, metabolic syndrome, and psoriasis. *J. Gastroenterol.* **2013**, *48*, 839–846. [CrossRef] [PubMed]

54.  Feagins, L.A.; Flores, A.; Arriens, C.; Park, C.; Crook, T.; Reimold, A.; Brown, G. Nonalcoholic fatty liver disease: A potential consequence of tumor necrosis factor-inhibitor therapy. *Eur. J. Gastroenterol. Hepatol.* **2015**, *27*, 1154–1160. [CrossRef] [PubMed]

55.  Del Giglio, M.; Gisondi, P.; Tessari, G.; Girolomoni, G. Weight reduction alone may not be sufficient to maintain disease remission in obese patients with psoriasis: A randomized, investigator-blinded study. *Dermatology* **2012** *224*, 31–37. [CrossRef] [PubMed]

56.  Jensen, P.; Zachariae, C.; Christensen, R.; Geiker, N.R.; Schaadt, B.K.; Stender, S.; Hansen, P.R.; Astrup, A.; Skov, L. Effect of weight loss on the severity of psoriasis: A randomized clinical study. *JAMA Dermatol.* **2013**, *149*, 795–801. [CrossRef] [PubMed]

57.  Gisondi, P.; del Giglio, M.; di Francesco, V.; Zamboni, M.; Girolomoni, G. Weight loss improves the response of obese patients with moderate-to-severe chronic plaque psoriasis to low-dose cyclosporine therapy: A randomized, controlled, investigator-blinded clinical trial. *Am. J. Clin. Nutr.* **2008**, *88*, 1242–1247. [PubMed]

58.  Al-Mutairi, N.; Nour, T. The effect of weight reduction on treatment outcomes in obese patients with psoriasis on biologic therapy: A randomized controlled prospective trial. *Expert Opin. Biol. Ther.* **2014**, *14*, 749–756. [CrossRef] [PubMed]

59.  Malhotra, A.; Shafiq, N.; Rajagopalan, S.; Dogra, S.; Malhotra, S. Thiazolidinediones for plaque psoriasis: A systematic review and meta-analysis. *Evid. Based Med.* **2012**, *17*, 171–176. [CrossRef] [PubMed]

60.  Nascimbeni, F.; Pais, R.; Bellentani, S.; Day, C.P.; Ratziu, V.; Loria, P.; Lonardo, A. From NAFLD in clinical practice to answers from guidelines. *J. Hepatol.* **2013**, *59*, 859–871. [CrossRef] [PubMed]

61.  Castera, L.; Vilgrain, V.; Angulo, P. Noninvasive evaluation of NAFLD. *Nat. Rev. Gastroenterol. Hepatol.* **2013**, *10*, 666–675. [CrossRef] [PubMed]

62.  Ballestri, S.; Romagnoli, D.; Nascimbeni, F.; Francica, G.; Lonardo, A. Role of ultrasound in the diagnosis and treatment of nonalcoholic fatty liver disease and its complications. *Expert Rev. Gastroenterol. Hepatol.* **2015**, *9*, 603–627. [CrossRef] [PubMed]

63.  Lonardo, A.; Ballestri, S.; Targher, G.; Loria, P. Diagnosis and management of cardiovascular risk in nonalcoholic fatty liver disease. *Expert Rev. Gastroenterol. Hepatol.* **2015**, *9*, 629–650. [CrossRef] [PubMed]

# 10

# Additive Effect of Non-Alcoholic Fatty Liver Disease on Metabolic Syndrome-Related Endothelial Dysfunction in Hypertensive Patients

Maria Perticone [1], Antonio Cimellaro [2], Raffaele Maio [3], Benedetto Caroleo [3], Angela Sciacqua [2], Giorgio Sesti [2] and Francesco Perticone [2,*]

[1]  Department of Experimental and Clinical Medicine, University Magna Græcia, Catanzaro 88100, Italy; mariaperticone@hotmail.com
[2]  Department of Medical and Surgical Sciences, University Magna Græcia, Catanzaro 88100, Italy; antocime@hotmail.it (A.C.); sciacqua@unicz.it (A.S.); sesti@unicz.it (G.S.)
[3]  Unit of Cardiovascular Diseases, Azienda Ospedaliera Mater Domini, Catanzaro 88100, Italy; raf_maio@yahoo.it (R.M.); benedettocaroleo@libero.it (B.C.)
*   Correspondence: perticone@unicz.it

Academic Editors: Amedeo Lonardo and Giovanni Targher

**Abstract:** Metabolic syndrome (MS) is characterized by an increased risk of incident diabetes and cardiovascular (CV) events, identifying insulin resistance (IR) and endothelial dysfunction as key elements. Moreover, non-alcoholic fatty liver disease (NAFLD) is bidirectionally linked with MS as a consequence of metabolic and inflammatory abnormalities. We addressed the question if the evolution in NAFLD might worsen endothelium-dependent vasodilating response in MS hypertensives. We recruited 272 Caucasian newly-diagnosed never-treated hypertensive outpatients divided into three groups according to the presence/absence of MS alone or in combination with NAFLD. MS and NAFLD were defined according to the National Cholesterol Education Program-Adult Treatment Panel III (NCEP-ATPIII) and non-invasive fatty liver index, respectively. We determined IR by using the homeostasis model assessment (HOMA) index. Vascular function, as forearm blood flow (FBF), was determined through strain-gauge plethysmography after intra-arterial infusion of acetylcholine (ACh) and sodium nitroprusside. MS+NAFLD+ group showed worse metabolic, inflammatory and vascular profiles compared with MS−NAFLD− and MS+NAFLD−. HOMA resulted in being the strongest predictor of FBF both in the MS+NAFLD− and in the MS+NAFLD+ groups, accounting for 20.5% and 33.2% of its variation, respectively. In conclusion, we demonstrated that MS+NAFLD+ hypertensives show a worse endothelium-dependent vasodilation compared with MS+NAFLD−, allowing for consideration of NAFLD as an early marker of endothelial dysfunction in hypertensives.

**Keywords:** endothelial dysfunction; non-alcoholic fatty liver disease; metabolic syndrome; cardiovascular disease and risk; arterial hypertension

## 1. Introduction

Metabolic syndrome (MS) is a clinical condition characterized by a clustering of hemodynamic and metabolic risk factors including raised blood pressure (BP), atherogenic dyslipidemia, raised fasting glucose and central obesity [1]. All of these factors are interrelated and associated with an increased risk for incident diabetes and cardiovascular (CV) diseases [2,3]. Although the pathogenesis of MS remains not completely clarified, insulin resistance (IR) is believed to play a pivotal pathophysiological role in its development [4].

It is well recognized that endothelial dysfunction, primarily characterized by a reduced nitric oxide (NO) bioavailability, is an early step in the continuum of the atherosclerotic process. In addition, there are several lines of evidence demonstrating that it is a strong and independent predictor of CV events in different settings of patients [5,6], and that it is able to predict the appearance and progression of subclinical organ damage [6–9]. On the other hand, some experimental and clinical data have demonstrated that NO-mediated vasodilation is impaired in patients with IR [10–12], representing a possible pathogenetic mechanism linking MS to increased CV risk.

Non-alcoholic fatty liver disease (NAFLD) is bidirectionally linked with MS (13) as a consequence of the inflammatory and metabolic processes characterizing this condition. In keeping with this, previously published data demonstrated a strong relationship between IR and NAFLD [13–16]. It is plausible that, in visceral obesity, present in the MS, the excess of portal or intra-peritoneal fat promotes the appearance and progression of NAFLD by directly increasing the flux of free fatty acids to the liver [16]. Moreover, we recently reported that hypertensive patients with NAFLD show a significantly reduced endothelium-dependent vasodilation compared with hypertensives without NAFLD [17], confirming that the presence of more risk factors in the same setting of patients differentiates the risk profile of each subject.

However, at this moment, there are no data demonstrating if NAFLD has an additive effect in worsening endothelial function in subjects with MS. Thus, we designed the present study with the aim to demonstrate the additive effect of both MS and NAFLD on endothelium-dependent vasodilating response in hypertensive subjects.

## 2. Results

### 2.1. Study Population

Characteristics of the whole study population, stratified according to the presence/absence of MS alone or in combination with NAFLD, are reported in Table 1. In comparison with MS+NAFLD− patients, subjects in the MS+NAFLD+ group had significantly higher body mass index (BMI) and waist circumference. With regards to hemodynamic parameters, MS+NAFLD+ group showed higher systolic BP and pulse pressure (PP) values. As expected, MS+NAFLD+ patients exhibited higher gamma-glutamyltransferase (GGT), aspartate aminotransferase (AST) and alanine aminotransferase (ALT) values, and a worse metabolic and inflammatory profile, compared to the MS+LS− group.

**Table 1.** Clinical, biochemical and hemodynamic characteristics of subjects in whole study population and in different groups.

| Variables | All (n = 272) | MS−NAFLD− (n = 101) | MS+NAFLD− (n = 78) | MS+NAFLD+ (n = 93) | p |
|---|---|---|---|---|---|
| Gender, M/F | 148/124 | 63/38 | 37/41 | 48/45 | 0.110 * |
| Age, years | 48.8 ± 9.3 | 47.2 ± 8.6 | 49.9 ± 10.3 | 49.9 ± 9.1 | 0.082 |
| Smoking, n (%) | 17 (17.3) | 17 (16.8) | 14 (17.9) | 16 (17.2) | 0.960 * |
| BMI, kg/m$^2$ | 30.1 ± 5.4 | 26.2 ± 2.5 | 31.2 ± 4.8 | 33.3 ± 5.6 ‡ | <0.0001 |
| Waist circumference, cm | 100.5 ± 14.2 | 90.2 ± 10.8 | 104.1 ± 13.2 | 108.5 ± 11.6 ‡ | <0.0001 |
| Systolic BP, mm Hg | 141 ± 17 | 129 ± 13 | 145 ± 17 | 150 ± 14 ‡ | <0.0001 |
| Diastolic BP, mm Hg | 89 ± 11 | 83 ± 10 | 92 ± 12 | 92 ± 10 | <0.0001 |
| PP, mm/Hg | 52 ± 14 | 46 ± 15 | 52 ± 13 | 59 ± 14 ‡ | <0.0001 |
| Total cholesterol, mg/dL | 197 ± 33 | 186 ± 26 | 204 ± 32 | 205 ± 37 | <0.0001 |
| HDL-cholesterol, mg/dL | 47 ± 14 | 53 ± 16 | 43 ± 10 | 43 ± 11 | <0.0001 |
| Triglyceride, mg/dL | 132 ± 63 | 107 ± 42 | 134 ± 65 | 156 ± 81 | <0.0001 |
| GGT, U/L | 31 ± 15 | 21 ± 7 | 26 ± 8 | 47 ± 11 ‡ | <0.0001 |
| AST, U/L | 37.7 ± 24.1 | 19.4 ± 4.6 | 30.8 ± 18.3 | 63.9 ± 20.9 ‡ | <0.0001 |
| ALT, U/L | 39.4 ± 27.4 | 18.8 ± 6.2 | 31.2 ± 16.5 | 69.2 ± 22.7 ‡ | <0.0001 |
| Serum Creatinine, mg/dL | 0.9 ± 0.2 | 0.9 ± 0.3 | 0.9 ± 0.2 | 0.9 ± 0.2 | 0.162 |
| e-GFR, mL/min/1.73 m$^2$ | 94.7 ± 20.6 | 97.1 ± 21.3 | 93.1 ± 18.7 | 92.9 ± 25.6 | 0.287 |
| FP glucose, mg/dL | 99.5 ± 19.6 | 90.1 ± 8.3 | 102.2 ± 21.9 | 107.9 ± 21.9 | <0.0001 |

**Table 1.** *Cont.*

| Variables | All (n = 272) | MS−NAFLD− (n = 101) | MS+NAFLD− (n = 78) | MS+NAFLD+ (n = 93) | p |
|---|---|---|---|---|---|
| FP insulin, mU/mL | 13.7 ± 6.3 | 10.3 ± 4.7 | 14.5 ± 6.0 | 16.8 ± 6.4 ‡ | <0.0001 |
| HOMA | 3.4 ± 1.9 | 2.3 ± 1.0 | 3.6 ± 1.5 | 4.5 ± 2.2 ‡ | <0.0001 |
| hs-CRP, mg/dL | 4.3 ± 2.7 | 3.2 ± 1.5 | 4.2 ± 3.0 | 5.7 ± 2.9 ‡ | <0.0001 |
| FBF, mL· 100· mL$^{-1}$ of tissue· min$^{-1}$ | | | | | |
| Basal | 3.1 ± 0.7 | 3.2 ± 0.9 | 3.0 ± 0.6 | 3.0 ± 0.7 | 0.238 |
| ACh, % of increase | 328 ± 141 | 413 ± 136 | 327 ± 127 | 236 ± 91 ‡ | <0.0001 |
| SNP, % of increase | 500 ± 120 | 507 ± 128 | 498 ± 121 | 496 ± 114 | 0.799 |

\* : X$^2$ test.    ‡ : = $p < 0.05$ by Bonferroni MS+NAFLD− Vs MS+NAFLD+.    ACh: acetylcholine; ALT alanine aminotransferase; AST: aspartate aminotransferase; BMI: body mass index; BP: blood pressure; PP: pulse pressure; hs-CRP: high sensitivity C-reactive protein; e-GFR: estimated glomerular filtration rate; FBF: forearm blood flow; FP: fasting plasma; GGT: gamma glutamyl transferase; HDL: high density lipoprotein; HOMA: homeostasis model assessment of insulin resistance; SNP: sodium nitroprusside.

## 2.2. Endothelium–Dependent and –Independent Vasodilation

The baseline forearm blood flow (FBF) did not differ among the three groups (Table 1). Intra-arterial infusion of achetylcholine (ACh) significantly increased FBF in a dose-dependent manner in all groups. The FBF values at the three incremental doses of ACh were 6.9 ± 3.0, 10.5 ± 4.6 and 16.3 ± 6.5 mL· 100 mL$^{-1}$ of tissue· min$^{-1}$, 5.2 ± 2.2, 8.1 ± 3.9 and 12.7 ± 4.3 mL· 100 mL$^{-1}$ of tissue· min$^{-1}$ and 4.8 ± 1.8, 6.9 ± 2.4 and 10.2 ± 3.7 mL· 100 mL$^{-1}$ of tissue· min$^{-1}$ for MS−NAFLD−, MS+NAFLD− and MS+NAFLD+ groups, respectively.

As expected, the endothelium-dependent maximal vasodilating response to ACh was significantly ($p < 0.0001$) reduced in both MS+NAFLD− and MS+NAFLD+ groups in comparison with MS−NAFLD− group (Figure 1). In addition, MS+NAFLD+ patients showed a worse ACh peak percent increase when compared to the MS+NAFLD− group (Table 1). On the contrary, all patients showed a normal endothelium-independent vasodilation to sodium nitroprusside (SNP) infusions, without any significant difference among groups.

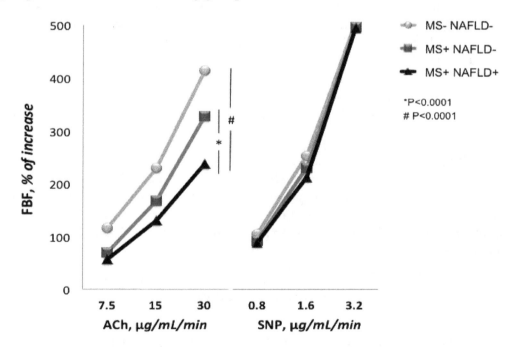

**Figure 1.** Responses of forearm blood flow (FBF) to intra-arterial infusions of acetylcholine (ACh) and sodium nitroprusside (SNP) in different groups.

Finally, in the logistic regression model (Figure 2), patients with both MS and NAFLD had the highest risk for decreased FBF (OR = 14.81; 95% CI = 6.99–31.38; $p < 0.0001$), whereas the group with MS alone had an almost doubled risk (OR = 2.53; 95% CI = 1.32–4.86; $p = 0.005$).

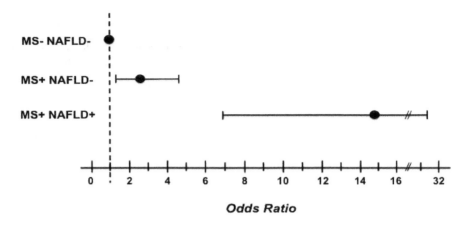

**Figure 2.** Graphic report of the logistic regression analysis for decreased forearm blood flow.

## 2.3. Correlational Analysis

A linear regression analysis was performed to test the correlation between FBF and different covariates in the whole study population and in different groups (Table 2). FBF was inversely correlated with homeostasis model assessment (HOMA) ($r = -0.584$, $p < 0.0001$), high sensitivity C-reactive protein (hs-CRP) ($r = -0.528$, $p < 0.0001$), waist circumference ($r = -0.521$, $p < 0.0001$), BMI ($r = -0.505$, $p < 0.0001$), PP ($r = -0.477$, $p < 0.0001$), systolic BP ($r = -0.466$, $p = <0.0001$) and age ($r = -0.319$; $p < 0.0001$).

In the MS-NAFLD- group, FBF was significantly correlated with PP ($r = -0.371$, $p < 0.0001$), systolic BP ($r = -0.361$, $p \leqslant 0.0001$), HOMA ($r = -0.362$, $p < 0.0001$), hs-CRP ($r = -0.329$, $p < 0.0001$), age ($r = -0.282$; $p = 0.002$), BMI ($r = -0.279$, $p = 0.002$) and waist circumference ($r = -0.186$, $p = 0.031$).

In patients with MS alone, the main covariates related with endothelial-dependent vasodilation were HOMA ($r = -0.464$, $p < 0.0001$), hs-CRP ($r = -0.446$, $p < 0.0001$), waist circumference ($r = -0.436$, $p < 0.0001$), BMI ($r = -0.406$, $p < 0.0001$), PP ($r = -0.344$, $p = 0.001$), age ($r = -0.305$; $p = 0.003$) and systolic BP ($r = -0.193$, $p = 0.045$). Finally, when considering MS and NAFLD together, FBF was inversely correlated with HOMA ($r = -0.616$, $p < 0.0001$), hs-CRP ($r = -0.522$, $p < 0.0001$), waist circumference ($r = -0.454$, $p < 0.0001$), BMI ($r = -0.414$, $p < 0.0001$), PP ($r = -0.344$, $p = 0.002$), systolic BP ($r = -0.273$, $p = 0.013$) age ($r = -0.249$; $p = 0.022$).

Variables reaching statistical significance, with the addition of smoking and gender as dichotomic values, were inserted in a stepwise multivariate linear regression model to determine the independent predictors of FBF (Table 3). In the whole population, HOMA was the strongest predictor of FBF, accounting for 33.7% ($p < 0.0001$) of its variation. In addition, the other independent predictors were: PP, waist circumference, hs-CRP, BMI and age accounting for 8.8%, 5.5%, 3.5%, 1.8%, 1.0% of its variation, respectively.

In subjects without MS and NAFLD, pulse pressure was the most important predictor of FBF, justifying about 12.9% ($p < 0.0001$) of its variation, followed by HOMA (9.9%), hs-CRP (6.8%) and age (4.2%).

Of interest, HOMA was the strongest predictor of FBF in patients with MS alone and MS in combination with NAFLD, accounting for 20.5% ($p < 0.0001$) and 33.2% ($p < 0.0001$) of its variation, respectively. Other independent predictors of the endothelial-dependent vasodilation in MS+NAFLD− group were waist circumference and hs-CRP accounting for a further 8.2% and 6.1% of its variation, respectively. Finally, in the MS+NAFLD+ group, hs-CRP, waist circumference and age add another 11.7%, 7.7% and 3.1% of FBF variation, respectively.

**Table 2.** Linear regression analysis on forearm blood flow (FBF) as a dependent variable in the whole study population and in different groups.

| Variables | All $n = 272$ | | MS−NAFLD− $n = 101$ | | MS+NAFLD− $n = 98$ | | MS+NAFLD+ $n = 73$ | |
|---|---|---|---|---|---|---|---|---|
| | $r$ | $p$ | $r$ | $p$ | $r$ | $p$ | $r$ | $p$ |
| Diastolic BP, mmHg | −0.138 | ns | 0.053 | ns | 0.122 | ns | 0.050 | ns |
| HDL cholesterol, mg/dL | 0.171 | ns | 0.125 | ns | −0.171 | ns | 0.001 | ns |
| Total cholesterol, mg/dL | −0.171 | ns | −0.094 | ns | 0.016 | ns | 0.007 | ns |
| Triglyceride, mg/dL | −0.202 | ns | −0.114 | ns | −0.005 | ns | 0.068 | ns |
| Age, years | −0.319 | <0.0001 | −0.282 | 0.002 | −0.305 | 0.003 | −0.249 | 0.022 |
| Systolic BP, mmHg | −0.466 | <0.0001 | −0.361 | <0.0001 | −0.193 | 0.045 | −0.273 | 0.013 |
| PP, mmHg | −0.477 | <0.0001 | −0.371 | <0.0001 | −0.344 | 0.001 | −0.344 | 0.002 |
| BMI, kg/m$^2$ | −0.505 | <0.0001 | −0.279 | 0.002 | −0.406 | <0.0001 | −0.414 | <0.0001 |
| Waist circumference, cm | −0.521 | <0.0001 | −0.186 | 0.031 | −0.436 | <0.0001 | −0.454 | <0.0001 |
| hs-CRP, mg/dL | −0.528 | <0.0001 | −0.329 | <0.0001 | −0.446 | <0.0001 | −0.522 | <0.0001 |
| HOMA | −0.584 | <0.0001 | −0.362 | <0.0001 | −0.464 | <0.0001 | −0.616 | <0.0001 |

BP: blood pressure; PP: pulse pressure; HDL: high-density lipoprotein; BMI: body mass index; hs-CRP: high-sensitivity C-reactive protein; HOMA: homeostasis model assessment of insulin resistance.

**Table 3.** Stepwise multiple regression analysis FBF as a dependent variable in the whole study population and in different groups.

| Variables | All ($n = 272$) | | MS−NAFLD− ($n = 101$) | | MS+NAFLD− ($n = 98$) | | MS+NAFLD+ ($n = 73$) | |
|---|---|---|---|---|---|---|---|---|
| | Partial $R^2$ (%) | $p$ | Partial $R^2$ (%) | $p$ | Partial $R^2$ (%) | $p$ | Partial $R^2$ (%) | $p$ |
| Age, years | 1.0 | 0.012 | 4.2 | 0.008 | - | - | 3.1 | 0.021 |
| BMI, kg/m$^2$ | 1.8 | 0.001 | - | - | - | - | - | - |
| hs-CRP, mg/dL | 3.5 | <0.0001 | 6.8 | 0.002 | 6.1 | 0.006 | 11.7 | <0.0001 |
| Waist circumference, cm | 5.5 | <0.0001 | - | - | 8.2 | 0.003 | 7.7 | 0.001 |
| PP, mmHg | 8.8 | <0.0001 | 12.9 | <0.0001 | - | - | - | - |
| HOMA | 33.7 | <0.0001 | 9.9 | <0.0001 | 20.5 | <0.0001 | 33.2 | <0.0001 |
| Total $R^2$ (%) | 54.3 | - | 33.8 | - | 34.8 | - | 55.7 | - |

BMI: body mass index; hs-CRP: high-sensitivity C-reactive protein; PP: pulse pressure; HOMA: homeostasis model assessment of insulin resistance.

## 3. Discussion

The results of our study, obtained in a well characterized cohort of newly-diagnosed never-treated hypertensive patients, demonstrate that the endothelium-dependent vasodilation, evaluated by strain-gauge plethysmography, was significantly reduced in MS+NAFLD+ patients in comparison with patients with only MS. Furthermore, MS+NAFLD+ patients showed a worse metabolic, inflammatory and hemodynamic profile. In particular, patients with NAFLD exhibited greater values of both BMI and waist circumference compared with those without; this is not surprising, since it is well known that obese subjects have a high risk for NAFLD [18] attributable, at least in part, to visceral fat accumulation and consequent increased flux of free fatty acids to the liver [16]. Moreover, the excessive intrahepatic triglyceride content further impairs insulin sensitivity of these subjects, thus creating a vicious circle explaining the observed metabolic and hemodynamic alterations. This is supported by the finding that, in the linear regression analysis, the main covariate related to FBF was PP in MS−NAFLD− group, while, in the other groups, FBF resulted primarily related to HOMA, regardless of the highest BP values. Moreover, HOMA resulted in being the strongest predictor of FBF both in the MS+NAFLD− and in the MS+NAFLD+ groups, accounting for 20.5% and 33.2% of its variation, respectively. These findings are in agreement with previously published data, confirming the presence of a relationship between impaired endothelium-dependent vasodilation and hypertension [5], as well as a negative effect of MS on vascular function. This is not surprising, since both the hemodynamic and metabolic risk factors configuring the MS are all associated with endothelial dysfunction and, consequently, with the risk of CV events. IR, a condition that can be considered the *leitmotiv* underlying the MS, plays a key role also in the appearance and progression of vascular damage, from the endothelial dysfunction to the atherosclerotic plaque. Moreover, IR is also strongly associated with NAFLD, a condition that can be considered as an epiphenomenon of the interaction between the inflammatory and metabolic factors featuring the MS. Since both endothelial dysfunction and IR are characterized by a reduced endothelial-NO synthase (eNOS)-derived NO bioavailability, it is plausible that the link between NAFLD and endothelial dysfunction could be represented by an altered NO balance. In fact, recent published data [19] demonstrated that NO produced by eNOS, plays a key role in liver physiology and pathophysiology, contributing to the maintenance of liver homeostasis; on the contrary, NO derived from inducible-NO synthase (iNOS) is particularly produced under many pathological conditions, and is able to modify many structural liver proteins. In several pathological conditions, such as IR, NO production is shifted from eNOS- to iNOS-derived, with consequent increase in reactive nitrogen species and free radicals. In particular, Pasarin *et al.* [20] demonstrated that the IR exhibited by a rat model of steatotic liver is particularly expressed at the liver endothelium, thus relating IR to iNOS induction; this IR precedes inflammation, fibrosis or other features of advanced liver disease. In keeping with this, it can be supposed that the impairment of both insulin-induced and ACh-dependent vasodilation seen in peripheral vessels of insulin resistant patients can be also observed in the liver vasculature, thus giving a plausible explanation of many events occurring in the disease progression from NAFLD to cirrhosis [21]. In fact, while insulin acts as a vasodilator agent in physiological conditions, throughout the mediation of NO bioavailability, this property resulted in impaired IR status, due to a combined defect in both insulin-mediated glucose transport and in insulin-stimulated endothelial vasodilation, derived from a fault in the phosphatidylinositol 3 kinase/Akt pathway. [22]. Moreover, the findings of the present study strengthen previously published data by our group [17], demonstrating a significant reduction in endothelium-dependent vasodilation evaluated by strain-gauge plethysmography in hypertensives with associated NAFLD, compared with hypertensives without NAFLD. All these data, taken together, endorse the close link between IR and NAFLD observed in other pathological conditions such as type-2 diabetes mellitus, obesity, and other metabolic alterations [14,23,24]. Finally, our data, obtained in a well-characterized population of hypertensive patients, are in agreement with those obtained by Targher and co-workers in diabetic patients, demonstrating that non-alcoholic fatty liver disease significantly increases CV risk in this setting of patients [25].

This study has several potential limitations. First of all, the small sample size and the cross-sectional design impose the data obtained to be confirmed in wider trials. Another limitation is that the diagnosis of NAFLD was performed by using the non-invasive fatty liver index (FLI) instead of liver biopsy that represents the gold standard. In fact, FLI is poorly correlated with liver histology [26], is no better than waist circumference in predicting NAFLD [27], and the pathophysiological information from the NAFLD arena cannot be directly extrapolated and applied to "liver steatosis" of undefined etiology (probably a mixture of alcoholic and nonalcoholic fatty liver disease), although some authors believe that steatosis *per se* may enhance CV risk [28]. Finally, in this study, we determined IR by using the HOMA index that does not allow for discrimination between peripheral or central IR.

In conclusion, we demonstrated that hypertensive patients with both MS and NAFLD show a worst endothelium-dependent vasodilation compared with hypertensives with MS alone, thus enhancing the crucial role of IR in the multifactorial pathway, in which cooperate both metabolic and hemodynamic factors, leading from endothelial dysfunction to the atherosclerotic plaque formation.

Thus, our results have an important clinical implication since allow to consider NAFLD not only as an organ damage consequent to IR, but also a simple and early marker of endothelial dysfunction in essential hypertension, contributing to better stratify CV risk in this setting of patients.

## 4. Materials and Methods

### 4.1. Study Population

The study population consisted of outpatients evaluated at the University Hospital of Catanzaro. We recruited 272 Caucasian newly-diagnosed never-treated hypertensive outpatients (148 males and 124 females) divided into three groups according with the presence or absence of MS alone or in combination with NAFLD (MS−NAFLD−, MS+NAFLD−, MS+NAFLD+). All patients participated in the CATAnzaro MEtabolic RIsk Factors Study (CATAMERIS) [29] and underwent physical examination and review of their medical history. None of the patients had history or clinical evidence of chronic hepatitis, alcoholism, coronary artery disease, valvular heart disease, peripheral vascular disease, coagulopathy, or any disease predisposing to vasculitis or Raynaud's phenomenon. A complete anthropometric assessment was performed by measurements of height, weight, and waist circumference according to a standardized protocol. BMI was calculated as kilograms per square meter, and the waist was measured at its smallest point with the abdomen relaxed.

The MS was defined according to NCEP-ATPIII [1]. The presence of NAFLD was detected calculating the non-invasive FLI, as suggested by Bedogni *et al.* [30], according to the formula:

$$FLI = (e^{\,0.953*\log e\,(triglyceride)\,+\,0.139*BMI\,+\,0.718*\log e\,(GGT)\,+\,0.053*waist\ circumference\,-\,15.745})/(1 + e^{\,0.953*\log e\,(triglyceride)\,+\,0.139*BMI\,+\,0.718*\log e\,(GGT)\,+\,0.053*waist\ circumference\,-\,15.745}) * 100.$$

FLI values ⩾60 are significant to rule in fatty liver as detected by ultrasonography. The protocol was approved by the Local Ethical Committee, and all participants gave their informed written consent before the study procedures. All the investigations of this research protocol were performed in accordance with the principles of the Declaration of Helsinki.

### 4.2. Biochemical Assays

All laboratory determinations were obtained after 12 fasting h. Enzymatic methods were used to measure fasting blood glucose, total and HDL-cholesterol, and triglyceride (Roche Diagnostics, Mannheim, Germany). ALT and AST levels were measured using the α-ketoglutarate reaction; GGT levels with the L-γ-glutamyl-3-carboxy-4-nitroaniliderate method. Serum insulin was measured through a highly specific radioimmunoassay using two monoclonal antibodies; intra-assay coefficient of variation (CofV) 2.1%, inter-assay CofV 2.9%. hs-CRP was measured by a high-sensitivity turbidimetric immunoassay (Behring, Marburg, Germany). Creatinine measurements were performed by use of the Jaffe methodology and the uricase/peroxidase (uricase/POD; Boehringer Mannheim,

Mannheim, Germany) method implemented in an auto-analyzer. Renal function was evaluated by estimated glomerular filtration rate (e-GFR) by using the Chronic Kidney Disease – Epidemiology (CKD-EPI) equation [31]. Insulin sensitivity was estimated by using the HOMA index, calculated according to the formula: HOMA = [insulin (µU/mL) × glucose (mmol/L)]/22.5. The HOMA index has a strict correlation with the measurement of insulin sensitivity obtained directly from the euglycemic clamp [32,33].

### 4.3. Blood Pressure Measurements

Clinical BP readings were obtained with a mercury sphygmomanometer in the left arm of patients lying supine, after 5 minutes of quiet rest. Each patient underwent a minimum of three BP measurements on three separate occasions at least two weeks apart. The average of the last two of three consecutive measurements obtained at intervals of three minutes was considered as baseline BP. Systolic and diastolic BP corresponded with the first appearance (phase I) and the disappearance (phase V) of Korotkfoff sounds, respectively. According to current guidelines, patients with a clinical BP ≥ 140 mmHg systolic and/or 90 mmHg diastolic were defined as hypertensive [34].

### 4.4. Forearm Blood Flow Measurements

All studies were performed at 09:00 A.M. after overnight fasting, with the subjects lying supine in a quiet air-conditioned room (22–24 °C). Subjects continued their regular diet, but were advised to stop caffeine, alcohol and smoking at least 24 h before the study. Forearm volume was determined by water displacement. A 20-gauge polyethylene catheter (Vasculon 2) was inserted, under local anesthesia and sterile conditions, into the brachial artery of the non-dominant arm for both BP evaluation (Baxter Healthcare Corp., Deerfield, IL, USA) and drug infusion. This arm was elevated above the level of the right atrium, and a mercury-filled elastic strain-gauge, connected to a plethysmograph (model EC-4, D.E. Hokanson, Issaquah, WA, USA) calibrated to measure the percent change in volume which was, in turn, connected to a chart recorder to obtain FBF measurements, was placed on the widest part of the forearm. To exclude venous outflow, a cuff placed on the upper arm was inflated to 40 mmHg with a rapid cuff inflator (model E-10, Hokanson, Issaquah, WA, USA). The hand blood flow was excluded by inflating a wrist cuff to BP values 1 min before each measurement. The antecubital vein in the opposite arm was cannulated. The FBF was measured as the slope of the change in the forearm volume [35]. The mean of at least three measurements was obtained at each time point.

### 4.5. Vascular Function

For the present study, we used the protocol previously described by Panza et al. [36], and subsequently used by our group [5–9,11,12,37]. For each patient, we obtained measurements of FBF and BP during intra-arterial infusion of saline, ACh and SNP at increasing doses. ACh (Sigma, Milan, Italy) was diluted with saline immediately before infusion. SNP (Malesci, Florence, Italy) was diluted in 5% glucose solution immediately before each infusion and protected from light with aluminium foil. To reach a stable baseline before data collection, all participants rested for 30 min after artery cannulation; measurements of FBF were repeated every 5 min until stable. We assessed endothelium-dependent and endothelium-independent vasodilation by a dose–response curve to intra-arterial ACh infusions (7.5, 15, and 30 µg/mL per min, each for 5 min) and SNP infusions (0.8, 1.6, and 3.2 µg/mL per min, each for 5 min), respectively. To avoid any bias related to drug infusion, the sequence of administration of ACh and SNP was randomized. The drug infusion rate, adjusted for the forearm volume of each subject, was 1 mL/min.

### 4.6. Statistical Analysis

Differences for clinical and biological data were compared by using analysis of variance (ANOVA), Bonferroni *post hoc* *t*-test and chi-square test, as appropriate. The vasodilating responses to ACh and SNP were compared by one-way ANOVA and, when analysis was significant, the Bonferroni *post hoc t*-test was applied. A logistic regression analysis was performed to test the risk for decreased FBF (defined by values $<300$ mL$\cdot$ 100 mL$^{-1}$ of tissue$\cdot$ min$^{-1}$) in presence of NAFLD and MS.

Linear regression analysis was performed to correlate FBF with the following covariates: age, waist circumference, BMI, systolic BP, diastolic BP, PP, total and LDL- and HDL-cholesterol, triglyceride, hs-CRP, HOMA. To define the independent predictors of FBF, variables reaching statistical significance were inserted in a stepwise multivariate linear regression model. Moreover, to avoid a possible colinearity, we considered only HOMA and not fasting glucose and insulin.

Parametric data are reported as mean $\pm$ SD. Significant differences were assumed to be at $p < 0.05$. All comparisons were performed using the statistical package SPSS 21.0 for Mac (Manufacturer, City, Country).

**Author Contributions:** Maria Perticone, Raffaele Maio and Francesco Perticone conceived and designed the experiments; Maria Perticone and Antonio Cimellaro performed the experiments; Antonio Cimellaro, Raffaele Maio and Angela Sciacqua analyzed the data; Maria Perticone, Benedetto Caroleo and Giorgio Sesti contributed reagents/materials/analysis tools; Maria Perticone and Francesco Perticone wrote the paper.

## Abbreviations

| | |
|---|---|
| MS | metabolic syndrome |
| CV | cardiovascular |
| IR | insulin resistance |
| NO | nitric oxide |
| NAFLD | non-alcoholic fatty liver disease |
| BMI | body mass index |
| PP | pulse pressure |
| BP | blood pressure |
| GGT | gamma-glutamyltransferase |
| AST | gamma-glutamyltransferase |
| ALT | alanine aminotransferase |
| FBF | forearm blood flow |
| ACh | achetylcholine |
| SNP | sodium nitroprusside |
| HOMA | homeostasis model assessment |
| hs-CRP | high sensitivity C-reactive protein |
| eNOS | endothelial-nitric oxide synthase |
| iNOS | inducible-nitric oxide synthase |
| FLI | fatty liver index |
| eGFR | estimated glomerular filtration rate |

## References

1.  Alberti, K.G.; Eckel, R.H.; Grundy, S.M.; Zimmet, P.Z.; Cleeman, J.I.; Donato, K.A.; Fruchart, J.C.; James, W.P.; Loria, C.M.; Smith, S.C., Jr.; *et al.* Harmonizing the metabolic syndrome: A joint interim statement of the International Diabetes Federation Task Force on Epidemiology and Prevention; National Heart, Lung, and Blood Institute; American Heart Association; World Heart Federation; International Atherosclerosis Society; and International Association for the study of obesity. *Circulation* **2009**, *120*, 1640–1645. [PubMed]

2.  Isomaa, B.; Almgren, P.; Tuomi, T.; Forsén, B.; Lahti, K.; Nissén, M.; Taskinen, M.R.; Groop, L. Cardiovascular morbidity and mortality associated with the metabolic syndrome. *Diabetes Care* **2001**, *24*, 683–689. [CrossRef] [PubMed]

3.  Lakka, H.M.; Laaksonen, D.E.; Lakka, T.A.; Niskanen, L.K.; Kumpusalo, E.; Tuomilehto, J.; Salonen, J.T. The metabolic syndrome and total and cardiovascular disease mortality in middle-aged men. *JAMA* **2002**, *288*, 2709–2716. [CrossRef] [PubMed]

4.   Hanley, A.J.; Karter, A.J.; Festa, A.; D'Agostino, R., Jr.; Wagenknecht, L.E.; Savage, P.; Tracy, R.P.; Saad, M.F.; Haffner, S. Factor analysis of metabolic syndrome using directly measured insulin sensitivity: The insulin resistance atherosclerosis study. *Diabetes* **2002**, *51*, 2642–2647. [CrossRef] [PubMed]

5.   Perticone, F.; Ceravolo, R.; Pujia, A.; Ventura, G.; Iacopino, S.; Scozzafava, A.; Ferraro, A.; Chello, M.; Mastroroberto, P.; Verdecchia, P.; *et al.* Prognostic significance of endothelial dysfunction in hypertensive patients. *Circulation* **2001**, *104*, 191–196. [CrossRef] [PubMed]

6.   Sciacqua, A.; Scozzafava, A.; Pujia, A.; Maio, R.; Borrello, F.; Andreozzi, F.; Vatrano, M.; Cassano, S.; Perticone, M.; Sesti, G.; *et al.* Interaction between vascular dysfunction and cardiac mass increases the risk of cardiovascular outcomes in essential hypertension. *Eur. Heart J.* **2005**, *26*, 921–927. [CrossRef] [PubMed]

7.   Perticone, F.; Maio, R.; Ceravolo, R.; Cosco, C.; Cloro, C.; Mattioli, P.L. Relationship between left ventricular mass and endothelium-dependent vasodilation in never-treated hypertensive patients. *Circulation* **1999**, *99*, 1991–1996. [CrossRef] [PubMed]

8.   Perticone, F.; Maio, R.; Perticone, M.; Miceli, S.; Sciacqua, A.; Tassone, E.J.; Shehaj, E.; Tripepi, G.; Sesti, G. Endothelial dysfunction predicts regression of hypertensive cardiac mass. *Int. J. Cardiol.* **2013**, *167*, 1188–1192. [CrossRef] [PubMed]

9.   Perticone, F.; Maio, R.; Perticone, M.; Sciacqua, A.; Shehaj, E.; Naccarato, P.; Sesti, G. Endothelial dysfunction and subsequent decline in glomerular filtration rate in hypertensive patients. *Circulation* **2010**, *122*, 379–384. [CrossRef] [PubMed]

10.  Reaven, G.M.; Lithell, H.; Landsberg, L. Hypertension and associated metabolic abnormalities-the role of insulin resistance and the sympathoadrenal system. *N. Engl. J. Med.* **1996**, *334*, 374–381. [PubMed]

11.  Perticone, F.; Sciacqua, A.; Scozzafava, A.; Ventura, G.; Laratta, E.; Pujia, A.; Federici, M.; Lauro, R.; Sesti, G. Impaired endothelial function in never-treated hypertensive subjects carrying the Arg972 polymorphism in the insulin receptor substrate-1 gene. *J. Clin. Endocrinol. Metab.* **2004**, *89*, 3606–3609. [CrossRef] [PubMed]

12.  Perticone, F.; Ceravolo, R.; Candigliota, M.; Ventura, G.; Iacopino, S.; Sinopoli, F.; Mattioli, P.L. Obesity and body fat distribution induce endothelial dysfunction by oxidative stress: protective effect of vitamin C. *Diabetes* **2001**, *50*, 159–165. [CrossRef] [PubMed]

13.  Yki-Järvinen, H. Non-alcoholic fatty liver disease as a cause and a consequence of metabolic syndrome. *Lancet Diabetes Endocrinol.* **2014**, *2*, 901–910. [CrossRef]

14.  Marchesini, G.; Brizi, M.; Bianchi, G.; Tomassetti, S.; Bugianesi, E.; Lenzi, M.; McCullough, A.J.; Natale, S.; Forlani, G.; Melchionda, N. Nonalcoholic fatty liver disease: A feature of the metabolic syndrome. *Diabetes* **2001**, *50*, 1844–1850. [CrossRef] [PubMed]

15.  Pagano, G.; Pacini, G.; Musso, G.; Gambino, R.; Mecca, F.; Depetris, N.; Cassader, M.; David, E.; Cavallo-Perin, P.; Rizzetto, M. Nonalcoholic steatohepatitis, insulin resistance, and metabolic syndrome: Further evidence for an etiologic association. *Hepatology* **2002**, *35*, 367–372. [CrossRef] [PubMed]

16.  Utzschneider, K.M.; Kahn, S.E. Review: The role of insulin resistance in nonalcoholic fatty liver disease. *J. Clin. Endocrinol. Metab.* **2006**, *91*, 4753–4761. [CrossRef] [PubMed]

17.  Sciacqua, A.; Perticone, M.; Miceli, S.; Laino, I.; Tassone, E.J.; Grembiale, R.D.; Andreozzi, F.; Sesti, G.; Perticone, F. Endothelial dysfunction and non-alcoholic liver steatosis in hypertensive patients. *Nutr. Metab. Cardiovasc Dis.* **2011**, *21*, 485–491. [CrossRef] [PubMed]

18.  Festi, D.; Colecchia, A.; Sacco, T.; Bondi, M.; Roda, E.; Marchesini, G. Hepatic steatosis in obese patients: Clinical aspects and prognostic significance. *Obes. Rev.* **2004**, *5*, 27–42. [CrossRef] [PubMed]

19.  Iwakir, Y.; Kim, M.Y. Nitric oxide in liver diseases. *Trends Pharmacol. Sci.* **2015**, *36*, 524–536. [CrossRef] [PubMed]

20.  Pasarín, M.; Abraldes, J.G.; Rodríguez-Vilarrupla, A.; La Mura, V.; García-Pagán, J.C.; Bosch, J. Insulin resistance and liver microcirculation in a rat model of early NAFLD. *J. Hepatol.* **2011**, *55*, 1095–1102. [CrossRef] [PubMed]

21.  Duncan, E.R.; Crossey, P.A.; Walker, S.; Anilkumar, N.; Poston, L.; Douglas, G.; Ezzat, V.A.; Wheatcroft, S.B.; Shah, A.M.; Kearney, M.T. Effect of endothelium-specific insulin resistance on endothelial function *in vivo*. *Diabetes* **2008**, *57*, 3307–3314. [CrossRef] [PubMed]

22.  Muniyappa, R.; Sowers, J.R. Role of insulin resistance in endothelial dysfunction. *Rev. Endocr. Metab. Disord.* **2013**, *14*, 5–12. [CrossRef] [PubMed]

23.  Marchesini, G.; Brizi, M.; Morselli-Labate, A.M.; Bianchi, G.; Bugianesi, E.; McCullough, A.J.; Forlani, G.; Melchionda, N. Association of non-alcoholic fatty liver disease to insulin resistance. *Am. J. Med.* **1999**, *107*, 450–455. [CrossRef]

24.  Angelico, F.; Del Ben, M.; Conti, R.; Francioso, S.; Feole, K.; Fiorello, S.; Cavallo, M.G.; Zalunardo, B.; Lirussi, F.; Alessandri, C.; *et al.* Insulin resistance, the metabolic syndrome and non-alcoholic fatty liver disease. *J. Clin. Endocrinol. Metab.* **2005**, *90*, 1578–1582. [CrossRef] [PubMed]

25.  Targher, G.; Bertolini, L.; Poli, F.; Rodella, S.; Scala, L.; Tessari, R.; Zenari, L.; Falezza, G. Nonalcoholic fatty liver disease and risk of future cardiovascular events among type 2 diabetic patients. *Diabetes* **2005**, *54*, 3541–3546. [PubMed]

26.  Fedchuk, L.; Nascimbeni, F.; Pais, R.; Charlotte, F.; Housset, C.; Ratziu, V. LIDO Study Group. Performance and limitations of steatosis biomarkers in patients with nonalcoholic fatty liver disease. *Aliment. Pharmacol. Ther.* **2014**, *40*, 1209–1222. [CrossRef] [PubMed]

27.  Motamed, N.; Sohrabi, M.; Ajdarkosh, H.; Hemmasi, G.; Maadi, M.; Sayeedian, F.S.; Pirzad, R.; Abedi, K.; Aghapour, S.; Fallahnezhad, M.; *et al.* Fatty liver index *vs.* waist circumference for predicting non-alcoholic fatty liver disease. *World J. Gastroenterol.* **2016**, *22*, 3023–3030. [CrossRef] [PubMed]

28.  Loria, P.; Marchesini, G.; Nascimbeni, F.; Ballestri, S.; Maurantonio, M.; Carubbi, F.; Ratziu, V.; Lonardo, A. Cardiovascular risk, lipidemic phenotype and steatosis. A comparative analysis of cirrhotic and non-cirrhotic liver disease due to varying etiology. *Atherosclerosis* **2014**, *232*, 99–109. [CrossRef] [PubMed]

29.  Succurro, E.; Marini, M.A.; Arturi, F.; Grembiale, A.; Lugarà, M.; Andreozzi, F.; Sciacqua, A.; Lauro, R.; Hribal, M.L.; Perticone, F.; *et al.* Elevated one-hour post-load plasma glucose levels identifies subjects with normal glucose tolerance but early carotid atherosclerosis. *Atherosclerosis* **2009**, *207*, 245–249. [CrossRef] [PubMed]

30.  Bedogni, G.; Bellentani, S.; Miglioli, L.; Masutti, F.; Passalacqua, M.; Castiglione, A.; Tiribelli, C. The Fatty Liver Index: A simple and accurate predictor of hepatic steatosis in the general population. *BMC Gastroenterol.* **2006**, *6*. [CrossRef] [PubMed]

31.  Levey, A.S.; Stevens, L.A.; Schmid, C.H.; Zhang, Y.L.; Castro, A.F., 3rd; Feldman, H.I.; Kusek, J.W.; Eggers, P.; van Lente, F.; Greene, T.; *et al.* A new equation to estimate glomerular filtration rate. *Ann. Intern. Med.* **2009**, *150*, 604–612. [CrossRef] [PubMed]

32.  Bonora, E.; Targher, G.; Alberiche, M.; Bonadonna, R.C.; Saggiani, F.; Zenere, M.B.; Monauni, T.; Muggeo, M. Homeostasis model assessment closely mirrors the glucose clamp technique in the assessment of insulin sensitivity: Studies in subjects with various degrees of glucose tolerance and insulin sensitivity. *Diabetes Care* **2000**, *23*, 57–63. [CrossRef] [PubMed]

33.  Matthews, D.R.; Hosker, J.P.; Rudenski, A.S.; Naylor, B.A.; Treacher, D.F.; Turner, R.C. Homeostasis model assessment: insulin resistance and beta-cell function from fasting plasma glucose and insulin concentrations in man. *Diabetologia* **1985**, *28*, 412–419. [CrossRef] [PubMed]

34.  Mancia, G.; Fagard, R.; Narkiewicz, K.; Redón, J.; Zanchetti, A.; Böhm, M.; Christiaens, T.; Cifkova, R.; de Backer, G.; Dominiczak, A.; *et al.* 2007 Guidelines for the management of arterial hypertension: the task force for the management of arterial hypertension of the european society of hypertension (ESH) and of the european society of cardiology (ESC). *Eur. Heart J.* **2007**, *28*, 1462–1536. [CrossRef] [PubMed]

35.  Whitney, R.J. Measurement of changes in human limb volume by means of a mercury-in-rubber strain gauge. *J. Physiol.* **1949**, *109*, 5.

36.  Panza, J.A.; Quyyumi, A.A.; Brush, J.E., Jr.; Epstein, S.E. Abnormal endothelium-dependent vascular relaxation in patients with essential hypertension. *N. Engl. J. Med.* **1990**, *323*, 22–27. [CrossRef] [PubMed]

37.  Perticone, F.; Sciacqua, A.; Maio, R.; Perticone, M.; Galiano Leone, G.; Bruni, R.; Di Cello, S.; Pascale, A.; Talarico, G.; Greco, L.; *et al.* Endothelial dysfunction, ADMA and insulin resistance in essential hypertension. *Int. J. Cardiol.* **2010**, *142*, 236–241. [CrossRef] [PubMed]

# 11

# A Guide to Non-Alcoholic Fatty Liver Disease in Childhood and Adolescence

Jonathan L. Temple [1], Paul Cordero [2,*], Jiawei Li [2], Vi Nguyen [2] and Jude A. Oben [2,3,*]

[1]   Faculty of Life Sciences and Medicine, King's College London, Strand, London WC2R 2LS, UK;
      jonathan.temple@kcl.ac.uk
[2]   Institute for Liver and Digestive Health, University College London, Rowland Hill Street,
      London NW3 2PF, UK; jiawei.li.10@ucl.ac.uk (J.L.); v.nguyen@ucl.ac.uk (V.N.)
[3]   Department of Gastroenterology and Hepatology, Guy's and St Thomas' Hospital, NHS Foundation Trust,
      Westminster Bridge Rd., London SE1 7EH, UK
*    Correspondence: paul.sanchez@ucl.ac.uk (P.C.); j.oben@ucl.ac.uk (J.A.O.);

Academic Editors: Amedeo Lonardo and Giovanni Targher

**Abstract:** Non-Alcoholic Fatty Liver Disease (NAFLD) is now the most prevalent form of chronic liver disease, affecting 10%–20% of the general paediatric population. Within the next 10 years it is expected to become the leading cause of liver pathology, liver failure and indication for liver transplantation in childhood and adolescence in the Western world. While our understanding of the pathophysiological mechanisms underlying this disease remains limited, it is thought to be the hepatic manifestation of more widespread metabolic dysfunction and is strongly associated with a number of metabolic risk factors, including insulin resistance, dyslipidaemia, cardiovascular disease and, most significantly, obesity. Despite this, "paediatric" NAFLD remains under-studied, under-recognised and, potentially, undermanaged. This article will explore and evaluate our current understanding of NAFLD in childhood and adolescence and how it differs from adult NAFLD, in terms of its epidemiology, pathophysiology, natural history, diagnosis and clinical management. Given the current absence of definitive radiological and histopathological diagnostic tests, maintenance of a high clinical suspicion by all members of the multidisciplinary team in primary and specialist care settings remains the most potent of diagnostic tools, enabling early diagnosis and appropriate therapeutic intervention.

**Keywords:** NAFLD; steatosis; obesity; children; adolescent

## 1. Introduction

Non-Alcoholic Fatty Liver Disease (NAFLD) encompasses a spectrum of chronic liver disease, characterised by excessive hepatic fat accumulation (steatosis) in the absence of significant alcohol consumption, occurring with or without hepatic inflammation and fibrosis [1]. Simple or bland hepatic steatosis describes the abnormal accumulation of fat in >5% of hepatocytes, without evidence of hepatocellular injury or fibrosis. A significant proportion of patients with hepatic steatosis, however, progress to a more advanced form of the disease, Non-Alcoholic Steatohepatitis (NASH), where steatosis coexists with hepatocellular injury and inflammation, which can precipitate hepatic necrosis, fibrosis and cirrhosis, as well as a significantly increased risk of hepatocellular carcinoma [1–3].

NAFLD is thought to be a hepatic manifestation of more widespread and underlying metabolic dysfunction and is strongly associated with a number of metabolic risk factors, including insulin resistance, dyslipidaemia, cardiovascular disease and, most significantly, obesity [2,4,5]. Our understanding of the pathophysiological mechanisms underpinning these relationships, however, remains incomplete.

While detailed clinico-pathological descriptions of NAFLD in adults can be found in the literature as far back as the 1850s, the first case of paediatric NAFLD was reported in 1983 by Moran *et al.* [6,7]. It is now the most prevalent form of chronic liver disease in childhood and adolescence, affecting approximately 10%–20% of the general paediatric population. Within the next 10 years, paediatric NAFLD is expected to become the most prevalent cause of liver pathology, liver failure and indication for liver transplantation in childhood and adolescence in the Western world [8–13].

Despite this, "paediatric" NAFLD remains under-studied, under-recognised and, potentially, undermanaged [14]. Important gaps remain in our overall approach to screening, diagnosis, management and follow-up, particularly during the transition between paediatric and adult clinical services [15]. More accurate epidemiological and pathophysiological data derived from larger longitudinal cohort studies are needed in order to better determine the true prevalence and natural history of paediatric NAFLD among different ethnic groups, aiding the selection and widespread implementation of more effective therapeutic interventions [13,16]. Recognition, first, of the occurrence of NAFLD in the paediatric population and, second, the differences in its clinical presentation, pathophysiology, histology and prognosis when compared to adult disease, is of critical importance.

## 2. Clinical Presentation of Paediatric Non-Alcoholic Fatty Liver Disease (NAFLD)

Although cases of paediatric NAFLD and NASH-related cirrhosis have been reported in patients as young as 2 and 8 years old, respectively, most usually present clinically above the age of 10 years. The mean age of diagnosis is 11–13 years old [11,12,17]. However, NAFLD often remains asymptomatic until significant damage to the liver and/or other systems has occurred or coincident acute liver injury manifests worse clinical outcomes than would otherwise be expected or NAFLD-associated comorbidities, including insulin resistance and Type II Diabetes Mellitus, develop. Diagnosis, therefore, is often incidental on physical examination or routine blood testing, accounting for approximately 7%–11% of abnormal liver function tests (LFTs) and 74% of liver biopsies in obese patients with metabolic risk factors [8,9].

Children may also report non-specific symptoms, including abdominal pain due to stretching of the liver capsule, fatigue, irritability, headaches and difficulty concentrating [12,14]. Hepatomegaly may be appreciated on manual palpation in up to 50% of cases but can be difficult to discern in obese patients. Acanthosis nigricans, a clinical marker of hyperinsulinemia that can manifest on the back of the neck, intertriginous areas or joints, has been reported in 33%–50% of children with biopsy-proven NAFLD [8,9,11,17,18].

A landmark study of 742 autopsy specimens from children in San Diego County (CA, USA) between 1993 and 2003 found evidence of NAFLD in 17.3% of children aged 15–19 years old [9]. This is consistent with other more recent studies [11,19,20], including one involving 995 adolescents aged 17 years old, which reported a prevalence of NAFLD of greater than 15% [21]. The true prevalence of paediatric NAFLD, however, is difficult to determine and may be even higher, given the marked variations in the populations studied, in terms of age, ethnicity, the diagnostic parameters applied and clinical bias with regards to the "appropriateness" of diagnosing NAFLD in children, as well as the general paucity of research.

Certainly, the prevalence of NAFLD in childhood and adolescence has greatly increased in recent decades, in the wake of rising levels of childhood obesity [22]. Paediatric NAFLD is strongly associated with a number of metabolic risk factors, including increased insulin resistance, dyslipidaemia, cardiovascular disease and, most significantly, visceral adiposity [12,22–24]. A number of studies now suggest the prevalence of NAFLD in overweight and obese youth to be up to 70%, compared to 7% in those of normal weight [25,26]. Severe obesity (>95th centile for age and gender-adjusted body mass index) is also associated with more adverse clinical outcomes and greater risk of progression to NASH and cirrhosis in childhood [14].

Below 3 years of age, obesity does not usually produce hepatic steatosis and, as such, its incidence may well indicate more severe underlying metabolic dysfunction with worse prognosis [17]. Therefore, 'brightness' of the liver on ultrasound or increased aminotransferases in this age group requires a detailed clinical workup, to exclude many rare metabolic or systemic diseases that may also present with hepatic steatosis, collectively referred to by some authors as the "NASH trash bin" [17].

While simple steatosis carries a minimal risk of cirrhosis and liver failure in adults, it appears to follow a more aggressive course in paediatric cases, with many children progressing to NASH and hepatic fibrosis either in childhood or early adulthood [27,28]. Paediatric patients with more advanced fibrosis on liver biopsy tend to have more hepatic complications and a worse prognosis, particularly regarding the risk of cirrhosis [29]. A high clinical suspicion should therefore be maintained, particularly in children more than 10 years old who are overweight or obese and have a waist circumference above the 95th centile, in the context of other metabolic risk factors, abnormal LFTs and a family history of severe NAFLD [17].

Some studies have suggested, however, that normal-weight individuals with NAFLD appear to present at a younger age than those who are overweight or obese and demonstrate a decreased association with components of the metabolic syndrome, such as hypertension and insulin resistance [30,31]. This has given rise to the controversial hypothesis that paediatric NAFLD might, in fact, represent a group of related but pathophysiologically distinct clinical phenomenologies.

## 2.1. NAFLD and Obesity

The single greatest risk factor for paediatric NAFLD is obesity, with an estimated prevalence in overweight and obese youth of 50%–80% compared to 2%–7% in children of normal weight [25,26]. A recent cross-sectional study of 182 obese sedentary children and adolescents demonstrated a positive correlation between increased abdominal fat and the incidence of NAFLD, independently of insulin resistance and dyslipidaemia [32]. Central obesity has also been shown to reliably predict evidence of NAFLD on ultrasound and aminotransferase elevation in a cohort of more than 11,000 obese patients aged 6–18 years old [33]. A further study by Manco et al. [34] reported that 92% of paediatric NAFLD patients had a Body Mass Index (BMI) higher than the 85th centile and 84% had a waist circumference greater than the 90th centile. Moreover, significant correlation between waist circumference, total fat mass and intra-abdominal adipose tissue and the incidence of NAFLD was also reported in a cross-sectional study of 145 patients aged 11–17 years [10]. Waist circumference may, therefore, represent an interesting and reliable screening tool in paediatric NAFLD.

While obesity is thought to cause an overabundance of circulating free fatty acids, increasing hepatic steatosis, as well as contributing to the development of insulin resistance, the exact pathophysiological mechanisms by which obesity increases the risk of paediatric NAFLD remain poorly understood [14,35]. Indeed, not all children who are obese develop NAFLD, suggesting that other factors may inform risk such as the preferential deposition of visceral, as opposed to subcutaneous, adipose tissue [6,36].

Visceral adipose tissue is the primary source of hepatic fat in adults, contributing 59% of the triglyceride found in the liver; the main component of fat accumulation in NAFLD [9]. Increasing evidence also suggests that adipose tissue fulfils important and distinct endocrine functions, producing multiple pro-inflammatory adipocytokines, including TNF-$\alpha$, IL-6, leptin and adiponectin, which are implicated in the clinical manifestation of NAFLD and its progression to NASH and cirrhosis [37,38]. Pentoxifylline, a phosphodiesterase inhibitor and non-specific TNF-$\alpha$ pathway antagonist, has been shown to promote a reduction in serum Alanine Aminotransferase (ALT) levels and improvement of the histological features of NASH in adult patients [12,39]. Other TNF-$\alpha$ inhibitors, such as infliximab, a selective chimeric monoclonal antibody against TNF-$\alpha$, and resveratrol, a polyphenol with anti-inflammatory activity, have shown interesting results in adult clinical trials [12,39].

Furthermore, abdominal visceral adipose tissue has peculiarities of its own, including higher lipolysis and greater release of adipokines [32]. There is also evidence to suggest that, as the adipose bed expands, adipocytes suffer from a micro-hypoxic environment, due to insufficiency of its vascular network, resulting in cell injury and death and consequent upregulation of the pro-inflammatory cascade [9]. Circulating adipokines also appear to promote specific patterns of lipid storage and metabolic stress, which in turn activate signalling cascades that induce oxidative stress and trigger a local and/or systemic inflammatory response [35]. However, visceral adipose mass is much less developed in children, compared with adults, though it accumulates rapidly with weight gain, particularly in males. It has, therefore, been suggested that subcutaneous adipose tissue, although less metabolically active than visceral adipose tissue, may play a greater role in paediatric NAFLD [6,36]. Indeed, recent reports describe specific differences in the distribution of subcutaneous adipose tissue between adolescents with NAFLD and those without. These differences are apparent from three years old but not at birth, suggesting that the first three years of life might represent a critical window in which various interactions between genetic, environmental, epigenetic and metabolic factors contribute to the future risk of NAFLD [6] (Figure 1).

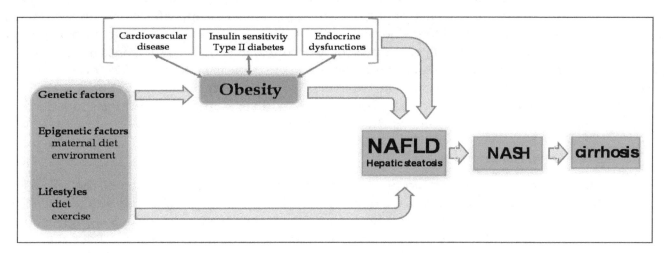

**Figure 1.** Obesity and Non-Alcoholic Fatty Liver Disease (NAFLD). Abbreviations: NAFLD: non-alcoholic fatty liver disease; NASH: non-alcoholic steatohepatitis.

## 2.2. Hepatic Complications of NAFLD

Non-Alcoholic Steatohepatitis (NASH) is commonly considered a more advanced form of NAFLD, where steatosis coexists with hepatocellular injury and inflammation, precipitating hepatic necrosis, fibrosis and cirrhosis and a significantly increased risk of hepatocellular carcinoma [1,19]. NASH significantly increases both overall and liver-related mortality, with the most common causes of death being cirrhosis and liver failure, neoplasia, sepsis, variceal haemorrhage and cardiovascular disease [11]. Long-term follow-up studies have shown that, in adults, NASH increases overall mortality by 35%–58% compared with age and sex-matched controls, while liver-related mortality is increased 9–10 fold [40–42]. NAFLD is, by far, the most common cause of hepatic fibrosis and cirrhosis in adults and children with unexplained or cryptogenic increases in serum alanine aminotransferase. However, advanced fibrosis can readily coexist with normal serum aminotransferase levels and has been reported in up to a third of patients with isolated simple steatosis [11].

### 2.2.1. Fibrosis

Approximately 25% of paediatric patients will progress to NASH, though the risk increases significantly in the context of obesity [43]. For example, a recent study of 24 severely obese bariatric adolescent patients found 63% had definitive NASH and a further 25% had "borderline" NASH [44]. Hepatic fibrosis has been documented retrospectively in more than one third of adult patients with NASH [11]. In a national multi-centre study, advanced fibrosis was reported at the time of diagnostic liver biopsy in nearly one in seven children with NAFLD [43]. Another study reported similar findings, with 17% of children with NAFLD having advanced fibrosis. After adjusting for fibrotic confounders, NASH appears to have a fibrotic potential similar to that of chronic Hepatitis C [11,45]. The main predictors of the severity of fibrosis are increasing age, BMI > 28–30 kg/m$^2$, hypertension, the degree of insulin resistance and diabetes [11]. Hepatic fibrosis also appears more prevalent in adolescents with severe obesity (83% *vs.* 29% in adults), further suggesting that paediatric patients, especially those who are obese, tend to follow a more aggressive clinical course than adults with NAFLD [14].

### 2.2.2. Cirrhosis

After 10 years, the risk of cirrhosis in adult patients with NASH is 15%–25%. Once cirrhosis is established, 30%–40% of these die within another 10 years [23]. Current evidence suggests that children have similar risks of progressing from NASH to decompensated end-stage liver disease, requiring transplantation [44].

End-stage NASH is a frequent and important cause of cryptogenic cirrhosis, mainly because hepatic fat accumulation and evidence of hepatocellular injury can disappear at this advanced stage; a phenomenon sometimes referred to as "burned out" NASH [11]. It has been shown that if a diagnosis of NASH were made on the basis of past or present exposure to metabolic risk factors, such as obesity, diabetes and hypertension, when histological signs are lacking, approximately 30%–75% of cryptogenic cirrhosis could be attributed to "burned-out" NASH. Liver failure is often the first presentation of patients with cirrhotic NASH and usually occurs after 7–10 years in adults but due to its quicker development, it may occur even more rapidly in paediatric cases [11].

### 2.2.3. Hepatocellular Carcinoma

Hepatocellular carcinoma can occur in both cirrhotic and, it appears, non-cirrhotic NASH. Its prevalence is greater still in obese or diabetic NAFLD patients [46,47]. In a study cohort of 285,884 boys and girls in Copenhagen who were followed for over three decades, higher body mass index (BMI) in childhood was associated with an increased risk of primary liver cancer in adulthood [48]. The hazard ratio (95% CI) of adult liver cancer was 1.20 (1.07–1.33) and 1.30 (1.16–1.46) per unit BMI $z$-score at 7 and 13 years, respectively. Similar associations were found for boys and girls for hepatocellular carcinoma only, across years of birth, and after accounting for diagnoses of viral hepatitis, alcohol-related disorders and biliary cirrhosis [48]. There is also, likely, a chronic underestimation of the proportion of NASH progressing towards end-stage liver disease, as many patients are no longer listed because of the co-occurrence of associated diseases, including obesity, cardiovascular disease and diabetes [11].

### 2.3. Extra-Hepatic Complications of NAFLD

While NAFLD is not a formal component of the diagnostic criteria for the metabolic syndrome, they do share common major risk factors, including central obesity, high serum triglycerides and high-density lipoprotein cholesterol (HDL-C), hypertension and insulin resistance, as well as altered glucose and lipid metabolism. Nearly 90% of NAFLD patients have at least one feature of the metabolic syndrome and up to 33% meet the complete diagnosis [4,18,49].

What is clear is that patient outcomes worsen when both conditions co-occur in an apparently synergistic manner [4,24,35,44] The presence of the metabolic syndrome, also, is a strong clinical predictor of NASH, particularly in overweight and obese paediatric patients [19,32]. This has led some to describe paediatric NAFLD in terms of either the hepatic manifestation or precursor of the metabolic syndrome [12,44,49]. Others, however, have suggested that both conditions may feed into one another, creating a vicious cycle of worsening metabolic disease, likely indicative of more widespread underlying metabolic dysfunction [35]. However, while we might infer that there exists significant overlap between the pathophysiological mechanisms that underlie these two conditions, their nature and extent remain poorly understood [4,18,49].

## 2.3.1. Cardiovascular Disease

NAFLD is an independent risk factor for coronary artery disease, as well as being strongly associated with a number of other cardiovascular risk factors, including multi-organ insulin resistance, dyslipidaemia and impaired flow-mediated vasodilatation [50]. Significant carotid atherosclerosis has been shown to occur 5–10 years earlier in patients with NAFLD than in those without and, in cases of biopsy proven NAFLD, hepatic steatosis is associated with increased carotid artery intima-media thickness and the presence of carotid plaques [11]. Biochemical surrogates of NAFLD, γ-glutamyl transferase (GGT) and ALT, predict the incidence of coronary artery disease and other cardiovascular disease, which is further elevated in NAFLD patients who suffer co-morbidly with diabetes mellitus [11]. Furthermore, in adults, NAFLD has been associated with myocardial insulin resistance, altered cardiac energy metabolism, abnormal left ventricular structure and impaired diastolic function; the duration and severity of these abnormalities in cardiac function likely contributing to the increased risk of heart failure and cardiovascular mortality in obese patients and, particularly, those with NAFLD [50]. Indeed, adult patients with NAFLD are at a significantly higher risk of cardiovascular mortality than the general population, with cardiovascular disease being the most common cause of death in NAFLD patients [11,44].

Cardiac functional abnormalities have also been reported in obese adolescents that were independent of traditional cardiac risk factors (*i.e.*, high systolic and diastolic pressures, total and low-density lipoprotein cholesterol and BMI) and correlated with insulin resistance [50]. One study assessing 50 children with biopsy-proven NAFLD using 24 h blood pressure monitoring and Doppler echocardiography parameters reported instances of cardiac dysfunction that were detectable in early NAFLD and were linked to no other cardiovascular or metabolic alteration other than liver damage. Left ventricular hypertrophy was present in 35% of patients, concentric remodelling in 14% and left atrial dilatation in 16%. Furthermore, children with simple steatosis showed lesser cardiac alterations than NASH patients [51]. Pacifico *et al.* [52] went on to demonstrate that even asymptomatic obese children with NAFLD exhibit early left ventricular diastolic and systolic dysfunctions, becoming more severe in patients with NASH. Hence, as NAFLD advances, the extent of cardiovascular dysfunction increases, with several other studies demonstrating greater endothelial dysfunction, an early proatherogenic lesion, and carotid intima thickness in NASH than in simple steatosis.

Elsewhere, Nobili *et al.* [53] have demonstrated that the severity of liver injury is strongly associated with the presence of a more atherogenic lipid profile, in terms of triglyceride/high density lipoprotein cholesterol (HDL), total cholesterol/HDL and low density lipoprotein (LDL)/HDL ratios. A further study of 548 children with a high triglycerides/HDL ratio reported an increased risk of insulin resistance that correlated independently, with more advanced NAFLD [54].

## 2.3.2. Insulin Resistance and Type II Diabetes Mellitus

Insulin Resistance (IR) is the most common metabolic abnormality associated with NAFLD and, perhaps, the most useful indicator of disease severity and progression in adults and children [19,49]. The severity of IR is strongly associated with the amount of hepatic fat accumulation, independently of global and intra-abdominal adiposity and the prevalence of NAFLD is greater in patients with hyperglycaemia and type II diabetes, with evidence of NAFLD present on ultrasound in up to 70% of clinical cases [14,32].

The key question remains, however, as to whether this relationship is causal or whether hepatic fat accumulation is, itself, a consequence of insulin resistance. On the one hand, hepatic steatosis and impairment reduces insulin clearance and, over time, greater insulin resistance [11]. Indeed, in NAFLD, steatosis and hepatic IR have been shown to occur in advance of peripheral IR, suggesting that the former is the primary defect in the development of the latter. Hepatic steatosis has, in turn, been shown to exacerbate insulin resistance by interfering with the phosphorylation of insulin receptor substrates, with the amount of hepatic steatosis correlating with the severity of IR [11,12].

On the other hand, insulin is an anabolic hormone that promotes glucose uptake in the liver, skeletal muscle and adipose tissue [9,10,12]. Increasing insulin resistance precipitates a reduction in glucose uptake by the liver and a compensatory increase in circulating levels of insulin. This drives increased hepatic and peripheral glycogenesis and lipogenesis, via sterol regulatory binding element (SREBP-1c) mediated upregulation of several prolipogenic genes, as well as impairing hepatocytic fatty acid metabolism [9,10,12]. As a result, circulating free fatty acids become increasingly abundant, most being taken up by the liver, where they are invariably processed into triglycerides and deposited within the cytoplasm of hepatocytes in large triglyceride-filled vacuoles, manifesting hepatic steatosis. As insulin resistance develops, high serum glucose levels also activate the carbohydrate responsive element binding protein, which further promotes lipogenesis and hepatic fat deposition [9].

It has also been suggested, therefore, that insulin resistance and hyperglycaemia may induce fibrosis directly or via upregulation of connective tissue growth factor, the generation of advanced glycation end products or through upregulation of pro-inflammatory cytokine production [11,55].

Controversially, others have sought to describe hepatic steatosis in terms of an adaptive, albeit imperfect, hepatic response to hepatic stress that forestalls the onset of NASH, albeit one that, in children, appears less effective and more prone to its own complications [9,11,56]. Indeed, Choi and Diehl suggested that the formation of lipid droplets may actually be protective by sequestering toxic free fatty acids in the form of triglycerides but, that when this buffer exceeds its capacity, certain free fatty acids begin to exert their toxic effect [57]. Work done in mice demonstrated that when triglyceride synthesis was inhibited, hepatic fat accumulation decreased but liver damage worsened, as measured by necroinflammation and fibrosis [58]. Conversely, up-regulation of diacylglycerol O-acyltransferase 2 (DGAT2) resulted in increased hepatic steatosis and was associated with a significant increase in liver inflammatory markers. Free fatty acids and their lipotoxic intermediates have been implicated in the promotion of inflammation, endoplasmic reticular stress, mitochondrial dysfunction and oxidant stress. These processes are injurious to hepatocytes, which, in turn, release pro-inflammatory cytokines and reactive oxygen species as they die, driving further hepatic inflammation [9]. Therefore, we are forced to consider whether steatosis, while a useful biomarker of ongoing injurious and fibrotic mechanisms resulting in disease progression, should be considered at all a therapeutic target and whether such interventions are in actual fact more damaging [11]. Instead, Wanless and Shiota [59] postulated that extracellular fat accumulation after hepatocyte necrosis might also impair hepatic blood flow through hepatic veins but this remains unproven.

2.3.3. Other Endocrine Disorders

There is evidence to suggest that other endocrine disorders, such as hypothyroidism, hypogonadism, hypopituitarism and polycystic ovary syndrome, independently of obesity, are important risk factors for NAFLD [11,60,61]. Several studies have addressed the association between thyroid dysfunction and NAFLD. Pacifico et al. [62] were the first to provide evidence of such a link between NAFLD, thyroid function and the metabolic syndrome in childhood, demonstrating a positive correlation between thyroid function tests, thyroid stimulating hormone (TSH) in particular, and the incidence of NAFLD in overweight and obese children, independently of visceral adiposity. Subsequently, Torun et al. [61] showed that TSH levels significantly increase in accordance with the extent of steatosis on ultrasound and ALT and BMI.

## 3. The Pathogenesis of NAFLD

Traditionally, the pathogenesis of NAFLD has been described in terms of a two-hit hypothesis, where hepatic steatosis sensitises the liver to the effects of oxidative stress and the action of various pro-inflammatory cytokines, which would, over time, drive the development of necroinflammation, fibrosis and, ultimately, cirrhosis [11,12]. However, increasing evidence of the complexity and inter-relatedness of numerous pathophysiological mechanisms, both hepatic and extra-hepatic, implicated in the development and progression of NAFLD, has precipitated a change in thinking.

The now widely accepted "multiple-hit model" instead approaches NAFLD in terms of a hepatic manifestation of more widespread metabolic dysfunction, brought about through the interaction of numerous genetic and environmental factors, as well as changes in cross-talk between different organs, including adipose tissue, the pancreas, gut and liver [4,6,12,44]. Obesity and insulin resistance have repeatedly been suggested as the first "true" hits.

The development of NAFLD in children, in particular, it seems is characterised by an intricate network of interactions between resident hepatic and recruited cells, such as Kupffer cells, T cells and hepatic stellate cells, which drive disease progression alongside other infiltrating inflammatory cell-derived factors released either as a direct result of hepatic steatosis, hepatocyte injury and apoptosis or as an indirect response to hepatic damage and/or gut-derived bacterial products acting on Toll-like pattern recognition (TLR) receptors [63,64]. Indeed, dysregulation of pro-inflammatory cytokines and adipokines are almost universally detected in NAFLD patients, while endoplasmic reticular, mitochondrial and cytokine-mediated oxidative stress and hepatocytic apoptosis appear to contribute to the development of NASH [65–67]. TLR antagonists may also, in time, prove effective therapeutic agents for NASH; a potential that mandates further study [12].

Hepatic Stellate cells are considered the main extracellular matrix-producing cells during NASH development and are activated following hepatocyte injury and apoptosis, mediating the development of hepatic fibrosis and, if activation is chronic, cirrhosis. Hepatic Progenitor Cells (HPC), the resident stem cell population within the liver, have recently been shown to be expanded in paediatric NAFLD [66]. They appear to play a role in the liver's response to oxidative stress, their levels correlating with fibrosis and NASH progression [66]. Furthermore, HPCs can undergo an epithelial-mesenchymal transition, resulting in a profibrogenic myofibroblast-like cell population, a process involving the Hedgehog signalling pathway [68].

Kupffer Cells are important regulators of the biological exchanges between hepatocytes and other liver cells, engaging and sustaining the action of neutrophils, natural killer T lymphocytes (NKT) and blood monocyte-derived macrophages, as well as phagocytosing and removing microorganisms, apoptotic cells and cell debris themselves, processing and presenting antigens to attract cytotoxic and regulatory T cells, contributing to adaptive immunity. Increasing evidence suggests that they fulfil many diverse roles in the pathogenesis and progression of NAFLD, including the regulation of immune tolerance and lipid homeostasis [63,69]. Indeed, Stienstra et al. [70] further demonstrated the integral role of Kupffer cells in regulating hepatic triglyceride storage and the promotion of hepatic steatosis via IL-1$\beta$-mediated suppression of perioxisome proliferator-activated receptor-$\alpha$ (PPAR-$\alpha$) activity, while others have reported that Kupffer cell depletion, in a murine experimental model of NASH, prevented hepatic fat accumulation and liver damage [63].

Several studies have described subsequent changes in the frequency and/or functionality of peripheral T cell subpopulations, manifesting an altered phenotype of infiltrating and circulating immune cells that appears to be distinct between adult and paediatric NASH [64]. Several studies have reported a predominance of CD8+ T cells over CD4+ and CD20+ subpopulations undergoing activation in paediatric NASH, in association with increased levels of IFN-$\gamma$ within the hepatic microenvironment, a high number of infiltrating neutrophils in correlation with Reactive Oxygen Species (ROS) generation in peripheral neutrophils and further alterations in the phenotype and functionality of circulating lymphocytes and neutrophils compared with age-matched controls. By contrast, CD8+ cells were a minor component of Natural Killer (NK) and NKT cells in adult NASH [19,64]. The molecular and immunological phenomenology of these systems both locally and systematically, in both paediatric and adult NASH, are complex and are only just beginning to be recognised, let alone understood.

Increasing evidence suggests that dysregulation of the autonomic nervous system innervation of the liver fulfils a critical role in the progression of simple steatosis to NASH and cirrhosis. Indeed, Hepatic Stellate Cell (HSC) autonomic receptors are reportedly upregulated in the livers of adult NAFLD patients and may represent another potential target for future anti-fibrotic therapies [71,72].

## 3.1. Genetics of Paediatric NAFLD

Over the last decade, with the advent of next-generation sequencing technologies, polymorphisms associated with the incidence and severity of paediatric NAFLD have been identified in numerous genes involved in lipid metabolism, insulin sensitivity, oxidative stress, regulation of the immune system and the development of fibrosis [4,73]. Furthermore, evidence of the strong genetic contribution to the pathogenesis of paediatric NAFLD comes from reports familial clustering of metabolic risk factors, including obesity, insulin resistance and type II diabetes. One study of children with biopsy-proven NAFLD, for example, reported that 59% of their siblings and 78% of their parents were found to have evidence of hepatic steatosis on MRI, significantly more than in relatives of age and BMI-matched children without NAFLD [74].

The prevalence and genetic variants associated with NAFLD also vary between different ethnic groups, likely affecting the heritability of metabolic risk factors that contribute to individual susceptibility to the disease [75]. Hispanic children demonstrate the highest prevalence of NAFLD (36%), greater than that of Afro-Caribbeans (14%), Asians (10.2%) and non-Hispanic whites (8.6%) despite these populations exhibiting similar obesity rates [13]. Hispanic patients have also been shown to be at higher risk of type II diabetes and tend to display more features of the metabolic syndrome than non-Hispanic whites, which may further contribute to their greater risk. It has also been suggested that differences in body fat distribution among Afro-Caribbean children, who notably have more subcutaneous fat and less visceral fat and consequently a lesser predisposition towards hepatic fat accumulation, may explain their lower prevalence of NAFLD. Indeed, visceral adiposity is less associated with NAFLD among Afro-Caribbean adolescents than among non-Hispanic whites. Furthermore, insulin resistance appears less tightly linked to visceral adiposity in Afro-Caribbean children with NAFLD and tends to be more associated with the extent and severity of liver damage. Conversely, the extent to which the relationship between insulin resistance and NAFLD severity varies between Hispanics and non-Hispanic whites appears negligible [13,75].

A recent genome-wide association study (GWAS) conducted by the Genetics of Obesity-Related Liver Disease Consortium identified robust associations between polymorphisms of the genes neurocan (NCAN), lysophospholipase-like 1 (LYPLAL1), glucokinase regulatory protein (GCKR) and protein phosphatase 1 regulatory subunit 3b (PPP1R3B) and NAFLD in adults of European ancestry [76]. However, Palmer et al. [16] reported that the allele frequency and effect size of PNPLA3 rs738409, NCAN rs2228603, LYPLAL1 rs12137855, GCKR rs780094 and PPP1R3B rs4240624 varied between adult patients of African and Hispanic ethnicity. Hernaez et al. [77] also reported a lack of consistency of these variants in the NHANES III study population of multiple ethnicities. Another GWAS conducted by Romeo et al. [78] also found that the PNPLA3 rs738409 variant was seen more commonly in Hispanics than in other ethnic groups and was associated with increased liver fat and hepatic inflammation, whereas PNPLA3 rs6006460 was seen more commonly in Afro-Caribbeans and correlated with lesser hepatic fat accumulation. This has been confirmed by another study of 83 obese children using MRI to quantify hepatic lipid content [79]. Further studies have also shown PNPLA3 rs738409 to be associated with greater hepatic steatosis and disease severity, as well as earlier clinical presentation [55,80].

The fat mass and obesity associated (FTO) gene variant rs9939609 has also been associated with increased risk of NAFLD and the Melanocortin 4 Receptor (MC4R) rs12970134 variant with increased ALT levels, independently of BMI, in children aged 7–18 years old with NAFLD [81]. Other genetic variants associated with NASH, hepatic fibrosis and the severity of liver damage in both adults and children have been described in genes involved in lipid metabolism, such as adiponutrin/patatin-like phospholipase domain-containing 3 (PNPLA3), Lipin 1 (LPIN1), adipoprotein C3 (APOC3), endocannabinoid receptor CB2, as well as the hereditary hemochromatosis (HFE) gene [55,82]. For example, PNPLA3 rs738409 has been associated with the presence and severity of hepatic steatosis in numerous studies, independently of insulin resistance or inflammatory changes, lobular inflammation and perivenular fibrosis in both adult and paediatric NAFLD [55,77,80,83]. Other genes associated with progression to NASH relate to oxidative stress and include the rs4880 variant of manganese-dependent superoxide dismutase (SOD2) gene, the rs1801278 variant of insulin receptor substrate-1 (IRS-1) and the rs3750861 variant of tumour suppressor gene Kruppel-like factor 6 (KLF-6) [55].

Our understanding of the mechanisms by which variation in these genes affects the incidence and progression of NAFLD, however, remains limited. PNPLA3, for example, is most robustly expressed in the liver. Its expression appears to be directly related to nutritional intake, being down-regulated in the fasting state and upregulated during feeding. *In vitro* and mouse models have shown that SREBP-1, which is activated by insulin, induces PNPLA3, which then promotes lipogenesis and modulates glucose homeostasis [84]. Additionally, cytochrome P450 oxidative enzyme family 2 subfamily E member 1 (CYP2E1) is a risk factor for oxidative stress and may be implicated in NAFLD [85,86]. Polymorphism of the cytokine Interleukin 6 (IL-6) have been associated with serum of liver damage markers [87]. Variants in the UGT1A1 gene (Gilbert syndrome) have also been shown to contribute to increased bilirubin levels, thus reducing the risk for NAFLD onset and development [88].

Accumulating evidence also suggests the involvement of the endocannabinoid system in NAFLD, which has many diverse roles in humans. For example, in studies of obese children with steatosis and biopsy-proven NAFLD, a functional variant of the otherwise hepatoprotective cannabinoid receptor 2 (CB2), Q63R, was associated with elevated serum aminotransferase levels [89]. Others have suggested that the CB2 Q63R variant fulfils a critical role in modulating hepatic inflammation in obese children, manifesting an increased susceptibility to liver damage in these patients [82].

Given that the effect of genetic variants tends to be more pronounced in children than in adults, due to a lack of confounding long-term environmental exposures, the investigation of relevant genetic variants associated with paediatric NAFLD, whilst not, at present, consequent to our clinical approach, may prove instructive for both paediatric and adult disease as our understanding of their pathophysiological role increases.

### 3.2. Maternal Diet, Intrauterine Growth and Neonatal Diet

In recent years, the critical role of maternal physiology and metabolism during the perinatal, foetal and even pre-conceptual phases of development in predisposing the unborn towards developing NAFLD within their own lifetimes and making it more likely that they will progress to NASH, has become ever more apparent [69,90–92].

This phenomenon, referred to as developmental programming, appears to be driven by the complex interaction of diverse communities of epigenetic modifications at key genes, which change the phenotypic characteristics of different cell types, hence the offspring's metabolic profile [93]. Recent evidence even suggests that, in addition to the effects of epigenetic programming upon first generation offspring, subsequent generations may also be affected [94].

A greater understanding of the molecular phenomenology underlying maternal epigenetic programming in obesity may well lead to the development of effective therapeutic interventions that may be targeted during key developmental windows to ameliorate the risk of maternal obesity and maternal diet to the unborn. Several studies have now demonstrated that controlled maternal weight loss prior to pregnancy is effective in reducing their offspring's lifetime risk of developing NAFLD, which is of particular relevance in the context of the rising global prevalence of obesity among women of childbearing age [94]. However, specific and coherent guidelines regarding when and how to effectively intervene in clinical practice have yet to be defined.

Several studies have also found an association between intrauterine growth restriction (IUGR) and obesity, dyslipidaemia, hepatic steatosis and steatohepatitis [4,95]. Although the pathogenic mechanisms underlying these relationships remain unclear, they are also thought to have their origins in adverse foetal epigenetic programming [93,94]. Similarly, while some studies have suggested that breastfeeding may be protective against the development of NASH in childhood, this likely depends greatly upon the physiological profile of the maternal source [4,96]. Others have also suggested that rapid weight gain, particularly in the first 3 months of post-natal life, rather than small birth size in and of itself, might increase the risk of NAFLD in childhood and later life, although further study is required to determine safe trends of neonatal weight gain [96].

### 3.3. Gender Differences and Puberty

In adults, numerous studies report that the prevalence of NAFLD, specifically simple steatosis, is twice as great in men as in women. While the exact reasons for these gender differences remain unclear, some have suggested that they might be explained by differences in fat distribution, serum lipid profile or a protective action of oestrogens and other hormonal differences between the sexes [14,97]. There are, however, no apparent gender differences in the risk of progression to NASH in adult or paediatric patients, although some studies have suggested that boys are more likely to develop a periportal paediatric pattern of NASH than girls [68].

However, in childhood and adolescence, gender differences appear to be more complex, with some studies supporting a higher risk in boys, similar to that in adults, while others do not. Instead, gender disparity with regards to NAFLD prevalence appears to increase with age and has been attributed to the physiological alterations that occur at the onset of puberty impacting the pathogenesis of this disease. Indeed, there is increasing evidence that associates rising levels of sex hormones during puberty with modification of diverse biological processes, including adipocyte development and function [4,24]. For example, animal studies have indicated that oestrogens reduce the severity of oxidative stress, impair hepatocellular mitochondrial function and inhibit hepatic stellate cell activation and fibrogenesis, which might significantly affect the development and progression of NAFLD by modifying the hepatic and systemic responses to hepatocellular injury [98–100]. Furthermore, the diminishing disparity in NAFLD prevalence between the genders, especially after middle age, has been widely noted, with some attributing it to hormonal changes that occur around menopause [101].

It has also been suggested that the rise in serum oestrogen levels in both boys and girls during puberty might also contribute to the reduced severity of NAFLD, particularly the more benign clinical course of simple steatosis, in adults. For example, in one study of 186 children with biopsy-proven NAFLD, after adjusting for confounders, patients at or beyond puberty were less likely to have high-grade steatosis, severe portal inflammation, borderline steatohepatitis (zone 1) or a high stage of fibrosis than patients who had not entered puberty [102]. There is also evidence to suggest that steatosis, inflammation and fibrosis are less severe during and after puberty among NAFLD patients [102].

### 3.4. Dysregulation of Hedgehog Signalling Pathway in NAFLD

Deregulation of the Hedgehog (Hh) Signalling Pathway, which morphologically orchestrates organogenesis during development, also appears to have a role in the pathogenesis and progression of NAFLD in adults and children [68]. While in the healthy adult this pathway is usually silent, it is reactivated when hepatic injury stimulates the production of Hh ligands, triggering the growth of various cell types involved in wound-healing, including resident hepatic immune cells, hepatic stellate cells and hepatic progenitor cells. While effective Hh signalling is necessary for injured mature livers to regenerate, prolongation or upregulation of this pathway's activity has been linked to chronic inflammation, fibrosis and liver cancer [68].

Others have demonstrated that damaged or ballooned hepatocytes produce Hh ligands in adults with NASH, whose previous levels correlated with numbers of Hh-responsive cells within the liver and the severity of inflammation and fibrosis [103]. Whether or not similar mechanisms exist in children remains unclear but highly plausible, given that children generally harbour greater numbers of Hh-producing cells and Hh-responsive cells than adults and that these populations have been shown to expand even in response to relatively minor parenchymal injury, which may make them especially vulnerable to insults that stimulate liver damage and may even go some way towards explaining why simple steatosis has a much less benign course in children than in adults and why advanced fibrosis/cirrhosis can occur relatively rapidly [68].

Moreover, as hepatic development is not completed until adolescence, changes in the clinical presentation and course of NAFLD prior to and during adolescence, the latter being more in line with the adult pattern of disease, may reflect changes in the liver's vulnerability to derangement of Hh pathway signalling [68]. It has even been suggested that age, gender and/or pubertal status may reciprocally influence Hh pathway activity in children, modulating the liver's response to steatosis and hepatocyte injury and hence the histological features of paediatric NAFLD [12,68]. For example, in contrast to the adult liver, the periportal compartment of prepubescent male livers, where fibrosis characteristic of paediatric NAFLD is observed on histological analysis, exhibits high Hh pathway activity. Hh-mediated repair responses also appear to be more robust and readily engaged in prepubescent boys with NAFLD, which may explain why they display a much greater disease prevalence than girls [68].

Hh pathway activation also stimulates hepatic stellate cells to become myofibroblastic and function as the major collagen matrix-producing cells in response to liver injury. There is further evidence to suggest that, even once liver injury has dissipated and these cells revert to a quiescent state, they remain "primed" to more readily reacquire their myofibroblastic and fibrogenic characteristics upon subsequent hepatic injury, which may further contribute to the aggressive pattern of paediatric NASH [104].

## 4. Making the Diagnosis

Paediatric NAFLD remains underdiagnosed due to a lack of recognition, under-appreciation of its associated complications or questions regarding the appropriateness of such a diagnosis in children by healthcare professionals. Far from being a process of exclusion, as it has often been described both clinically and in the literature, the diagnosis of NAFLD should be actively considered in all overweight or obese children >10 years old, particularly in the context of hypertension, evidence of hepatomegaly, acanthosis nigricans, insulin resistance and Type II diabetes mellitus [8,12,17,19,60].

Differential diagnosis should first be based on the clinical features, then on blood tests, imaging techniques, and, finally, liver biopsy (Figure 2), which is currently considered the gold standard for the diagnosis of NAFLD [17], facilitating differentiation between simple steatosis and NASH, determining the presence and severity of hepatic fibrosis and providing prognostic information regarding the potential for disease progression [11,19,49]. Any evidence of hepatic steatosis in children <10 years old, with or without elevated liver function tests (LFTs), hepatomegaly or splenomegaly, is of particular concern and should be assessed comprehensively and expediently in order to exclude other aetiologies, including infectious hepatitis, autoimmune hepatitis, Wilson's disease, haemochromatosis, $\alpha$-1 antitrypsin deficiency and other monogenic causes of impaired fatty acid metabolism or lysosomal or peroxisomal storage. Despite being much less common in the paediatric population, Alcohol-induced Fatty Liver Disease must also be excluded and should not be discounted out of hand, even in young children [9,11,19,43,49].

Positive serum autoantibodies (anti-mitochondrial and anti-nuclear) are often present in paediatric NAFLD patients (~20%), even in the absence of autoimmune hepatitis, although their clinical significance remains unclear [12]. NAFLD is also often associated with abnormalities in iron metabolism, raising intra-hepatic free iron alongside mildly elevated serum ferritin and transferrin, in the absence of genetic haemochromatosis, seemingly mediated by pro-inflammatory adipokines. As such, liver biopsy is required in order to assess hepatic iron concentration and exclude significant hepatic injury and fibrosis, in patients with suspected NAFLD who demonstrate persistently elevated serum ferritin and increased transferrin saturation, especially in the context of homozygote or heterozygote C282Y mutations in the HFE gene [4,19,105]. Furthermore, due to its high prevalence, NAFLD can readily co-occur with other chronic liver diseases, worsening clinical outcomes that, otherwise, can be improved by concurrently treating the metabolic risk factors underlying NAFLD, such as obesity and insulin resistance [11,19].

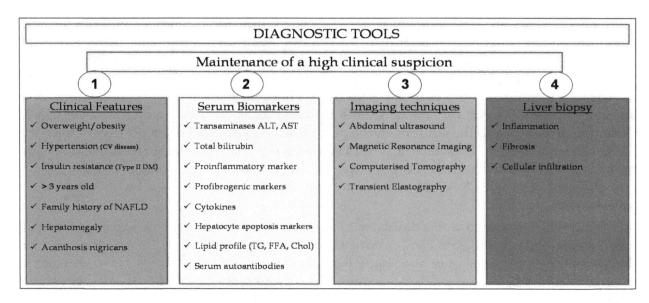

**Figure 2.** Diagnostic tools for children and adolescent NAFLD. Abbreviations: NAFLD: non-alcoholic fatty liver disease; DM: diabetes mellitus; ALT: alanine aminotransferase; AST: aspartate aminotransferase; TG: triglycerides; FFA: free fatty acids; Chol: cholesterol.

Although possessing limited sensitivity, abdominal ultrasound and liver function tests remain the first choice in diagnosing NAFLD in children [11,19]. As such, while not recommended in the general paediatric population, biannual screening for elevated serum alanine aminotransferase (ALT) and aspartate aminotransferase (AST) should be undertaken in all obese patients above 10 years old, as well as those whose BMI falls between the 85th and 94th centiles and have associated metabolic risk factors. However, as a result of the pathophysiological and clinical differences between paediatric and adult NAFLD, diagnostic algorithms and risk prediction scores, such as the NAFLD activity score, which were developed for use in adults, are of limited utility in children and should not be relied upon [9,29]. Furthermore, radiological and histopathological findings should be interpreted with caution, as serum aminotransferase levels remain normal in the majority of paediatric cases, irrespective of disease severity and the often negligible levels of hepatic steatosis in advanced paediatric NASH rendering hepatic ultrasound insensitive. Even liver biopsy is not always reliable in paediatric NAFLD due to steatotic lesioning within the liver being less diffuse and characterised by much more subtle histopathological changes [17,19,106].

In the absence of definitive radiological and histopathological diagnostic tests, maintenance of a high clinical suspicion in both primary and specialist care settings and by all members of the multidisciplinary team remains the most potent of diagnostic tools, enabling early diagnosis and appropriate therapeutic intervention designed to stymie disease progression.

### 4.1. Alternative Classification System

The term 'Non-alcoholic', although originally intended to clearly differentiate the aetiology of this disease from Alcohol-Induced Fatty Liver Disease, is often extremely unhelpful and perpetuates the false assumption among healthcare professionals that paediatric NAFLD represents a diagnosis of exclusion. Furthermore, what constitutes the threshold of "significant" alcohol consumption, particularly in paediatric cases, remains moot. Others have, therefore, suggested the adoption of "Obesity-induced Liver Disease" as a replacement term but this could also prove misleading, given that, while obesity is the single greatest risk factor for this disease, NAFLD can develop in normo-weight children [27,35,107]. Such terminology is also likely to be the focus of significant social stigma, which is of particular concern in younger and more emotionally and psychologically vulnerable patients, potentially affecting their engagement with clinical services.

In light of the significant pathophysiological overlap between NAFLD and Alcohol-induced Fatty Liver Disease, it may be more helpful to think of "Fatty" Liver Disease or, less pejoratively, "Steatotic" Liver Disease (SLD) in terms of "primary", "secondary", "mixed" and "complex" aetiological subtypes. As such, "Primary" or "Type 1" SLD would encompass what is currently referred to as "Non-alcoholic Fatty Liver Disease", which represents the phenotypic manifestation of underlying metabolic dysfunction in the absence of other causes of liver injury. "Secondary" or "Type 2" SLD would describe pathology resulting from a number of medical or surgical conditions or drug intake, including alcohol. In such cases where metabolic dysfunction and significant alcohol consumption coincide, the term "Mixed" or "Type 3" SLD could be used and, where Steatotic Liver Disease coincides with another form of chronic liver disease, such as autoimmune hepatitis, "Complex" or "Type 4" SLD. Thus, by appropriately reviewing the clinical nomenclature, we might better emphasise the importance of the diagnostic, pathophysiological, therapeutic and prognostic relationships between NAFLD and other chronic liver diseases in childhood and adolescence, as well as clearly directing intervention to improve clinical outcomes.

### 4.2. Serum Biomarkers for Liver Damage

Elevated levels of various circulating biomarkers have been described in patients with NAFLD, including AST and ALT, cytokeratin 18 (CK-18) fragments, apolipoprotein A1, total bilirubin, hyaluronic acid, C-reactive protein, fibroblast growth factor-21, interleukin 1 receptor antagonist, adiponectin, and TNF-$\alpha$ [83]. However, at present, there remains no readily available biomarker that reliably differentiates between simple steatosis and NASH.

Aminotransferases, AST and ALT, are the most commonly referenced serum biomarkers for liver damage in a wide variety of liver diseases, including NAFLD. They are easily obtained, low in cost and elevated levels have been associated across numerous studies with the presence and severity of NAFLD in adults [9,11,22,101]. Furthermore, in one multicentre study of 176 children, AST and GGT were predictive of both NAFLD and NASH but lacked the discriminatory power to accurately and reliably delineate cases of NASH from simple steatosis [108]. However, consensus as to what constitutes "normal" aminotransferase levels in children has yet to be established. Indeed, another study of 502 18–64 year olds with NAFLD demonstrated progressive decline of ALT levels with advancing age, while AST remained stable, suggesting that ALT elevation in childhood may be less diagnostically useful than in adult disease [101]. Most importantly, several studies have reported that up to two thirds of children with NASH did not display elevated serum ALT and AST levels, even in more advanced disease [109–112]. While normal AST and ALT levels do not exclude severe liver damage or fibrosis in paediatric NAFLD, when elevated they should inspire a high level of clinical suspicion, particularly in overweight or obese patients with a family history of NAFLD and, thus, may still be of significant use as a screening tool [9,74].

Elevated serum CK-18 fragments, markers of hepatocyte apoptosis, have demonstrated robust association with the incidence and severity of NASH in both adults and children [113]. Wieckowska et al. [114], for example, reported a strong positive correlation between CK-18 in plasma obtained from patients with suspected NAFLD at the time of liver biopsy and hepatic damage. Plasma CK-18 levels were also markedly increased in patients with NASH compared to those with simple steatosis, and were capable of accurately predicting NASH. These observations have been reproduced in subsequent studies, collectively suggesting CK18 levels to have a sensitivity of 78% and specificity of 87% for steatohepatitis in patients with NAFLD [115]. However, CK-18 would likely only be of use once the diagnosis of NAFLD had been made, as hepatocyte apoptosis is not unique to NAFLD. Furthermore, despite its significant clinical potential, CK-18 is not, at the present time, readily available and a standardised cut-off has yet to be established.

Total Bilirubin was also found by Puri et al. [116] to inversely correlate with the prevalence of NASH in children, which it is thought may reflect some anti-oxidative protective effect of bilirubin within the liver.

Finally, serum lipid profile, including total cholesterol, while potentially reflective of abnormal lipid metabolism that may contribute to NASH, has yet to be adequately investigated in paediatric liver disease. As such, its sensitivity, specificity and clinical utility remain unclear [53,117]. However, analysis of molecular lipid concentrations in blood samples taken from 679 adults found that those with NAFLD displayed increased triglycerols with low carbon number and double-bond content, while lysophosphotidylcholines and either phospholipids were diminished [118]. A serum lipid signature comprising these three molecular lipids had a sensitivity of 69.1% and a specificity of 73.8% in the subsequent validation series. Further investigation is required to validate these results in children, however.

### 4.3. Abdominal Ultrasound

Abdominal ultrasound is the most commonly used imaging modality for NAFLD, both clinically and in research [10,12]. It has been shown to be an effective means of identifying pure hepatic steatosis and mild NASH in children and has led to a great increase in findings of NAFLD in recent years. Its relatively low cost, wide availability and safety also make it an ideal screening tool [10,17]. In NAFLD, the liver is usually enlarged and appears echogenic, or "bright", which indicates fatty accumulation within the parenchyma. However, it is unable to quantify the true extent of steatosis and its sensitivity diminishes significantly in cases where hepatic fat accumulation remains below 30%, in individuals who are severely obese (BMI > 40) and in severe NASH [9,44,119]. Ultrasound is unable to reliably differentiate between simple steatosis and steatohepatitis or exclude fibrosis. Accurately differentiating between focal steatosis or steatohepatitis and hepatic tumours or inflammatory vascular conditions is also challenging, given their close resemblance to one another on ultrasound and the potential for steatosis to obscure the imaging of other hepatic lesions [106,119]. However, while the focal manifestations of NAFLD may be characterised by poorly delineated margins and similar contrast enhancement with normal liver parenchyma, they do not exert a mass effect on the surrounding tissue and, at least in adults, favour certain topographical configurations, mainly occurring adjacent to the falciform ligament or ligamentum venosum, in the porta hepatis and gallbladder. Whether such distributions of focal fatty lesions hold true in paediatric NAFLD, however, remains to be established [11,119]. Furthermore, atypical focal fatty liver sparing can also mimic hepatic neoplasia, manifesting round or oval-shaped phenomena with clear margins. The diagnostic efficacy of abdominal ultrasound is also greatly dependent upon operator proficiency and lacks standard methods of interpretation for paediatric NAFLD, underscoring the importance of considering the wider clinical picture throughout the diagnostic process and selection of appropriate therapeutic intervention.

### 4.4. Magnetic Resonance Imaging

Unlike abdominal ultrasound, MRI exhibits high sensitivity and specificity for paediatric NAFLD and is able to differentiate, even in severely obese patients, between simple steatosis and NASH [17,20]. It is also able to quantify the distribution and severity of even mild steatosis and fibrosis throughout the entire liver and with moderate to strong correlation with histological grading in children and adults [28,120,121]. However, the relatively high cost of MRI, as well as the need for sedation in young children prohibits widespread use in clinical practice and, as such, it remains primarily a research tool. It is also, at present, unable to assess the extent of inflammation or cirrhosis in the liver parenchyma but rather identifies the consequences of chronic liver disease, such as hepatosplenomegaly and portal hypertension.

### 4.5. Other Imaging Techniques

While Computerised Tomography (CT) offers greater sensitivity than abdominal ultrasound in detecting the presence and extent of hepatic fat accumulation in NAFLD, the high radiation exposure it encumbers prohibits routine use in young children [20,121]. Furthermore, it also lacks the sensitivity required to detect mild steatosis and small changes in fat content over time.

Transient Elastography is able to detect hepatic fibrosis in paediatric NAFLD, using a technique similar to abdominal ultrasound to measure hepatic "stiffness" non-invasively. However, at present, it cannot reliably determine the extent or severity of hepatic fibrosis, particularly in its early stages, as both steatosis and inflammatory activity also marginally increase liver stiffness. This technique also suffers from diminished sensitivity and specificity in severely obese patients [122,123].

## 4.6. Liver Biopsy and Histopathology

Liver biopsy remains the gold standard for diagnosing NAFLD, differentiating between simple steatosis and NASH and determining the severity of liver damage, inflammation and fibrosis [19,29]. It also allows the clinician to rule out other causes of liver pathology, especially in cases of significant liver damage where abdominal ultrasound demonstrates reduced sensitivity and specificity. However, it is invasive and, as such, carries significant risks that render it unsuitable for use as a screening tool, particularly in children. It is also expensive and subject to sampling error, where subsequent histopathological analysis is unrepresentative of the liver as a whole. As such, even a normal liver biopsy cannot fully exclude NAFLD and should always be considered in context of the wider clinical picture.

The key decision pertains as to when biopsy is indicated and when it is not. In each case, the clinician must weigh the potential risks associated with biopsy against the likelihood that it will impact clinical management. Ideally, this would mean that we should only biopsy children who are at significant risk of NASH. However, our incomplete understanding of the natural history of this disease, at present, confounds any attempt to reliably stratify patients according to such risk, as the alteration of clinical outcomes based on the severity of histology at baseline remains unknown [124]. Nevertheless, current guidelines published by the American Association for the Study of Liver Diseases (AASLD) recommend that liver biopsy should only be undertaken in patients younger than 10 years old with a family history of severe NAFLD, the presence of hepatosplenomegaly at physical examination and abnormal laboratory results, encompassing transaminasaemia, insulin resistance, absence of autoantibodies and inconclusive results from biochemical tests for severe/progressive liver disease [19].

While children with NAFLD may exhibit the same morphological lesions as adults, these are often more subtle and can be absent altogether [44]. Hepatocyte ballooning, for example, which describes the enlargement of hepatocyte diameter by a factor of 1.5–2 and the main morphological feature of hepatocellular damage in adult NASH, is often not observed in paediatric cases. Similarly, the distinctive clarification and rarefication of hepatocyte cytoplasm and the inclusion therein of eosinophilic cytoskeletal peptide aggregates, referred to as Mallory Denk bodies, so characteristic of adult NASH, is relatively uncommon [11,12,19].

The distribution of fatty accumulation and fibrotic lesioning within the liver also differs between paediatric and adult disease. Adult NAFLD is characterised by microvacuolar periportal or panacinar hepatocellular steatosis, portal inflammation, portal fibrosis and perisinusoidal fibrosis. In contrast, paediatric NAFLD is characterised by macrovacuolar, azonal hepatocellular steatosis, portal inflammation and portal fibrosis [44,125].

Inflammation is characteristic of NASH across all age groups and comprises mixed inflammatory cells which infiltrate the hepatic parenchyma, including lymphocytes, histiocytes, Kupffer cells (KC) and granulocytes [63,64]. While, in adults, lobular inflammation is nearly universal and portal inflammation associated with more severe/advanced cases of NASH, portal inflammation is more typical of paediatric cases, providing further evidence that childhood disease follows a more severe course [125]. Furthermore, while isolated steatosis or steatosis with lobular inflammation without signs of hepatocellular injury are considered part of the wider spectrum of NAFLD in adults and insufficient evidence to suggest NASH, in children, where signs of hepatocellular injury are less obvious, this distinction is less clear. However, Schwimmer and others go on to describe both patterns of

NAFLD in children, suggesting that factors other than age might determine the histological appearance of the disease [125]. Although the mechanistic underpinnings of this phenomenon remain unclear, Swiderska-Syn *et al.* [68] hypothesised that the Hedgehog pathway, which is involved in the fibro-ductal response, may effect such differences.

## 4.7. Non-Invasive Diagnostic Scoring Systems

The invasiveness, cost, morbidity and impracticality of liver biopsy in at-risk patients and especially in children has driven the development of non-invasive clinical risk prediction scores. However, many have yet to be validated in the paediatric population. Non-invasive hepatic fibrosis scores, AST/ALT, NFS and Fib-4 or AST/platelet ratio were developed for use in adults but have performed poorly in diagnosing significant fibrosis in children with NAFLD [29,126]. The paediatric NAFLD fibrosis index (PNFI) is calculated from the patient's age, waist circumference and triglyceride levels and aims to predict liver fibrosis in children [126]. However, although it provides a good positive predictive value, its negative predictive value for ruling out fibrosis is sub-optimal. Several studies have suggested that the enhanced liver fibrosis (ELF) score, an algorithmic composite of serum markers of liver fibrosis, including hyaluronic acid, amino terminal propeptide of collagen type III and the tissue inhibitor of metalloproteinase, can be used to accurately predict fibrosis in children with NAFLD [126,127]. While the potential of these scores is great, their clinical utility remains, at present, unclear.

## 5. Management of Paediatric NAFLD

There is, currently, a lack of consensus as to how NAFLD in childhood and adolescence should be managed in clinical practice [65]. However, it is clear that effective therapeutic strategies should recognise that this is a multifactorial disease in which metabolic dysfunction is widespread, multifaceted, interdependent and is founded upon the interaction between numerous genetic and environmental forces. As such, therapeutic intervention should be adapted to each patient in context of their existing co-morbidities and how they might best be managed, including obesity, hyperlipidaemia, insulin resistance, Type II diabetes mellitus and cardiovascular disease. High clinical suspicion, enabling appropriate referral to paediatric gastroenterology, early diagnosis and intervention, has consistently been shown to be effective in improving overall quality of life for the patient, as well as reducing their long-term cardiovascular and hepatic morbidity and mortality [14,24,128].

First-line interventions should focus on appropriately reducing central obesity and insulin resistance, primarily through dietary modification and increased physical exercise in order to effect therapeutic weight loss [129]. Depending on the extent of hepatic fibrosis, patients with NASH may also benefit from pharmacological therapies designed to slow or reverse disease progression [24]. Unlike in adults, where simple steatosis appears benign and, thus, pharmacological intervention is not recommended, in children the evidence suggests that it tends to follow a more aggressive course and, as such, pharmacological intervention, although not currently recommended, may be prudent before the transition to NASH occurs (Figure 3).

An approach that combines reducing visceral adiposity, insulin resistance and hyperinsulinemia with the prevention or reversal of hepatocellular damage appear to be the most successful rather than employing one or other of these strategies in isolation. The efficacy of any intervention should be assessed after a six-month period and, if ineffective, additional therapeutic options might then be considered, including pharmacological therapy or surgical intervention [24,65,128,130,131]. The development of comprehensive, evidence-based and internationally accepted clinical guidelines specifically for paediatric NAFLD will depend upon rectification of the current paucity of research and lack of robust epidemiological data. Nevertheless, they should emphasise the importance of the multidisciplinary team and the effective management of metabolic risk factors, as well as improving the interconnectedness of diverse health disciplines, especially during the transition from paediatric to adult clinical services and in those patients at the extreme end of the obesity spectrum, in whom non-surgical therapies for weight loss are currently non-existent.

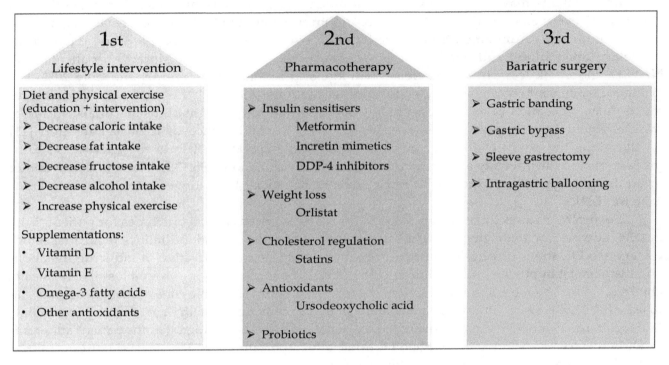

**Figure 3.** Management of paediatric NAFLD.

Sleep shortage as a result of lifestyle, as well as major sleep disorders, such as sleep apnea and insomnia, have also been associated with NAFLD and may benefit from more active clinical consideration and therapeutic intervention. While the nature of these pathological relationships, remains the subject of much debate, various metabolic or endocrine effects in the context of obesity are thought to play a role [30].

## 5.1. Diet and Physical Exercise

Western diet, which is characterised by a hyper-caloric intake high in fats and simple sugars, precipitates a rapid increase in post-prandial plasma glucose and insulin levels, increasing hepatic *de novo*-lipogenesis, steatosis, insulin resistance, central obesity and the risk of NAFLD [21,132]. The Western Australian Pregnancy (Raine) Cohort Study ($n$ = 995), for example, found that a Western dietary pattern at 14 years old was associated with an increased frequency of NAFLD at 17 years, independent of sex, dietary misreporting, family income, frequency of physical activity and sedentary behaviour [132]. As most paediatric patients with NAFLD are obese, addressing their obesity by means of dietary modifications, including reduction of caloric, fat and fast-release carbohydrate intake, as well as increasing physical exercise in order to effect weight loss should be considered the first-line of any effective interventional strategy. Indeed, current AASLD guidelines recommend limiting overall dietary fat intake to less than 5% of total caloric intake, while limiting trans-fats to <1% and saturated fats to <7% [74].

Numerous studies have shown that even a moderate reduction in weight, 5% in steatosis and 10% in NASH, has the potential to reduce hepatic steatosis, improve insulin sensitivity and significantly improve clinical outcomes in adults [14,19,44]. However, its effectiveness in patients with pre-existing NASH-induced hepatic fibrosis remains uncertain. Although few in number, paediatric studies seem to support these findings. One study in children with biopsy-proven NAFLD demonstrated that a reduction of 20% or more over 12 months precipitated significant improvement in serum ALT and steatosis in 68% of children [133]. Another study of 53 paediatric patients with NAFLD also reported significant reduction of steatosis, inflammation and hepatocyte ballooning on liver biopsy following similar lifestyle interventions [131].

Improvements may even be possible in a much shorter timeframe. Indeed, a recent Danish study of 117 obese children demonstrated marked improvement in their insulin sensitivity, liver fat accumulation and serum aminotransferase levels in two thirds of the cohort after only ten weeks of dietary intervention and one hour of moderate exercise daily [134]. Moreover, patients with NAFLD undertook less physical exercise than age and sex-matched controls and only 20%–33% of them met current recommendations for physical activity [135–137]. Physical activity correlates inversely with hepatic steatosis, independently of changes in body weight or dietary intake, increases insulin sensitivity and reduces central obesity, even in the absence of dietary alteration [11]. Furthermore, the extent of these changes appears, while apparent even in the short-term, to be proportional to the intensity and duration of lifestyle modification [135,138]. There is also evidence in adults to suggest that vigorous exercise is more beneficial than longer intervals of moderate exercise [139].

The minimum amount of weight loss necessary to improve clinical outcomes for patients with NASH, however, remains unclear. The current lack of specific clinical guidelines regarding which dietary modifications or physical exercise regimes would be most effective in inducing metabolic and histological improvement in children with NAFLD, beyond achieving weight loss in overweight children, perturbs a more systematic and evidence-based approach to the clinical management of this disease [19,24,65]. That said, any diet, whether alone or in conjunction with increased physical activity, that facilitates weight loss can effectively reduce hepatic steatosis, provided that the patient adheres to it. Early dietary intervention in childhood is especially important, given that dietary patterns formed in childhood tend to be retained into adulthood [132].

Lifestyle modification, however, can be difficult for younger patients to engage with and maintain long-term, particularly in the context of negative perceptions of dietary intervention and the prescription of physical exercise in children, among patients and their parents [9]. As such, lifestyle intervention should be tailored towards patients as individuals, taking account of the cultural and socioeconomic determinants of diet and exercise habits, as well as differences in patient perceptions of obesity and body image, particularly in adolescence, before setting clear and achievable goals derived by the patient and clinician in partnership. The adoption of similar lifestyle modifications by family members and, in some cases, behavioural therapy may aid compliance [15]. More effective and straightforward tools for monitoring day-to-day quality and quantity of dietary intake and physical activity in childhood, as well as greater efforts to educate and provide guidance for parents and their children regarding maintaining a healthy diet and the importance of physical activity are needed [140].

5.1.1. Dietary Fructose

Besides the control of total caloric intake, the consumption of certain micronutrients, such as fructose, which is a constituent of sucrose, corn syrup, fruit juice, soft-drinks and various sweeteners, should also be reduced. Unlike glucose, fructose is metabolised exclusively in the liver and is preferentially shunted into the *de novo*-lipogenesis pathway via glyceraldehyde-3-phosphate, contributing to increased triglyceride synthesis and hepatic steatosis [141,142]. It has also been suggested that fructose may interact with nuclear transcription factors, such as sterol response element binding protein-1c, precipitating alterations in the expression of genes involved in liver glycolysis and lipogenesis [143]. It may also promote liver injury in NAFLD by causing bacterial overgrowth and increased intestinal permeability, precipitating endotoxemia and subsequent initiation of inflammation but this has yet to be proven [142,143].

In adults and in rodents, fructose has also been associated, particularly in the context of a high-fat diet, with a higher risk of NAFLD and increased liver fibrosis [21,44,142]. Moreover, the severity of hepatic steatosis and inflammation in rats fed fructose-enriched diets tends to be more severe than in controls [144]. Human studies also report greater fructose consumption in adult NAFLD patients and greater soft drink consumption and fasting serum triglyceride levels in children with NAFLD relative to controls [142]. Indeed, fructose consumption has dramatically increased in recent years and has also been associated with increased central obesity, dyslipidaemia and insulin resistance, all independent risk factors for NAFLD [27,145].

### 5.1.2. Vitamin D

Vitamin D plasma levels have also been shown to inversely correlate with NASH and fibrosis in children and adolescents [146,147]. Furthermore, Vitamin D deficiency is more common in obese patients than those of normal weight and was shown to be associated with the incidence of NAFLD, liver steatosis, necroinflammation and fibrosis in adults [146,148].

Vitamin D receptors regulate the expression of numerous genes, some of which are involved in glucose and lipid metabolism, and are widely distributed throughout the liver [146,148]. In rats exposed to obesogenic diet, Vitamin D deficiency exacerbates NAFLD through the activation of Toll-like receptors and is associated with insulin resistance, hepatic inflammatory markers and oxidative stress [149].

Growing evidence also suggests that low serum Vitamin D is associated with insulin resistance and Type II diabetes and that appropriate Vitamin D supplementation can improve insulin sensitivity [150]. However, in the Western Australian Pregnancy (Raine) Cohort, others have reported the association of low Vitamin D levels with evidence of NAFLD on ultrasound at 17 years of age was independent of adiposity and insulin resistance [146]. As such, screening for Vitamin D deficiency in adolescents otherwise considered at high risk of NAFLD may be appropriate. Further clinical and experimental investigation of this phenomenon, as well as the benefits of dietary supplementation, is warranted [146].

### 5.1.3. ω-3 Fatty Acids

Experimental models in animals and adults have shown that long chain ω-3 fatty acids, known important regulators of hepatic gene transcription, can decrease hepatic steatosis, improve insulin sensitivity and cardiovascular disease and decrease markers of inflammation [24,151,152].

Elsewhere, dietary depletion of polyunsaturated fats, such as ω-3, has been associated with the pathogenesis of NAFLD, while its progression has been associated with high circulating and hepatic levels of saturated fatty acids and industrial trans-fats. As such, limiting daily consumption of foods high in saturated fatty acids, while supplementing ω-3 intake may have a role in NAFLD treatment [9,153,154].

It is thought that the beneficial effects of ω-3 supplementation may be secondary to their known anti-inflammatory, antithrombotic, antiarrhythmic, hypolipidaemic and vasodilatory properties. There is evidence to suggest that they might also improve lipid profiles, lowering triglyceride serum levels, decreasing insulin resistance, hepatic steatosis and cytokine synthesis [153]. For example, dietary supplementation with docosahexaenoic acid (DHA), the major dietary long-chain polyunsaturated (ω-3) fatty acid, which exerts a potent anti-inflammatory effect through the G protein-coupled receptor 120 (GPR-120), has been associated with significant improvement in the histological parameters of NAFLD, including NAFLD activity score, hepatocyte ballooning and steatosis in children, after 18 months [154]. Interestingly, hepatic progenitor cell proliferation was also reduced in correlation with these same histological parameters, as were the numbers of inflammatory macrophages on biopsy, while GPR-120 expression in hepatocytes was markedly increased. As such, it was suggested that DHA might also modulate hepatic progenitor cell activation, hepatocyte survival and macrophage polarisation through interaction with GPR-120 and NF-κB repression [154]. Another study also described that, after 6 months of ω-3 supplementation, hepatic echogenicity and insulin sensitivity were significantly improved in children with NAFLD, although no change in serum ALT or BMI was observed [155]. More recently, another RCT reported the use of probiotics and ω-3 fatty acids showed encouraging early results, with improvement of serum liver enzymes but without validating liver histology [156]. AASLD guidelines currently state that it would be premature to recommend ω-3 fatty acids for the specific treatment of NAFLD or NASH but they may be considered first-line therapeutic agents to treat hypertriglyceridaemia in patients with NAFLD [19].

### 5.2. Alcohol

Heavy alcohol consumption is a risk factor for chronic liver disease and should be avoided in patients with simple steatosis and NASH [19]. There is even evidence to suggest that regular consumption of smaller quantities of alcohol (below 20 g/day) may be harmful [30]. However, there are no studies reporting the effect of ongoing alcohol consumption on disease severity or natural history of NAFLD or the risk of liver cancer in childhood and adolescence in the long-term.

### 5.3. Bariatric Surgery

Bariatric surgery has been shown to significantly improve weight and comorbid disease in patients with NAFLD. It encompasses a range of restrictive procedures, which promote satiety and delayed gastric emptying, including adjustable gastric banding and sleeve gastrectomy, malabsorptive procedures, including biliopancreatic diversion, and combinatorial procedures, such as Roux-en-Y gastric bypass [11,14,19,157].

At present, bariatric surgery is only recommended for severely obese adolescents with significant steatohepatitis in whom therapeutic lifestyle intervention has been unsuccessful [14,157]. In such patients, it has been shown to significantly reduce the extent and severity of hepatic injury, steatosis and systemic inflammation, as well as having broader metabolic benefits, improving insulin sensitivity, positively modifying levels of circulating adipokines and the intestinal microbiome, particularly in the case of malabsorptive procedures [14]. Furthermore, it has been suggested that malabsorptive procedures might also have additional effects on gut hormone profiles, reducing ghrelin, enhancing Glucagon-like peptide-1 (GLP1) secretion and facilitating early ileal exposure to nutrients, alongside reduced expression of peptide YY (PYY) and oxyntomodulin obesity-related genes and altered bile metabolism [14,158].

However, despite a large body of evidence suggesting histological improvement secondary to weight loss in adults, bariatric surgery in NASH patients of any age group remains controversial [11,12,14,19,159]. Indeed, a lack of randomised controlled studies, small sample sizes variable inclusion criteria, incomplete longitudinal follow-up and lack of clear identification of confounding factors, such as insulin resistance led the Cochrane meta-analysis to conclude that the impact of bariatric surgery on NASH in childhood and adolescence is unconvincing [160]. As such, current AASLD guidelines state that while bariatric surgery is not contraindicated in otherwise eligible obese patients, it is "not an established option for NASH treatment" [19].

Reports of de novo progression of NASH and even hepatic fibrosis and cirrhosis following bariatric surgery are also highly controversial [14]. Although some have sought to attribute this phenomenon to a state of "heightened metabolic stress", in other surgical series, massive weight loss was shown to improve steatohepatitis and fibrosis. In this case, overall improvement was found to be dependent on the degree of insulin resistance, although long-term histological outcomes were not assessed [14,161].

Given the more aggressive nature of simple steatosis in paediatric disease, some have suggested that more earnest clinical intervention to reduce weight loss, including consideration of bariatric surgery, may be beneficial, even before the transition to steatohepatitis, in patients who are severely obese [12,28,159,160]. Further standardisation of eligibility criteria for surgery in the paediatric population, as well as studies on the safety and long-term efficacy of this approach, are warranted.

### 5.4. Pharmacological Intervention

Our understanding of the molecular pathogenesis of NAFLD remains limited and so current pharmacological intervention consists of strategies aimed at decreasing the incidence and severity of metabolic risk factors, such as obesity, insulin resistance, dyslipidaemia, as well as some drugs that target the major molecular pathways involved in the pathogenesis and progression of this disease of which we are aware, such as decreasing hepatic damage mediated by oxidative stress [67].

The aim of therapy is to forestall and, in some cases, reverse the progression of NAFLD to end-stage liver disease [11,162]. In particular, there remains a need for effective pharmacological therapies for children who do not adhere to or are unresponsive to lifestyle modification, in order to avoid severe organ damage [9,12].

Given the more aggressive clinical course of paediatric as opposed to adult NAFLD, targeted pharmacological intervention, although not presently recommended, may be prudent even before evidence of the transition to NASH is observed [11,14,19,28,68].

Collaboration between hepatologists and other relevant specialties, including endocrinology, paediatrics, dietetics, cardiology and primary care should be encouraged in order to optimise treatment, particularly in the current absence of clear clinical guidelines for pharmacological intervention in paediatric NAFLD.

## 5.4.1. Insulin Sensitizers

Insulin resistance and Type II diabetes mellitus are strongly associated with the incidence, severity and progression of NAFLD in the paediatric population. As such, drugs that can improve insulin sensitivity have a key role in the prognostication and therapeutic management of this disease, potentially reversing even advanced liver damage and hepatic fibrosis, improving long-term clinical outcomes [24].

Metformin, an oral insulin-sensitising agent, lowers hepatic glucose production and promotes glucose uptake in the periphery and, when given in 500 mg doses twice daily for 24 weeks, has been shown to reduce hepatic steatosis on magnetic resonance spectroscopy and ALT levels in non-diabetic children with biopsy-proven NASH [163]. That said, while the Treatment of NAFLD in Children (TONIC) trial, in which a large non-diabetic paediatric cohort was used to compare metformin with Vitamin E therapy, found metformin to be no more effective than a placebo in achieving a sustained decrease in ALT levels, it did show significant improvement in hepatocyte ballooning [164]. Current AASLD guidelines do not recommend the prescription of metformin for NAFLD in non-diabetic paediatric patients [19]. Its effectiveness at doses higher than 500 mg twice daily, however, remains unknown. Moreover, specific guidelines for prescribing metformin in children and adolescents with NAFLD and Type II Diabetes are needed.

Pioglitazone, a Peroxisome-Proliferator Activated Receptor-$\gamma$ (PPARg) agonist, increases insulin sensitivity and reduces hepatic fat content by promoting the redistribution of triacylglycerols from the liver and muscle to adipose tissue [19,24]. Therefore, while they have shown great promise in studies of adult NAFLD, their use often results in weight gain. Their safety and therapeutic efficacy in children, however, has yet to be determined and, indeed, there is a general reluctance to prescribe thiazolidinediones in paediatric patients, due to the potential side effects of long-term therapy, which include cardiotoxicity, fluid retention, osteoporosis and, as in adults, obesity [24].

Only glitazones have consistently shown some benefit in the treatment of patients with NASH in randomised-controlled trials [19,128]. Recent research suggests that pioglitazone can improve hepatic steatosis and inflammation, as well as reducing aminotransferase levels and histological evidence of hepatocyte injury in patients with biopsy-proven NASH [24,165,166]. However, the majority of patients in these trials were non-diabetic and, furthermore, the treatment had no apparent effect on the extent or severity of hepatic fibrosis.

Incretin mimetics and dipeptidyl peptidase-4 (DPP-4) inhibitors, which increase insulin secretion, decrease fatty acid oxidation and lipogenesis and improve hepatic glucose metabolism, may also have a role in NAFLD therapeutics [12,165–167]. DPP-4 is an enzyme implicated in the degradation of circulating GLP1, an incretin secreted in response to food intake that stimulates insulin secretion and inhibits glucagon release. Studies conducted in animals and adult humans have demonstrated the efficacy of GLP-1 receptor agonists, which were resistant to DPP-4 degradation, and DPP-4 inhibitors [12,167–169].

Suppressors of the renin-angiotensin system, such as losartan, reportedly improve insulin sensitivity and adipokine production/release and prevent hepatic stellate cell activation by exerting preventative effects on hepatic inflammation and fibrogenesis [12,168,170]. However, because of their contraindications, there is no available data on their therapeutic effects in children.

### 5.4.2. Weight Loss Drugs

Orlistat, an enteric lipase inhibitor, is the only FDA approved therapy for weight loss in adolescents. It is moderately effective in achieving short-term weight loss but is limited in young patients due to adverse gastrointestinal side effects. However, despite several studies reporting improved ALT levels and hepatic steatosis in patients with NAFLD, others have failed to demonstrate histological improvement on biopsy. As such, their use in NAFLD remains controversial [171,172].

### 5.4.3. Statins

Patients with simple steatosis and NASH are at increased risk of cardiovascular disease, with several studies having demonstrated this to be the most common cause of death in NAFLD. Effective therapeutic intervention in NAFLD, therefore, should encompass stratification of patients in terms of cardiovascular risk factors, including dyslipidaemia, and the appropriate clinical management thereof [11,19,27].

Despite general reluctance to prescribe statins to treat dyslipidaemia in patients with suspected or established chronic liver disease and the not uncommon occurrence of elevated aminotransferases in patients receiving statins, serious liver injury as a direct consequence of their use is rarely seen in clinical practice. Indeed, the risk of serious hepatic injury in patients with chronic liver disease, including NAFLD, does not appear to exceed that of patients without [173,174]. The evidence in children, however, remains less certain.

Several studies have thus far reported that statins can significantly improve liver biochemistries and cardiovascular outcomes in patients with elevated liver enzymes likely due to NAFLD. However, there remain no randomised-controlled trials with histological endpoints to support this either in simple steatosis or in NASH [11,174]. While current AASLD guidelines state that statins can be used to treat dyslipidaemia in adult patients with simple steatosis and NASH [19], their prescription in paediatric patients remains controversial.

### 5.5. Antioxidant Therapies

Oxidative stress is considered a key mechanism of hepatocellular injury and the progression of simple steatosis to NASH in children [88,175]. Given that, within hepatocytes, reactive oxygen species (ROS) are mostly generated in the mitochondria, some have suggested that, in hepatic steatosis, increased intracellular fatty acid levels may act as an overabundant substrate for mitochondrial malfunctioning, increasing ROS and, downstream, inflammatory cytokine and adipokine production, as well as, via their oxidation by peroxisomal acyl-CoA oxidases, the production of hydrogen peroxide, another reactive oxygen species [176,177].

Ordinarily, various enzymatic antioxidant mechanisms protect the liver from such oxidative injury, which in NAFLD, it seems, are simply overwhelmed. Therefore, the employ of antioxidant therapies would be expected to break this chain of lipid peroxidation and restore the endogenous antioxidant/oxidant equilibrium, halting the progression of NASH [148,178].

## 5.6. Vitamin E

Vitamin E therapy has been shown to reduce histological evidence of hepatic steatosis, inflammation and hepatocyte ballooning, as well as a reduction in aminotransferase levels in patients with NASH [148]. It has even been associated with the clinical resolution of steatohepatitis in adult NAFLD patients, although it does not appear to affect the extent or severity of hepatic fibrosis once it is established [179]. Studies in children have also reported improvement of liver function and glucose metabolism following a 12-month regime of Vitamin E (600 IU/day) and ascorbic acid (500 mg/day) in combination with dietary modification and physical exercise [133].

More recently, the NASH Clinical Research Network's Treatment of NAFLD children (TONIC) trial, reported a modest benefit on hepatocyte ballooning following Vitamin E therapy in combination with similar lifestyle modifications in 8–17 year olds with biopsy proven NASH [164]. While aminotransferase levels were unaffected, statistically significant improvement of the NAS score and resolution of NASH with Vitamin E therapy was also observed over the following two years [164]. However, whether similar improvements can still be achieved in the absence of concurrent lifestyle modification remains controversial, as does the appropriate dosing of antioxidant therapies, including Vitamin E, in children. Indeed, there is some concern as to whether or not Vitamin E therapy increases all-cause mortality, as well as the risk of certain cancers, when administered in high doses [180].

While the most recent EASL guidelines advocate Vitamin E as a first-line pharmacotherapy in non-diabetic adults with biopsy proven NASH, the AASLD 2005 guidelines suggest that although Vitamin E also appears to be beneficial in non-diabetic children with NASH, confirmatory studies are needed before its use can be recommended in clinical practice. Furthermore, due to a similar lack of evidence, its use is not supported in diabetic patients with NASH, NAFLD without liver biopsy, NASH cirrhosis or cryptogenic cirrhosis at any age [11,19,148,162].

## 5.7. Ursodeoxycholic Acid

Ursodeoxycholic acid is one of the most widely used cytoprotective and antioxidant agents, able to protect hepatocytes from bile salt-mediated mitochondrial injury, as well as activating anti-apoptotic signalling pathways, fulfilling diverse immunomodulatory functions, in theory, stabilising cellular and organelle membranes in patients with NASH [24,181,182].

In children, a randomised controlled trial of ursodeoxycholic acid in combination with vitamin E therapy induced long-term improvements in liver function tests [183]. However, in another study of obese children with NAFLD, it was ineffective both alone and when combined with dietary intervention in decreasing serum ALT or the appearance of steatosis on ultrasound [184]. In another study in children, high doses of this acid induced a significant reduction in aminotransferase levels, although this was not the case with lower doses [185]. That said, its histological impact and therapeutic dose-threshold, as well as its effect on disease progression remains unclear. For example, in another study, two years of low-dose ursodeoxycholic acid in combination with vitamin E therapy was reported to improve biochemical and histological biomarkers [186]. Thus, the potential of ursodeoxycholic acid for reversing liver damage in paediatric NAFLD requires further attention.

## 5.8. Probiotic Therapy

Persistent cross-talk among the gut, the immune system and the liver appears to play an increasingly pivotal role in the pathogenesis and progression of NAFLD [63,64,154]. Emerging evidence suggests that specific nutrients are capable of increasing intestinal permeability to bacterial endotoxins, which, in turn, stimulate an immune-mediated inflammatory response from liver-resident cells, precipitating a profibrogenic phenotype. Several studies have also shown that the composition of the gut microbiome differs in NASH patients differs from that of obese patients without NASH and normoweight controls, specifically displaying a greater abundance of gram-negative bacteria [56,149].

Loguercio *et al.* [187] reported reduced hepatic injury and improved liver function tests following probiotic treatment in patients with various forms of chronic liver disease, including NAFLD. More recently, probiotic therapy in obese children with lactobacillus has been associated with significant improvement in serum aminotransferases and anti-peptidoglycan polysaccharide antibody levels, irrespective of BMI and visceral fat [188]. Further studies, have suggested that probiotics may reduce liver inflammation and improve gut epithelial barrier function. Probiotic therapy, therefore, represents a promising tool for the treatment of NAFLD in children by restoring the normal balance of gut microbiota [12,189].

Farnesoid X receptors (FXR), which are expressed in the bowel and liver, have also been implicated in the pathogenesis of NAFLD by mediating control of lipid and glucose homeostasis and bacterial flora growth and may, therefore, represent a novel therapeutic target [12,190].

## 6. Conclusions

Non-Alcoholic Fatty Liver Disease (NAFLD) is now the most common form of chronic liver disease, affecting 10%–20% of the general paediatric population and 50%–80% of those who are obese [27,35]. Within the next 10 years, it is expected to become the leading cause of liver pathology, liver failure and indication for liver transplantation in childhood and adolescence in the Western world [19,29,49,117]. Despite this, "paediatric" NAFLD remains under-studied, under-recognised and, potentially, undermanaged. Important gaps remain in our overall approach to screening, diagnosis, management and follow-up, particularly during the transition between paediatric and adult clinical services and in those patients at the extreme end of the obesity spectrum, in whom non-surgical therapies for weight loss are currently non-existent [9,11,44].

The importance of raising clinical and public awareness of NAFLD in childhood and adolescence, as well as addressing widespread misconceptions regarding its prevalence, natural history and prognosis among healthcare professionals at all stages of their training and in light of emerging evidence, cannot be overstated. The strong association between paediatric NAFLD and metabolic risk factors, including insulin resistance, dyslipidaemia, cardiovascular disease and, most significantly, obesity, highlights the need for greater interconnectedness and collaboration between diverse clinical specialties and the potential for significantly improving patient outcomes through targeted dietary modification, reduction of caloric intake, increased physical exercise and, where appropriate, pharmacological therapy [9,21,67,131].

The current paucity of research in paediatric NAFLD has perpetuated a limited understanding of its pathophysiology and hampered the selection and development of more effective therapeutic interventions since this disease was first described in children in the mid-1970s. More accurate epidemiological data derived from longitudinal and larger cohort studies will be needed in order to determine the true prevalence of NAFLD in childhood and adolescence and allow the development of more accurate risk prediction scores to augment clinical screening and surveillance, as well as comprehensive clinical guidelines specifically for the diagnosis and management of paediatric disease, which are currently lacking.

By appropriately reviewing the nomenclature, we might better emphasise the importance of the clinicopathological relationships between NAFLD and other chronic liver diseases in childhood and adolescence.

In the absence of definitive radiological and histopathological diagnostic tests, maintenance of a high clinical suspicion in both primary and specialist care settings and by all members of the multidisciplinary team remains the most potent of diagnostic tools, enabling early diagnosis and appropriate therapeutic intervention.

**Acknowledgments:** This work has been funded by the Welcome Trust and the Obesity Action Campaign. We also acknowledge all the researchers that contribute to the understanding of this field.

## Abbreviations

| | |
|---|---|
| LD | Linear dichroism |
| AASLD | American Association for the Study of Liver Diseases |
| ALT | Alanine Aminotransferase |
| AMPK | AMP-activated Protein Kinase |
| APOC3 | Adipoprotein C3 |
| AST | Aspartate Aminotransferase |
| BMI | Body Mass Index |
| CB2 | Cannabinoid Receptor 2 |
| CK-18 | Cytokeratin 18 |
| CT | Computerized Tomography |
| CYP2E1 | Cytochrome P450 family 2 subfamily E member 1 |
| DGAT2 | Diacylglycerol O-Acyltransferase 2 |
| DHA | Docosahexaenoic Acid |
| DPP-4 | Incretin Mimetics and Dipeptidyl Peptidase-4 |
| EASL | European Association for the Study of the Liver |
| ELF | Enhanced Liver Fibrosis |
| FTO | Fat Mass and Obesity associated |
| FXR | Farnesoid X Receptor |
| GCKR | Glucokinase Regulatory Protein |
| GGT | $\gamma$-glutamyl Transferase |
| GLP1 | Glucagon-Like Peptide-1 |
| GRP-120 | G Protein-coupled Receptor 120 |
| GWAS | Genome-Wide Association Study |
| HDL | High-Density Lipoprotein |
| HPC | Hepatic Progenitor Cells |
| HSC | Hepatic Stellate Cells |
| IL-6 | Interleukin 6 |
| IR | Insulin Resistance |
| IRS-1 | Insulin Receptor Substrate-1 |
| IUGR | Intrauterine Growth Restriction |
| KC | Kupffer Cells |
| KLF-6 | Kruppel-Like Factor 6 |
| LDL | Low Density Lipoprotein |
| LFTs | Liver Function Tests |
| LPIN1 | Lipin 1 |
| LYPLAL1 | Lysophospholipase-Like 1 |
| MC4R | Melanocortin 4 Receptor |
| NAFLD | Non-Alcoholic Fatty Liver Disease |
| NASH | Non-Alcoholic Steatohepatitis |
| NCAN | Neurocan |
| NKT | Natural Killer T lymphocytes |
| PNFI | Pediatric NAFLD Fibrosis Index |
| PNPLA3 | Adiponutrin/Patatin-like Phospholipase Domain-containing 3 |
| PPARg | Peroxisome-Proliferator Activated Receptor-$\gamma$ |
| PPP1R3B | Protein Phosphatase 1 Regulatory Subunit 3b |
| PYY | Peptide YY |
| ROS | Reactive Oxygen Species |
| SLD | Steatotic Liver Disease |
| SOD2 | Manganese-dependent Superoxide Dismutase |
| SREBP1c | Sterol Regulatory Binding Element |
| TNF-$\alpha$ | Tumor Necrosis Factor $\alpha$ |
| TONIC | Treatment of NAFLD in Children |

# References

1.  Angulo, P. Nonalcoholic fatty liver disease. *N. Engl. J. Med.* **2002**, *346*, 1221–1231. [CrossRef] [PubMed]
2.  Lawlor, D.A.; Callaway, M.; Macdonald-Wallis, C.; Anderson, E.; Fraser, A.; Howe, L.D.; Day, C.; Sattar, N. Nonalcoholic fatty liver disease, liver fibrosis, and cardiometabolic risk factors in adolescence: A cross-sectional study of 1874 general population adolescents. *J. Clin. Endocrinol. Metab.* **2014**, *99*, E410–E417. [CrossRef] [PubMed]
3.  Alexander, J.; Torbenson, M.; Wu, T.T.; Yeh, M.M. Non-alcoholic fatty liver disease contributes to hepatocarcinogenesis in non-cirrhotic liver: A clinical and pathological study. *J. Gastroenterol. Hepatol.* **2013**, *28*, 848–854. [CrossRef] [PubMed]
4.  Alisi, A.; Cianfarani, S.; Manco, M.; Agostoni, C.; Nobili, V. Non-alcoholic fatty liver disease and metabolic syndrome in adolescents: Pathogenetic role of genetic background and intrauterine environment. *Ann. Med.* **2012**, *44*, 29–40. [CrossRef] [PubMed]
5.  Perticone, M.; Cimellaro, A.; Maio, R.; Caroleo, B.; Sciacqua, A.; Sesti, G.; Perticone, F. Additive effect of non-alcoholic fatty liver disease on metabolic syndrome-related endothelial dysfunction in hypertensive patients. *Int. J. Mol. Sci.* **2016**, *17*. [CrossRef] [PubMed]
6.  Ayonrinde, O.T.; Olynyk, J.K.; Marsh, J.A.; Beilin, L.J.; Mori, T.A.; Oddy, W.H.; Adams, L.A. Childhood adiposity trajectories and risk of nonalcoholic fatty liver disease in adolescents. *J. Gastroenterol. Hepatol.* **2015**, *30*, 163–171. [CrossRef] [PubMed]
7.  Moran, J.R.; Ghishan, F.K.; Halter, S.A.; Greene, H.L. Steatohepatitis in obese children: A cause of chronic liver dysfunction. *Am. J. Gastroenterol.* **1983**, *78*, 374–377. [PubMed]
8.  Marcason, W. What are the current guidelines for pediatric non-alcoholic fatty liver disease? *J. Acad. Nutr. Diet.* **2013**, *113*, 1772. [CrossRef] [PubMed]
9.  Mencin, A.A.; Lavine, J.E. Advances in pediatric nonalcoholic fatty liver disease. *Pediatr. Clin. N. Am.* **2011**, *58*, 1375–1392. [CrossRef] [PubMed]
10. Monteiro, P.A.; Antunes Bde, M.; Silveira, L.S.; Christofaro, D.G.; Fernandes, R.A.; Freitas Junior, I.F. Body composition variables as predictors of nafld by ultrasound in obese children and adolescents. *BMC Pediatr.* **2014**, *14*, 25. [CrossRef] [PubMed]
11. Ratziu, V.; Bellentani, S.; Cortez-Pinto, H.; Day, C.; Marchesini, G. A position statement on NAFLD/NASH based on the EASL 2009 special conference. *J. Hepatol.* **2010**, *53*, 372–384. [CrossRef] [PubMed]
12. Berardis, S.; Sokal, E. Pediatric non-alcoholic fatty liver disease: An increasing public health issue. *Eur. J. Pediatr.* **2014**, *173*, 131–139. [CrossRef] [PubMed]
13. Schwimmer, J.B.; Deutsch, R.; Kahen, T.; Lavine, J.E.; Stanley, C.; Behling, C. Prevalence of fatty liver in children and adolescents. *Pediatrics* **2006**, *118*, 1388–1393. [CrossRef] [PubMed]
14. Holterman, A.; Gurria, J.; Tanpure, S.; DiSomma, N. Nonalcoholic fatty liver disease and bariatric surgery in adolescents. *Semin. Pediatr. Surg.* **2014**, *23*, 49–57. [CrossRef] [PubMed]
15. Vajro, P.; Ferrante, L.; Lenta, S.; Mandato, C.; Persico, M. Management of adults with paediatric-onset chronic liver disease: Strategic issues for transition care. *Dig. Liver Dis.* **2014**, *46*, 295–301. [CrossRef] [PubMed]
16. Palmer, N.D.; Musani, S.K.; Yerges-Armstrong, L.M.; Feitosa, M.F.; Bielak, L.F.; Hernaez, R.; Kahali, B.; Carr, J.J.; Harris, T.B.; Jhun, M.A.; *et al.* Characterization of european ancestry nonalcoholic fatty liver disease-associated variants in individuals of african and hispanic descent. *Hepatology* **2013**, *58*, 966–975. [CrossRef] [PubMed]
17. Vajro, P.; Lenta, S.; Socha, P.; Dhawan, A.; McKiernan, P.; Baumann, U.; Durmaz, O.; Lacaille, F.; McLin, V.; Nobili, V. Diagnosis of nonalcoholic fatty liver disease in children and adolescents: Position paper of the espghan hepatology committee. *J. Pediatr. Gastroenterol. Nutr.* **2012**, *54*, 700–713. [CrossRef] [PubMed]
18. Boyraz, M.; Hatipoglu, N.; Sari, E.; Akcay, A.; Taskin, N.; Ulucan, K.; Akcay, T. Non-alcoholic fatty liver disease in obese children and the relationship between metabolic syndrome criteria. *Obes. Res. Clin. Pract.* **2014**, *8*, e356–e363. [CrossRef] [PubMed]
19. Chalasani, N.; Younossi, Z.; Lavine, J.E.; Diehl, A.M.; Brunt, E.M.; Cusi, K.; Charlton, M.; Sanyal, A.J. The diagnosis and management of non-alcoholic fatty liver disease: Practice guideline by the American association for the study of liver diseases, American college of gastroenterology, and the American gastroenterological association. *Am. J. Gastroenterol.* **2012**, *107*, 811–826. [CrossRef] [PubMed]

20. Deng, J.; Fishbein, M.H.; Rigsby, C.K.; Zhang, G.; Schoeneman, S.E.; Donaldson, J.S. Quantitative MRI for hepatic fat fraction and T2* measurement in pediatric patients with non-alcoholic fatty liver disease. *Pediatr. Radiol.* **2014**, *44*, 1379–1387. [CrossRef] [PubMed]

21. Liccardo, D.; Alisi, A.; Porta, G.; Nobili, V. Is there any link between dietary pattern and development of nonalcoholic fatty liver disease in adolescence? An expert review. *Expert Rev. Gastroenterol. Hepatol.* **2013**, *7*, 601–604. [CrossRef] [PubMed]

22. Lerret, S.M.; Garcia-Rodriguez, L.; Skelton, J.; Biank, V.; Kilway, D.; Telega, G. Predictors of nonalcoholic steatohepatitis in obese children. *Gastroenterol. Nurs.* **2011**, *34*, 434–437. [CrossRef] [PubMed]

23. Navarro-Jarabo, J.M.; Ubina-Aznar, E.; Tapia-Ceballos, L.; Ortiz-Cuevas, C.; Perez-Aisa, M.A.; Rivas-Ruiz, F.; Andrade, R.J.; Perea-Milla, E. Hepatic steatosis and severity-related factors in obese children. *J. Gastroenterol. Hepatol.* **2013**, *28*, 1532–1538. [CrossRef] [PubMed]

24. Alisi, A.; Nobili, V. Non-alcoholic fatty liver disease in children now: Lifestyle changes and pharmacologic treatments. *Nutrition* **2012**, *28*, 722–726. [CrossRef] [PubMed]

25. Ozhan, B.; Ersoy, B.; Kiremitci, S.; Ozkol, M.; Taneli, F. Insulin sensitivity indices: Fasting *versus* glucose-stimulated indices in pediatric non-alcoholic fatty liver disease. *Eur. Rev. Med. Pharmacol. Sci.* **2015**, *19*, 3450–3458. [PubMed]

26. Anderson, E.L.; Howe, L.D.; Jones, H.E.; Higgins, J.P.; Lawlor, D.A.; Fraser, A. The prevalence of non-alcoholic fatty liver disease in children and adolescents: A systematic review and meta-analysis. *PLoS ONE* **2015**, *10*, e0140908. [CrossRef] [PubMed]

27. Kelsey, M.M.; Zaepfel, A.; Bjornstad, P.; Nadeau, K.J. Age-related consequences of childhood obesity. *Gerontology* **2014**, *60*, 222–228. [CrossRef] [PubMed]

28. Regnell, S.E.; Peterson, P.; Trinh, L.; Broberg, P.; Leander, P.; Lernmark, A.; Mansson, S.; Elding Larsson, H. Magnetic resonance imaging reveals altered distribution of hepatic fat in children with type 1 diabetes compared to controls. *Metabolism* **2015**, *64*, 872–878. [CrossRef] [PubMed]

29. Mansoor, S.; Yerian, L.; Kohli, R.; Xanthakos, S.; Angulo, P.; Ling, S.; Lopez, R.; Christine, C.K.; Feldstein, A.E.; Alkhouri, N. The evaluation of hepatic fibrosis scores in children with nonalcoholic fatty liver disease. *Dig. Dis. Sci.* **2015**, *60*, 1440–1447. [CrossRef] [PubMed]

30. Trovato, F.M.; Martines, G.F.; Brischetto, D.; Catalano, D.; Musumeci, G.; Trovato, G.M. Fatty liver disease and lifestyle in youngsters: Diet, food intake frequency, exercise, sleep shortage and fashion. *Liver Int.* **2016**, *36*, 427–433. [CrossRef] [PubMed]

31. Younossi, Z.M.; Stepanova, M.; Negro, F.; Hallaji, S.; Younossi, Y.; Lam, B.; Srishord, M. Nonalcoholic fatty liver disease in lean individuals in the United States. *Medicine* **2012**, *91*, 319–327. [CrossRef] [PubMed]

32. Silveira, L.S.; Monteiro, P.A.; Antunes Bde, M.; Seraphim, P.M.; Fernandes, R.A.; Christofaro, D.G.; Freitas Junior, I.F. Intra-abdominal fat is related to metabolic syndrome and non-alcoholic fat liver disease in obese youth. *BMC Pediatr.* **2013**, *13*, 115. [CrossRef] [PubMed]

33. Kelishadi, R.; Cook, S.R.; Adibi, A.; Faghihimani, Z.; Ghatrehsamani, S.; Beihaghi, A.; Salehi, H.; Khavarian, N.; Poursafa, P. Association of the components of the metabolic syndrome with non-alcoholic fatty liver disease among normal-weight, overweight and obese children and adolescents. *Diabetol. Metab. Syndr.* **2009**, *1*, 29. [CrossRef] [PubMed]

34. Manco, M.; Bedogni, G.; Marcellini, M.; Devito, R.; Ciampalini, P.; Sartorelli, M.R.; Comparcola, D.; Piemonte, F.; Nobili, V. Waist circumference correlates with liver fibrosis in children with non-alcoholic steatohepatitis. *Gut* **2008**, *57*, 1283–1287. [CrossRef] [PubMed]

35. Alterio, A.; Alisi, A.; Liccardo, D.; Nobili, V. Non-alcoholic fatty liver and metabolic syndrome in children: A vicious circle. *Horm. Res. Paediatr.* **2014**, *82*, 283–289. [CrossRef] [PubMed]

36. Mager, D.R.; Yap, J.; Rodriguez-Dimitrescu, C.; Mazurak, V.; Ball, G.; Gilmour, S. Anthropometric measures of visceral and subcutaneous fat are important in the determination of metabolic dysregulation in boys and girls at risk for nonalcoholic fatty liver disease. *Nutr. Clin. Pract.* **2013**, *28*, 101–111. [CrossRef] [PubMed]

37. Boyraz, M.; Cekmez, F.; Karaoglu, A.; Cinaz, P.; Durak, M.; Bideci, A. Relationship of adipokines (adiponectin, resistin and RBP4) with metabolic syndrome components in pubertal obese children. *Biomark. Med.* **2013**, *7*, 423–428. [CrossRef] [PubMed]

38. Sayin, O.; Tokgoz, Y.; Arslan, N. Investigation of adropin and leptin levels in pediatric obesity-related nonalcoholic fatty liver disease. *J. Pediatr. Endocrinol. Metab.* **2014**, *27*, 479–484. [CrossRef] [PubMed]

39. Li, W.; Zheng, L.; Sheng, C.; Cheng, X.; Qing, L.; Qu, S. Systematic review on the treatment of pentoxifylline in patients with non-alcoholic fatty liver disease. *Lipids Health Dis.* **2011**, *10*, 49. [CrossRef] [PubMed]

40. Adams, L.A.; Lymp, J.F.; St Sauver, J.; Sanderson, S.O.; Lindor, K.D.; Feldstein, A.; Angulo, P. The natural history of nonalcoholic fatty liver disease: A population-based cohort study. *Gastroenterology* **2005**, *129*, 113–121. [CrossRef] [PubMed]

41. Ekstedt, M.; Franzen, L.E.; Mathiesen, U.L.; Thorelius, L.; Holmqvist, M.; Bodemar, G.; Kechagias, S. Long-term follow-up of patients with NAFLD and elevated liver enzymes. *Hepatology* **2006**, *44*, 865–873. [CrossRef] [PubMed]

42. Ong, J.P.; Pitts, A.; Younossi, Z.M. Increased overall mortality and liver-related mortality in non-alcoholic fatty liver disease. *J. Hepatol.* **2008**, *49*, 608–612. [CrossRef] [PubMed]

43. Schwimmer, J.B.; Newton, K.P.; Awai, H.I.; Choi, L.J.; Garcia, M.A.; Ellis, L.L.; Vanderwall, K.; Fontanesi, J. Paediatric gastroenterology evaluation of overweight and obese children referred from primary care for suspected non-alcoholic fatty liver disease. *Aliment. Pharmacol. Ther.* **2013**, *38*, 1267–1277. [CrossRef] [PubMed]

44. Holterman, A.X.; Guzman, G.; Fantuzzi, G.; Wang, H.; Aigner, K.; Browne, A.; Holterman, M. Nonalcoholic fatty liver disease in severely obese adolescent and adult patients. *Obesity* **2013**, *21*, 591–597. [CrossRef] [PubMed]

45. Charlotte, F.; Le Naour, G.; Bernhardt, C.; Poynard, T.; Ratziu, V.; Group, L.S. A comparison of the fibrotic potential of nonalcoholic fatty liver disease and chronic hepatitis C. *Hum. Pathol.* **2010**, *41*, 1178–1185. [CrossRef] [PubMed]

46. Caldwell, S.H.; Crespo, D.M.; Kang, H.S.; Al-Osaimi, A.M. Obesity and hepatocellular carcinoma. *Gastroenterology* **2004**, *127*, S97–S103. [CrossRef] [PubMed]

47. El-Serag, H.B.; Hampel, H.; Javadi, F. The association between diabetes and hepatocellular carcinoma: A systematic review of epidemiologic evidence. *Clin. Gastroenterol. Hepatol.* **2006**, *4*, 369–380. [CrossRef] [PubMed]

48. Berentzen, T.L.; Gamborg, M.; Holst, C.; Sorensen, T.I.; Baker, J.L. Body mass index in childhood and adult risk of primary liver cancer. *J. Hepatol.* **2014**, *60*, 325–330. [CrossRef] [PubMed]

49. Atabek, M.E.; Selver Eklioglu, B.; Akyurek, N. Which metabolic syndrome criteria best predict non-alcoholic fatty liver disease in children? *Eat. Weight Disord.* **2014**, *19*, 495–501. [CrossRef] [PubMed]

50. Singh, G.K.; Vitola, B.E.; Holland, M.R.; Sekarski, T.; Patterson, B.W.; Magkos, F.; Klein, S. Alterations in ventricular structure and function in obese adolescents with nonalcoholic fatty liver disease. *J. Pediatr.* **2013**, *162*, 1160–1168. [CrossRef] [PubMed]

51. Fintini, D.; Chinali, M.; Cafiero, G.; Esposito, C.; Giordano, U.; Turchetta, A.; Pescosolido, S.; Pongiglione, G.; Nobili, V. Early left ventricular abnormality/dysfunction in obese children affected by NAFLD. *Nutr. Metab. Cardiovasc. Dis.* **2014**, *24*, 72–74. [CrossRef] [PubMed]

52. Pacifico, L.; Di Martino, M.; de Merulis, A.; Bezzi, M.; Osborn, J.F.; Catalano, C.; Chiesa, C. Left ventricular dysfunction in obese children and adolescents with nonalcoholic fatty liver disease. *Hepatology* **2014**, *59*, 461–470. [CrossRef] [PubMed]

53. Nobili, V.; Alkhouri, N.; Bartuli, A.; Manco, M.; Lopez, R.; Alisi, A.; Feldstein, A.E. Severity of liver injury and atherogenic lipid profile in children with nonalcoholic fatty liver disease. *Pediatr. Res.* **2010**, *67*, 665–670. [CrossRef] [PubMed]

54. Pacifico, L.; Bonci, E.; Andreoli, G.; Romaggioli, S.; Di Miscio, R.; Lombardo, C.V.; Chiesa, C. Association of serum triglyceride-to-HDL cholesterol ratio with carotid artery intima-media thickness, insulin resistance and nonalcoholic fatty liver disease in children and adolescents. *Nutr. Metab. Cardiovasc. Dis.* **2014**, *24*, 737–743. [CrossRef] [PubMed]

55. Nobili, V.; Donati, B.; Panera, N.; Vongsakulyanon, A.; Alisi, A.; Dallapiccola, B.; Valenti, L. A 4-polymorphism risk score predicts steatohepatitis in children with nonalcoholic fatty liver disease. *J. Pediatr. Gastroenterol. Nutr.* **2014**, *58*, 632–636. [CrossRef] [PubMed]

56. Yuan, J.; Baker, S.S.; Liu, W.; Alkhouri, R.; Baker, R.D.; Xie, J.; Ji, G.; Zhu, L. Endotoxemia unrequired in the pathogenesis of pediatric nonalcoholic steatohepatitis. *J. Gastroenterol. Hepatol.* **2014**, *29*, 1292–1298. [CrossRef] [PubMed]

57. Choi, S.S.; Diehl, A.M. Hepatic triglyceride synthesis and nonalcoholic fatty liver disease. *Curr. Opin. Lipidol.* **2008**, *19*, 295–300. [CrossRef] [PubMed]

58. Yamaguchi, K.; Yang, L.; McCall, S.; Huang, J.; Yu, X.X.; Pandey, S.K.; Bhanot, S.; Monia, B.P.; Li, Y.X.; Diehl, A.M. Inhibiting triglyceride synthesis improves hepatic steatosis but exacerbates liver damage and fibrosis in obese mice with nonalcoholic steatohepatitis. *Hepatology* **2007**, *45*, 1366–1374. [CrossRef] [PubMed]

59. Wanless, I.R.; Shiota, K. The pathogenesis of nonalcoholic steatohepatitis and other fatty liver diseases: A four-step model including the role of lipid release and hepatic venular obstruction in the progression to cirrhosis. *Semin. Liver Dis.* **2004**, *24*, 99–106. [PubMed]

60. Morandi, A.; Maffeis, C. Predictors of metabolic risk in childhood obesity. *Horm. Res. Paediatr.* **2014**, *82*, 3–11. [CrossRef] [PubMed]

61. Torun, E.; Ozgen, I.T.; Gokce, S.; Aydin, S.; Cesur, Y. Thyroid hormone levels in obese children and adolescents with non-alcoholic fatty liver disease. *J. Clin. Res. Pediatr. Endocrinol.* **2014**, *6*, 34–39. [CrossRef] [PubMed]

62. Pacifico, L.; Bonci, E.; Ferraro, F.; Andreoli, G.; Bascetta, S.; Chiesa, C. Hepatic steatosis and thyroid function tests in overweight and obese children. *Int. J. Endocrinol.* **2013**, *2013*, 381014. [CrossRef] [PubMed]

63. De Vito, R.; Alisi, A.; Masotti, A.; Ceccarelli, S.; Panera, N.; Citti, A.; Salata, M.; Valenti, L.; Feldstein, A.E.; Nobili, V. Markers of activated inflammatory cells correlate with severity of liver damage in children with nonalcoholic fatty liver disease. *Int. J. Mol. Med.* **2012**, *30*, 49–56. [PubMed]

64. Ferreyra Solari, N.E.; Inzaugarat, M.E.; Baz, P.; de Matteo, E.; Lezama, C.; Galoppo, M.; Galoppo, C.; Chernavsky, A.C. The role of innate cells is coupled to a Th1-polarized immune response in pediatric nonalcoholic steatohepatitis. *J. Clin. Immunol.* **2012**, *32*, 611–621. [CrossRef] [PubMed]

65. Barshop, N.J.; Sirlin, C.B.; Schwimmer, J.B.; Lavine, J.E. Review article: Epidemiology, pathogenesis and potential treatments of paediatric non-alcoholic fatty liver disease. *Aliment. Pharmacol. Ther.* **2008**, *28*, 13–24. [CrossRef] [PubMed]

66. Nobili, V.; Carpino, G.; Alisi, A.; Franchitto, A.; Alpini, G.; de Vito, R.; Onori, P.; Alvaro, D.; Gaudio, E. Hepatic progenitor cells activation, fibrosis, and adipokines production in pediatric nonalcoholic fatty liver disease. *Hepatology* **2012**, *56*, 2142–2153. [CrossRef] [PubMed]

67. Yoon, H.J.; Cha, B.S. Pathogenesis and therapeutic approaches for non-alcoholic fatty liver disease. *World J. Hepatol.* **2014**, *6*, 800–811. [CrossRef] [PubMed]

68. Swiderska-Syn, M.; Suzuki, A.; Guy, C.D.; Schwimmer, J.B.; Abdelmalek, M.F.; Lavine, J.E.; Diehl, A.M. Hedgehog pathway and pediatric nonalcoholic fatty liver disease. *Hepatology* **2013**, *57*, 1814–1825. [CrossRef] [PubMed]

69. Mouralidarane, A.; Soeda, J.; Visconti-Pugmire, C.; Samuelsson, A.M.; Pombo, J.; Maragkoudaki, X.; Butt, A.; Saraswati, R.; Novelli, M.; Fusai, G.; *et al.* Maternal obesity programs offspring nonalcoholic fatty liver disease by innate immune dysfunction in mice. *Hepatology* **2013**, *58*, 128–138. [CrossRef] [PubMed]

70. Stienstra, R.; Saudale, F.; Duval, C.; Keshtkar, S.; Groener, J.E.; van Rooijen, N.; Staels, B.; Kersten, S.; Muller, M. Kupffer cells promote hepatic steatosis via interleukin-1β-dependent suppression of peroxisome proliferator-activated receptor α activity. *Hepatology* **2010**, *51*, 511–522. [CrossRef] [PubMed]

71. Morgan, M.L.; Sigala, B.; Soeda, J.; Cordero, P.; Nguyen, V.; McKee, C.; Mouraliderane, A.; Vinciguerra, M.; Oben, J.A. Acetylcholine induces fibrogenic effects via M2/M3 acetylcholine receptors in non-alcoholic steatohepatitis and in primary human hepatic stellate cells. *J. Gastroenterol. Hepatol.* **2016**, *31*, 475–483. [CrossRef] [PubMed]

72. Sigala, B.; McKee, C.; Soeda, J.; Pazienza, V.; Morgan, M.; Lin, C.I.; Selden, C.; Vander Borght, S.; Mazzoccoli, G.; Roskams, T.; *et al.* Sympathetic nervous system catecholamines and neuropeptide y neurotransmitters are upregulated in human nafld and modulate the fibrogenic function of hepatic stellate cells. *PLoS ONE* **2013**, *8*, e72928. [CrossRef] [PubMed]

73. Shang, X.R.; Song, J.Y.; Liu, F.H.; Ma, J.; Wang, H.J. Gwas-identified common variants with nonalcoholic fatty liver disease in Chinese children. *J. Pediatr. Gastroenterol. Nutr.* **2015**, *60*, 669–674. [CrossRef] [PubMed]

74. Schwimmer, J.B.; Celedon, M.A.; Lavine, J.E.; Salem, R.; Campbell, N.; Schork, N.J.; Shiehmorteza, M.; Yokoo, T.; Chavez, A.; Middleton, M.S.; *et al.* Heritability of nonalcoholic fatty liver disease. *Gastroenterology* **2009**, *136*, 1585–1592. [CrossRef] [PubMed]

75. Deboer, M.D.; Wiener, R.C.; Barnes, B.H.; Gurka, M.J. Ethnic differences in the link between insulin resistance and elevated ALT. *Pediatrics* **2013**, *132*, e718–e726. [CrossRef] [PubMed]

76. Lin, Y.C.; Chang, P.F.; Chang, M.H.; Ni, Y.H. Genetic variants in GCKR and PNPLA3 confer susceptibility to nonalcoholic fatty liver disease in obese individuals. *Am. J. Clin. Nutr.* **2014**, *99*, 869–874. [CrossRef] [PubMed]

77.  Hernaez, R.; McLean, J.; Lazo, M.; Brancati, F.L.; Hirschhorn, J.N.; Borecki, I.B.; Harris, T.B.; Genetics of Obesity-Related Liver Disease (GOLD) Consortium; Nguyen, T.; Kamel, I.R.; *et al.* Association between variants in or near PNPLA3, GCKR, and PPP1R3B with ultrasound-defined steatosis based on data from the third national health and nutrition examination survey. *Clin. Gastroenterol. Hepatol.* **2013**, *11*, 1183–1190. [CrossRef] [PubMed]

78.  Romeo, S.; Kozlitina, J.; Xing, C.; Pertsemlidis, A.; Cox, D.; Pennacchio, L.A.; Boerwinkle, E.; Cohen, J.C.; Hobbs, H.H. Genetic variation in *PNPLA3* confers susceptibility to nonalcoholic fatty liver disease. *Nat. Genet.* **2008**, *40*, 1461–1465. [CrossRef] [PubMed]

79.  Santoro, N.; Kursawe, R.; D'Adamo, E.; Dykas, D.J.; Zhang, C.K.; Bale, A.E.; Cali, A.M.; Narayan, D.; Shaw, M.M.; Pierpont, B.; *et al.* A common variant in the patatin-like phospholipase 3 gene (*PNPLA3*) is associated with fatty liver disease in obese children and adolescents. *Hepatology* **2010**, *52*, 1281–1290. [CrossRef] [PubMed]

80.  Mangge, H.; Baumgartner, B.G.; Zelzer, S.; Pruller, F.; Schnedl, W.J.; Reininghaus, E.Z.; Haybaeck, J.; Lackner, C.; Stauber, R.; Aigner, E.; *et al.* Patatin-like phospholipase 3 (*rs738409*) gene polymorphism is associated with increased liver enzymes in obese adolescents and metabolic syndrome in all ages. *Aliment. Pharmacol. Ther.* **2015**, *42*, 99–105. [CrossRef] [PubMed]

81.  Guan, L.; Shang, X.R.; Liu, F.H.; Song, J.Y.; Ma, J.; Wang, H.J. Association of INSIG2 rs9308762 with alt level independent of BMI. *J. Pediatr. Gastroenterol. Nutr.* **2014**, *58*, 155–159. [CrossRef] [PubMed]

82.  Rossi, F.; Bellini, G.; Alisi, A.; Alterio, A.; Maione, S.; Perrone, L.; Locatelli, F.; Miraglia del Giudice, E.; Nobili, V. Cannabinoid receptor type 2 functional variant influences liver damage in children with non-alcoholic fatty liver disease. *PLoS ONE* **2012**, *7*, e42259. [CrossRef] [PubMed]

83.  Hyysalo, J.; Mannisto, V.T.; Zhou, Y.; Arola, J.; Karja, V.; Leivonen, M.; Juuti, A.; Jaser, N.; Lallukka, S.; Kakela, P.; *et al.* A population-based study on the prevalence of NASH using scores validated against liver histology. *J. Hepatol.* **2014**, *60*, 839–846. [CrossRef] [PubMed]

84.  Qiao, A.; Liang, J.; Ke, Y.; Li, C.; Cui, Y.; Shen, L.; Zhang, H.; Cui, A.; Liu, X.; Liu, C.; *et al.* Mouse patatin-like phospholipase domain-containing 3 influences systemic lipid and glucose homeostasis. *Hepatology* **2011**, *54*, 509–521. [CrossRef] [PubMed]

85.  Weltman, M.D.; Farrell, G.C.; Hall, P.; Ingelman-Sundberg, M.; Liddle, C. Hepatic cytochrome P450 2E1 is increased in patients with nonalcoholic steatohepatitis. *Hepatology* **1998**, *27*, 128–133. [CrossRef] [PubMed]

86.  Weltman, M.D.; Farrell, G.C.; Liddle, C. Increased hepatocyte CYP2E1 expression in a rat nutritional model of hepatic steatosis with inflammation. *Gastroenterology* **1996**, *111*, 1645–1653. [CrossRef]

87.  Sugimoto, Y.; Wakai, K.; Nakagawa, H.; Suma, S.; Sasakabe, T.; Sakamoto, T.; Takashima, N.; Suzuki, S.; Ogawa, S.; Ohnaka, K.; *et al.* Associations between polymorphisms of interleukin-6 and related cytokine genes and serum liver damage markers: A cross-sectional study in the Japan Multi-Institutional Collaborative Cohort (J-MICC) study. *Gene* **2015**, *557*, 158–162. [CrossRef] [PubMed]

88.  Lin, Y.C.; Chang, P.F.; Hu, F.C.; Chang, M.H.; Ni, Y.H. Variants in the *UGT1A1* gene and the risk of pediatric nonalcoholic fatty liver disease. *Pediatrics* **2009**, *124*, e1221–e1227. [CrossRef] [PubMed]

89.  Rossi, F.; Bellini, G.; Nobili, B.; Maione, S.; Perrone, L.; del Giudice, E.M. Association of the cannabinoid receptor 2 (Cb2) Gln63Arg polymorphism with indices of liver damage in obese children: An alternative way to highlight the CB2 hepatoprotective properties. *Hepatology* **2011**, *54*, 1102. [CrossRef] [PubMed]

90.  Cordero, P.; Milagro, F.I.; Campion, J.; Martinez, J.A. Supplementation with methyl donors during lactation to high-fat-sucrose-fed dams protects offspring against liver fat accumulation when consuming an obesogenic diet. *J. Dev. Orig. Health Dis.* **2014**, *5*, 385–395. [CrossRef] [PubMed]

91.  Cordero, P.; Milagro, F.I.; Campion, J.; Martinez, J.A. Maternal methyl donors supplementation during lactation prevents the hyperhomocysteinemia induced by a high-fat-sucrose intake by dams. *Int. J. Mol. Sci.* **2013**, *14*, 24422–24437. [CrossRef] [PubMed]

92.  Mouralidarane, A.; Soeda, J.; Sugden, D.; Bocianowska, A.; Carter, R.; Ray, S.; Saraswati, R.; Cordero, P.; Novelli, M.; Fusai, G.; *et al.* Maternal obesity programs offspring non-alcoholic fatty liver disease through disruption of 24-h rhythms in mice. *Int. J. Obes.* **2015**, *39*, 1339–1348. [CrossRef] [PubMed]

93.  Cordero, P.; Li, J.; Oben, J.A. Epigenetics of obesity: Beyond the genome sequence. *Curr. Opin. Clin. Nutr. Metab. Care* **2015**, *18*, 361–366. [CrossRef] [PubMed]

94. Cordero, P.; Li, J.; Temple, J.L.; Nguyen, V.; Oben, J.A. Epigenetic mechanisms of maternal obesity effects on the descendants. In *Parental Obesity: Intergenerational Programming and Consequences*; Green, L.R., Hester, R.L., Eds.; Springer-Verlag New York: New York, NY, USA, 2016.

95. Alisi, A.; Panera, N.; Agostoni, C.; Nobili, V. Intrauterine growth retardation and nonalcoholic fatty liver disease in children. *Int. J. Endocrinol.* **2011**, *2011*, 269853. [CrossRef] [PubMed]

96. Breij, L.M.; Kerkhof, G.F.; Hokken-Koelega, A.C. Accelerated infant weight gain and risk for nonalcoholic fatty liver disease in early adulthood. *J. Clin. Endocrinol. Metab.* **2014**, *99*, 1189–1195. [CrossRef] [PubMed]

97. Amarapurkar, D.; Kamani, P.; Patel, N.; Gupte, P.; Kumar, P.; Agal, S.; Baijal, R.; Lala, S.; Chaudhary, D.; Deshpande, A. Prevalence of non-alcoholic fatty liver disease: Population based study. *Ann. Hepatol.* **2007**, *6*, 161–163. [PubMed]

98. Hanada, S.; Snider, N.T.; Brunt, E.M.; Hollenberg, P.F.; Omary, M.B. Gender dimorphic formation of mouse mallory-denk bodies and the role of xenobiotic metabolism and oxidative stress. *Gastroenterology* **2010**, *138*, 1607–1617. [CrossRef] [PubMed]

99. Kozlov, A.V.; Duvigneau, J.C.; Hyatt, T.C.; Raju, R.; Behling, T.; Hartl, R.T.; Staniek, K.; Miller, I.; Gregor, W.; Redl, H.; *et al.* Effect of estrogen on mitochondrial function and intracellular stress markers in rat liver and kidney following trauma-hemorrhagic shock and prolonged hypotension. *Mol. Med.* **2010**, *16*, 254–261. [CrossRef] [PubMed]

100. Yasuda, M.; Shimizu, I.; Shiba, M.; Ito, S. Suppressive effects of estradiol on dimethylnitrosamine-induced fibrosis of the liver in rats. *Hepatology* **1999**, *29*, 719–727. [CrossRef] [PubMed]

101. Goh, G.B.; Pagadala, M.R.; Dasarathy, J.; Unalp-Arida, A.; Pai, R.K.; Yerian, L.; Khiyami, A.; Sourianarayanane, A.; Sargent, R.; Hawkins, C.; *et al.* Age impacts ability of aspartate-alanine aminotransferase ratio to predict advanced fibrosis in nonalcoholic fatty liver disease. *Dig. Dis. Sci.* **2015**, *60*, 1825–1831. [CrossRef] [PubMed]

102. Suzuki, A.; Abdelmalek, M.F.; Schwimmer, J.B.; Lavine, J.E.; Scheimann, A.O.; Unalp-Arida, A.; Yates, K.P.; Sanyal, A.J.; Guy, C.D.; Diehl, A.M.; *et al.* Association between puberty and features of nonalcoholic fatty liver disease. *Clin. Gastroenterol. Hepatol.* **2012**, *10*, 786–794. [CrossRef] [PubMed]

103. Rangwala, F.; Guy, C.D.; Lu, J.; Suzuki, A.; Burchette, J.L.; Abdelmalek, M.F.; Chen, W.; Diehl, A.M. Increased production of sonic hedgehog by ballooned hepatocytes. *J. Pathol.* **2011**, *224*, 401–410. [CrossRef] [PubMed]

104. Li, T.; Leng, X.S.; Zhu, J.Y.; Wang, G. Suppression of hedgehog signaling regulates hepatic stellate cell activation and collagen secretion. *Int. J. Clin. Exp. Pathol.* **2015**, *8*, 14574–14579. [PubMed]

105. Hernaez, R.; Yeung, E.; Clark, J.M.; Kowdley, K.V.; Brancati, F.L.; Kao, W.H. Hemochromatosis gene and nonalcoholic fatty liver disease: A systematic review and meta-analysis. *J. Hepatol.* **2011**, *55*, 1079–1085. [CrossRef] [PubMed]

106. Wu, S.; Tu, R.; Liu, G.; Huang, L.; Guan, Y.; Zheng, E. Focal fatty sparing usually does not arise in preexisting nonalcoholic diffuse homogeneous fatty liver. *J. Ultrasound Med.* **2014**, *33*, 1447–1452. [CrossRef] [PubMed]

107. Bellentani, S.; Saccoccio, G.; Masutti, F.; Croce, L.S.; Brandi, G.; Sasso, F.; Cristanini, G.; Tiribelli, C. Prevalence of and risk factors for hepatic steatosis in Northern Italy. *Ann. Intern. Med.* **2000**, *132*, 112–117. [CrossRef] [PubMed]

108. Patton, H.M.; Lavine, J.E.; van Natta, M.L.; Schwimmer, J.B.; Kleiner, D.; Molleston, J.; Nonalcoholic Steatohepatitis Clinical Research Network. Clinical correlates of histopathology in pediatric nonalcoholic steatohepatitis. *Gastroenterology* **2008**, *135*, 1961–1971. [CrossRef] [PubMed]

109. Fracanzani, A.L.; Valenti, L.; Bugianesi, E.; Andreoletti, M.; Colli, A.; Vanni, E.; Bertelli, C.; Fatta, E.; Bignamini, D.; Marchesini, G.; *et al.* Risk of severe liver disease in nonalcoholic fatty liver disease with normal aminotransferase levels: A role for insulin resistance and diabetes. *Hepatology* **2008**, *48*, 792–798. [CrossRef] [PubMed]

110. Mofrad, P.; Contos, M.J.; Haque, M.; Sargeant, C.; Fisher, R.A.; Luketic, V.A.; Sterling, R.K.; Shiffman, M.L.; Stravitz, R.T.; Sanyal, A.J. Clinical and histologic spectrum of nonalcoholic fatty liver disease associated with normal ALT values. *Hepatology* **2003**, *37*, 1286–1292. [CrossRef] [PubMed]

111. Vernon, G.; Baranova, A.; Younossi, Z.M. Systematic review: The epidemiology and natural history of non-alcoholic fatty liver disease and non-alcoholic steatohepatitis in adults. *Aliment. Pharmacol. Ther.* **2011**, *34*, 274–285. [CrossRef] [PubMed]

112. Wilson, H.K.; Monster, A.C. New technologies in the use of exhaled breath analysis for biological monitoring. *Occup. Environ. Med.* **1999**, *56*, 753–757. [CrossRef] [PubMed]

113. Feldstein, A.E.; Alkhouri, N.; de Vito, R.; Alisi, A.; Lopez, R.; Nobili, V. Serum cytokeratin-18 fragment levels are useful biomarkers for nonalcoholic steatohepatitis in children. *Am. J. Gastroenterol.* **2013**, *108*, 1526–1531. [CrossRef] [PubMed]

114. Wieckowska, A.; Zein, N.N.; Yerian, L.M.; Lopez, A.R.; McCullough, A.J.; Feldstein, A.E. *In vivo* assessment of liver cell apoptosis as a novel biomarker of disease severity in nonalcoholic fatty liver disease. *Hepatology* **2006**, *44*, 27–33. [CrossRef] [PubMed]

115. Musso, G.; Gambino, R.; Cassader, M.; Pagano, G. Meta-analysis: Natural history of non-alcoholic fatty liver disease (NAFLD) and diagnostic accuracy of non-invasive tests for liver disease severity. *Ann. Med.* **2011**, *43*, 617–649. [CrossRef] [PubMed]

116. Puri, K.; Nobili, V.; Melville, K.; Corte, C.D.; Sartorelli, M.R.; Lopez, R.; Feldstein, A.E.; Alkhouri, N. Serum bilirubin level is inversely associated with nonalcoholic steatohepatitis in children. *J. Pediatr. Gastroenterol. Nutr.* **2013**, *57*, 114–118. [CrossRef] [PubMed]

117. Eng, K.; Lopez, R.; Liccardo, D.; Nobili, V.; Alkhouri, N. A non-invasive prediction model for non-alcoholic steatohepatitis in paediatric patients with non-alcoholic fatty liver disease. *Dig. Liver Dis.* **2014**, *46*, 1008–1013. [CrossRef] [PubMed]

118. Oresic, M.; Hyotylainen, T.; Kotronen, A.; Gopalacharyulu, P.; Nygren, H.; Arola, J.; Castillo, S.; Mattila, I.; Hakkarainen, A.; Borra, R.J.; et al. Prediction of non-alcoholic fatty-liver disease and liver fat content by serum molecular lipids. *Diabetologia* **2013**, *56*, 2266–2274. [CrossRef] [PubMed]

119. Yilmaz, Y.; Ergelen, R.; Akin, H.; Imeryuz, N. Noninvasive detection of hepatic steatosis in patients without ultrasonographic evidence of fatty liver using the controlled attenuation parameter evaluated with transient elastography. *Eur. J. Gastroenterol. Hepatol.* **2013**, *25*, 1330–1334. [CrossRef] [PubMed]

120. Schwimmer, J.B.; Middleton, M.S.; Behling, C.; Newton, K.P.; Awai, H.I.; Paiz, M.N.; Lam, J.; Hooker, J.C.; Hamilton, G.; Fontanesi, J.; et al. Magnetic resonance imaging and liver histology as biomarkers of hepatic steatosis in children with nonalcoholic fatty liver disease. *Hepatology* **2015**, *61*, 1887–1895. [CrossRef] [PubMed]

121. Tovo, C.V.; de Mattos, A.Z.; Coral, G.P.; Branco, F.S.; Suwa, E.; de Mattos, A.A. Noninvasive imaging assessment of non-alcoholic fatty liver disease: Focus on liver scintigraphy. *World J. Gastroenterol.* **2015**, *21*, 4432–4439. [PubMed]

122. Kim, K.M.; Choi, W.B.; Park, S.H.; Yu, E.; Lee, S.G.; Lim, Y.S.; Lee, H.C.; Chung, Y.H.; Lee, Y.S.; Suh, D.J. Diagnosis of hepatic steatosis and fibrosis by transient elastography in asymptomatic healthy individuals: A prospective study of living related potential liver donors. *J. Gastroenterol.* **2007**, *42*, 382–388. [CrossRef] [PubMed]

123. Nobili, V.; Vizzutti, F.; Arena, U.; Abraldes, J.G.; Marra, F.; Pietrobattista, A.; Fruhwirth, R.; Marcellini, M.; Pinzani, M. Accuracy and reproducibility of transient elastography for the diagnosis of fibrosis in pediatric nonalcoholic steatohepatitis. *Hepatology* **2008**, *48*, 442–448. [CrossRef] [PubMed]

124. Ovchinsky, N.; Moreira, R.K.; Lefkowitch, J.H.; Lavine, J.E. Liver biopsy in modern clinical practice: A pediatric point-of-view. *Adv. Anat. Pathol.* **2012**, *19*, 250–262. [CrossRef] [PubMed]

125. Schwimmer, J.B.; Behling, C.; Newbury, R.; Deutsch, R.; Nievergelt, C.; Schork, N.J.; Lavine, J.E. Histopathology of pediatric nonalcoholic fatty liver disease. *Hepatology* **2005**, *42*, 641–649. [CrossRef] [PubMed]

126. Mansoor, S.; Collyer, E.; Alkhouri, N. A comprehensive review of noninvasive liver fibrosis tests in pediatric nonalcoholic fatty liver disease. *Curr. Gastroenterol. Rep.* **2015**, *17*, 23. [CrossRef] [PubMed]

127. Nobili, V.; Parkes, J.; Bottazzo, G.; Marcellini, M.; Cross, R.; Newman, D.; Vizzutti, F.; Pinzani, M.; Rosenberg, W.M. Performance of ELF serum markers in predicting fibrosis stage in pediatric non-alcoholic fatty liver disease. *Gastroenterology* **2009**, *136*, 160–167. [CrossRef] [PubMed]

128. Musso, G.; Gambino, R.; Cassader, M.; Pagano, G. A meta-analysis of randomized trials for the treatment of nonalcoholic fatty liver disease. *Hepatology* **2010**, *52*, 79–104. [CrossRef] [PubMed]

129. Nobili, V.; Marcellini, M.; Devito, R.; Ciampalini, P.; Piemonte, F.; Comparcola, D.; Sartorelli, M.R.; Angulo, P. Nafld in children: A prospective clinical-pathological study and effect of lifestyle advice. *Hepatology* **2006**, *44*, 458–465. [CrossRef] [PubMed]

130. DeVore, S.; Kohli, R.; Lake, K.; Nicholas, L.; Dietrich, K.; Balistreri, W.F.; Xanthakos, S.A. A multidisciplinary clinical program is effective in stabilizing BMI and reducing transaminase levels in pediatric patients with NAFLD. *J. Pediatr. Gastroenterol. Nutr.* **2013**, *57*, 119–123. [CrossRef] [PubMed]

131. Nobili, V.; Manco, M.; Devito, R.; Di Ciommo, V.; Comparcola, D.; Sartorelli, M.R.; Piemonte, F.; Marcellini, M.; Angulo, P. Lifestyle intervention and antioxidant therapy in children with nonalcoholic fatty liver disease: A randomized, controlled trial. *Hepatology* **2008**, *48*, 119–128. [CrossRef] [PubMed]

132. Oddy, W.H.; Herbison, C.E.; Jacoby, P.; Ambrosini, G.L.; O'Sullivan, T.A.; Ayonrinde, O.T.; Olynyk, J.K.; Black, L.J.; Beilin, L.J.; Mori, T.A.; et al. The western dietary pattern is prospectively associated with nonalcoholic fatty liver disease in adolescence. *Am. J. Gastroenterol.* **2013**, *108*, 778–785. [CrossRef] [PubMed]

133. Nobili, V.; Manco, M.; Devito, R.; Ciampalini, P.; Piemonte, F.; Marcellini, M. Effect of Vitamin E on aminotransferase levels and insulin resistance in children with non-alcoholic fatty liver disease. *Aliment. Pharmacol. Ther.* **2006**, *24*, 1553–1561. [CrossRef] [PubMed]

134. Gronbaek, H.; Lange, A.; Birkebaek, N.H.; Holland-Fischer, P.; Solvig, J.; Horlyck, A.; Kristensen, K.; Rittig, S.; Vilstrup, H. Effect of a 10-week weight loss camp on fatty liver disease and insulin sensitivity in obese Danish children. *J. Pediatr. Gastroenterol. Nutr.* **2012**, *54*, 223–228. [CrossRef] [PubMed]

135. Zelber-Sagi, S.; Nitzan-Kaluski, D.; Goldsmith, R.; Webb, M.; Zvibel, I.; Goldiner, I.; Blendis, L.; Halpern, Z.; Oren, R. Role of leisure-time physical activity in nonalcoholic fatty liver disease: A population-based study. *Hepatology* **2008**, *48*, 1791–1798. [CrossRef] [PubMed]

136. Barlow, S.E.; Expert, C. Expert committee recommendations regarding the prevention, assessment, and treatment of child and adolescent overweight and obesity: Summary report. *Pediatrics* **2007**, *120*, S164–S192. [CrossRef] [PubMed]

137. Haukeland, J.W.; Konopski, Z.; Eggesbo, H.B.; von Volkmann, H.L.; Raschpichler, G.; Bjoro, K.; Haaland, T.; Loberg, E.M.; Birkeland, K. Metformin in patients with non-alcoholic fatty liver disease: A randomized, controlled trial. *Scand. J. Gastroenterol.* **2009**, *44*, 853–860. [CrossRef] [PubMed]

138. Krasnoff, J.B.; Painter, P.L.; Wallace, J.P.; Bass, N.M.; Merriman, R.B. Health-related fitness and physical activity in patients with nonalcoholic fatty liver disease. *Hepatology* **2008**, *47*, 1158–1166. [CrossRef] [PubMed]

139. Kistler, K.D.; Brunt, E.M.; Clark, J.M.; Diehl, A.M.; Sallis, J.F.; Schwimmer, J.B.; Group, N.C.R. Physical activity recommendations, exercise intensity, and histological severity of nonalcoholic fatty liver disease. *Am. J. Gastroenterol.* **2011**, *106*, 460–468. [CrossRef] [PubMed]

140. Niblett, P. Statistics on Obesity, Physical Activity and Diet—England, 2015. Available online: http://www.hscic.gov.uk/catalogue/PUB16988 (accessed on 14 June 2016).

141. Jin, R.; Le, N.A.; Liu, S.; Farkas Epperson, M.; Ziegler, T.R.; Welsh, J.A.; Jones, D.P.; McClain, C.J.; Vos, M.B. Children with nafld are more sensitive to the adverse metabolic effects of fructose beverages than children without NAFLD. *J. Clin. Endocrinol. Metab.* **2012**, *97*, E1088–E1098. [CrossRef] [PubMed]

142. O'Sullivan, T.A.; Oddy, W.H.; Bremner, A.P.; Sherriff, J.L.; Ayonrinde, O.T.; Olynyk, J.K.; Beilin, L.J.; Mori, T.A.; Adams, L.A. Lower fructose intake may help protect against development of nonalcoholic fatty liver in adolescents with obesity. *J. Pediatr. Gastroenterol. Nutr.* **2014**, *58*, 624–631. [CrossRef] [PubMed]

143. Spruss, A.; Bergheim, I. Dietary fructose and intestinal barrier: Potential risk factor in the pathogenesis of nonalcoholic fatty liver disease. *J. Nutr. Biochem.* **2009**, *20*, 657–662. [CrossRef] [PubMed]

144. Kawasaki, T.; Igarashi, K.; Koeda, T.; Sugimoto, K.; Nakagawa, K.; Hayashi, S.; Yamaji, R.; Inui, H.; Fukusato, T.; Yamanouchi, T. Rats fed fructose-enriched diets have characteristics of nonalcoholic hepatic steatosis. *J. Nutr.* **2009**, *139*, 2067–2071. [CrossRef] [PubMed]

145. Kar, S.; Khandelwal, B. Fast foods and physical inactivity are risk factors for obesity and hypertension among adolescent school children in east district of sikkim, india. *J. Nat. Sci. Biol. Med.* **2015**, *6*, 356–359. [CrossRef] [PubMed]

146. Black, L.J.; Jacoby, P.; Ping-Delfos, S.; Chan, W.; Mori, T.A.; Beilin, L.J.; Olynyk, J.K.; Ayonrinde, O.T.; Huang, R.C.; Holt, P.G.; et al. Low serum 25-hydroxyvitamin D concentrations associate with non-alcoholic fatty liver disease in adolescents independent of adiposity. *J. Gastroenterol. Hepatol.* **2014**, *29*, 1215–1222. [CrossRef] [PubMed]

147. Nobili, V.; Giorgio, V.; Liccardo, D.; Bedogni, G.; Morino, G.; Alisi, A.; Cianfarani, S. Vitamin D levels and liver histological alterations in children with nonalcoholic fatty liver disease. *Eur. J. Endocrinol.* **2014**, *170*, 547–553. [CrossRef] [PubMed]

148. Li, J.; Cordero, P.; Nguyen, V.; Oben, J.A. The role of vitamins in the pathogenesis of non-alcoholic fatty liver disease. *Integr. Med. Insights* **2016**, *11*, 19–25. [CrossRef] [PubMed]

149. Roth, C.L.; Elfers, C.T.; Figlewicz, D.P.; Melhorn, S.J.; Morton, G.J.; Hoofnagle, A.; Yeh, M.M.; Nelson, J.E.; Kowdley, K.V. Vitamin D deficiency in obese rats exacerbates nonalcoholic fatty liver disease and increases hepatic resistin and toll-like receptor activation. *Hepatology* **2012**, *55*, 1103–1111. [CrossRef] [PubMed]

150. George, P.S.; Pearson, E.R.; Witham, M.D. Effect of Vitamin D supplementation on glycaemic control and insulin resistance: A systematic review and meta-analysis. *Diabet. Med.* **2012**, *29*, e142–e150. [CrossRef] [PubMed]

151. Flachs, P.; Rossmeisl, M.; Bryhn, M.; Kopecky, J. Cellular and molecular effects of *n*-3 polyunsaturated fatty acids on adipose tissue biology and metabolism. *Clin. Sci.* **2009**, *116*, 1–16. [CrossRef] [PubMed]

152. Masterton, G.S.; Plevris, J.N.; Hayes, P.C. Review article: ω-3 fatty acids—A promising novel therapy for non-alcoholic fatty liver disease. *Aliment. Pharmacol. Ther.* **2010**, *31*, 679–692. [CrossRef] [PubMed]

153. Janczyk, W.; Socha, P.; Lebensztejn, D.; Wierzbicka, A.; Mazur, A.; Neuhoff-Murawska, J.; Matusik, P. ω-3 fatty acids for treatment of non-alcoholic fatty liver disease: Design and rationale of randomized controlled trial. *BMC Pediatr.* **2013**, *13*, 85. [CrossRef] [PubMed]

154. Nobili, V.; Carpino, G.; Alisi, A.; de Vito, R.; Franchitto, A.; Alpini, G.; Onori, P.; Gaudio, E. Role of docosahexaenoic acid treatment in improving liver histology in pediatric nonalcoholic fatty liver disease. *PLoS ONE* **2014**, *9*, e88005. [CrossRef] [PubMed]

155. Nobili, V.; Bedogni, G.; Alisi, A.; Pietrobattista, A.; Rise, P.; Galli, C.; Agostoni, C. Docosahexaenoic acid supplementation decreases liver fat content in children with non-alcoholic fatty liver disease: Double-blind randomised controlled clinical trial. *Arch. Dis. Child.* **2011**, *96*, 350–353. [CrossRef] [PubMed]

156. Nobili, V.; Alkhouri, N.; Alisi, A.; Della Corte, C.; Fitzpatrick, E.; Raponi, M.; Dhawan, A. Nonalcoholic fatty liver disease: A challenge for pediatricians. *JAMA Pediatr.* **2015**, *169*, 170–176. [CrossRef] [PubMed]

157. Loy, J.J.; Youn, H.A.; Schwack, B.; Kurian, M.; Ren Fielding, C.; Fielding, G.A. Improvement in nonalcoholic fatty liver disease and metabolic syndrome in adolescents undergoing bariatric surgery. *Surg. Obes. Relat. Dis.* **2015**, *11*, 442–449. [CrossRef] [PubMed]

158. Peterli, R.; Steinert, R.E.; Woelnerhanssen, B.; Peters, T.; Christoffel-Courtin, C.; Gass, M.; Kern, B.; von Fluee, M.; Beglinger, C. Metabolic and hormonal changes after laparoscopic Roux-en-Y gastric bypass and sleeve gastrectomy: A randomized, prospective trial. *Obes. Surg.* **2012**, *22*, 740–748. [CrossRef] [PubMed]

159. Sasaki, A.; Nitta, H.; Otsuka, K.; Umemura, A.; Baba, S.; Obuchi, T.; Wakabayashi, G. Bariatric surgery and non-alcoholic fatty liver disease: Current and potential future treatments. *Front. Endocrinol.* **2014**, *5*, 164. [CrossRef] [PubMed]

160. Chavez-Tapia, N.C.; Tellez-Avila, F.I.; Barrientos-Gutierrez, T.; Mendez-Sanchez, N.; Lizardi-Cervera, J.; Uribe, M. Bariatric surgery for non-alcoholic steatohepatitis in obese patients. *Cochrane Database Syst. Rev.* **2010**, *1*. [CrossRef]

161. Lassailly, G.; Caiazzo, R.; Buob, D.; Pigeyre, M.; Verkindt, H.; Labreuche, J.; Raverdy, V.; Leteurtre, E.; Dharancy, S.; Louvet, A.; *et al.* Bariatric surgery reduces features of nonalcoholic steatohepatitis in morbidly obese patients. *Gastroenterology* **2015**, *149*, 379–388. [CrossRef] [PubMed]

162. Nanda, K. Non-alcoholic steatohepatitis in children. *Pediatr. Transpl.* **2004**, *8*, 613–618. [CrossRef] [PubMed]

163. Schwimmer, J.B.; Middleton, M.S.; Deutsch, R.; Lavine, J.E. A phase 2 clinical trial of metformin as a treatment for non-diabetic paediatric non-alcoholic steatohepatitis. *Aliment. Pharmacol. Ther.* **2005**, *21*, 871–879. [CrossRef] [PubMed]

164. Lavine, J.E.; Schwimmer, J.B.; van Natta, M.L.; Molleston, J.P.; Murray, K.F.; Rosenthal, P.; Abrams, S.H.; Scheimann, A.O.; Sanyal, A.J.; Chalasani, N.; *et al.* Effect of Vitamin E or metformin for treatment of nonalcoholic fatty liver disease in children and adolescents: The tonic randomized controlled trial. *JAMA* **2011**, *305*, 1659–1668. [CrossRef] [PubMed]

165. Belfort, R.; Harrison, S.A.; Brown, K.; Darland, C.; Finch, J.; Hardies, J.; Balas, B.; Gastaldelli, A.; Tio, F.; Pulcini, J.; *et al.* A placebo-controlled trial of pioglitazone in subjects with nonalcoholic steatohepatitis. *N. Engl. J. Med.* **2006**, *355*, 2297–2307. [CrossRef] [PubMed]

166. Sanyal, A.J.; Chalasani, N.; Kowdley, K.V.; McCullough, A.; Diehl, A.M.; Bass, N.M.; Neuschwander-Tetri, B.A.; Lavine, J.E.; Tonascia, J.; Unalp, A.; *et al.* Pioglitazone, Vitamin E, or placebo for nonalcoholic steatohepatitis. *N. Engl. J. Med.* **2010**, *362*, 1675–1685. [CrossRef] [PubMed]

167. Lee, J.; Hong, S.W.; Rhee, E.J.; Lee, W.Y. GLP-1 receptor agonist and non-alcoholic fatty liver disease. *Diabetes Metab. J.* **2012**, *36*, 262–267. [CrossRef] [PubMed]

168. Duvnjak, M.; Tomasic, V.; Gomercic, M.; Smircic Duvnjak, L.; Barsic, N.; Lerotic, I. Therapy of nonalcoholic fatty liver disease: Current status. *J. Physiol. Pharmacol.* **2009**, *60*, 57–66. [PubMed]

169. Tilg, H.; Moschen, A. Update on nonalcoholic fatty liver disease: Genes involved in nonalcoholic fatty liver disease and associated inflammation. *Curr. Opin. Clin. Nutr. Metab. Care* **2010**, *13*, 391–396. [CrossRef] [PubMed]

170. Georgescu, E.F. Angiotensin receptor blockers in the treatment of NASH/NAFLD: Could they be a first-class option? *Adv. Ther.* **2008**, *25*, 1141–1174. [CrossRef] [PubMed]

171. Carter, R.; Mouralidarane, A.; Ray, S.; Soeda, J.; Oben, J. Recent advancements in drug treatment of obesity. *Clin. Med.* **2012**, *12*, 456–460. [CrossRef]

172. Harrison, S.A.; Fecht, W.; Brunt, E.M.; Neuschwander-Tetri, B.A. Orlistat for overweight subjects with nonalcoholic steatohepatitis: A randomized, prospective trial. *Hepatology* **2009**, *49*, 80–86. [CrossRef] [PubMed]

173. Wierzbicki, A.S.; Oben, J. Nonalcoholic fatty liver disease and lipids. *Curr. Opin. Lipidol.* **2012**, *23*, 345–352. [CrossRef] [PubMed]

174. Tziomalos, K.; Athyros, V.G.; Paschos, P.; Karagiannis, A. Nonalcoholic fatty liver disease and statins. *Metabolism* **2015**, *64*, 1215–1223. [CrossRef] [PubMed]

175. Desai, S.; Baker, S.S.; Liu, W.; Moya, D.A.; Browne, R.W.; Mastrandrea, L.; Baker, R.D.; Zhu, L. Paraoxonase 1 and oxidative stress in paediatric non-alcoholic steatohepatitis. *Liver Int.* **2014**, *34*, 110–117. [CrossRef] [PubMed]

176. Li, Z.; Berk, M.; McIntyre, T.M.; Gores, G.J.; Feldstein, A.E. The lysosomal-mitochondrial axis in free fatty acid-induced hepatic lipotoxicity. *Hepatology* **2008**, *47*, 1495–1503. [CrossRef] [PubMed]

177. Koliaki, C.; Szendroedi, J.; Kaul, K.; Jelenik, T.; Nowotny, P.; Jankowiak, F.; Herder, C.; Carstensen, M.; Krausch, M.; Knoefel, W.T.; *et al.* Adaptation of hepatic mitochondrial function in humans with non-alcoholic fatty liver is lost in steatohepatitis. *Cell Metab.* **2015**, *21*, 739–746. [CrossRef] [PubMed]

178. Guo, H.; Zhong, R.; Liu, Y.; Jiang, X.; Tang, X.; Li, Z.; Xia, M.; Ling, W. Effects of bayberry juice on inflammatory and apoptotic markers in young adults with features of non-alcoholic fatty liver disease. *Nutrition* **2014**, *30*, 198–203. [CrossRef] [PubMed]

179. Ji, H.F.; Sun, Y.; Shen, L. Effect of Vitamin E supplementation on aminotransferase levels in patients with nafld, nash, and chc: Results from a meta-analysis. *Nutrition* **2014**, *30*, 986–991. [CrossRef] [PubMed]

180. Bjelakovic, G.; Nikolova, D.; Gluud, C. Antioxidant supplements and mortality. *Curr. Opin. Clin. Nutr. Metab. Care* **2014**, *17*, 40–44. [CrossRef] [PubMed]

181. Ratziu, V. Treatment of NASH with ursodeoxycholic acid: Pro. *Clin. Res. Hepatol. Gastroenterol.* **2012**, *36*, S41–S45. [CrossRef]

182. Xiang, Z.; Chen, Y.P.; Ma, K.F.; Ye, Y.F.; Zheng, L.; Yang, Y.D.; Li, Y.M.; Jin, X. The role of ursodeoxycholic acid in non-alcoholic steatohepatitis: A systematic review. *BMC Gastroenterol.* **2013**, *13*, 140. [CrossRef] [PubMed]

183. Pietu, F.; Guillaud, O.; Walter, T.; Vallin, M.; Hervieu, V.; Scoazec, J.Y.; Dumortier, J. Ursodeoxycholic acid with Vitamin E in patients with nonalcoholic steatohepatitis: Long-term results. *Clin. Res. Hepatol. Gastroenterol.* **2012**, *36*, 146–155. [CrossRef] [PubMed]

184. Vajro, P.; Franzese, A.; Valerio, G.; Iannucci, M.P.; Aragione, N. Lack of efficacy of ursodeoxycholic acid for the treatment of liver abnormalities in obese children. *J. Pediatr.* **2000**, *136*, 739–743. [CrossRef]

185. Van de Meeberg, P.C.; Houwen, R.H.; Sinaasappel, M.; Heijerman, H.G.; Bijleveld, C.M.; Vanberge-Henegouwen, G.P. Low-dose versus high-dose ursodeoxycholic acid in cystic fibrosis-related cholestatic liver disease. Results of a randomized study with 1-year follow-up. *Scand. J. Gastroenterol.* **1997**, *32*, 369–373. [CrossRef] [PubMed]

186. Dufour, J.F.; Oneta, C.M.; Gonvers, J.J.; Bihl, F.; Cerny, A.; Cereda, J.M.; Zala, J.F.; Helbling, B.; Steuerwald, M.; Zimmermann, A.; *et al.* Randomized placebo-controlled trial of ursodeoxycholic acid with Vitamin E in nonalcoholic steatohepatitis. *Clin. Gastroenterol. Hepatol.* **2006**, *4*, 1537–1543. [CrossRef] [PubMed]

187. Loguercio, C.; Federico, A.; Tuccillo, C.; Terracciano, F.; D'Auria, M.V.; de Simone, C.; del Vecchio Blanco, C. Beneficial effects of a probiotic VSL#3 on parameters of liver dysfunction in chronic liver diseases. *J. Clin. Gastroenterol.* **2005**, *39*, 540–543. [PubMed]

188. Vajro, P.; Mandato, C.; Licenziati, M.R.; Franzese, A.; Vitale, D.F.; Lenta, S.; Caropreso, M.; Vallone, G.; Meli, R. Effects of lactobacillus rhamnosus strain GG in pediatric obesity-related liver disease. *J. Pediatr. Gastroenterol. Nutr.* **2011**, *52*, 740–743. [CrossRef] [PubMed]

189. Machado, M.V.; Cortez-Pinto, H. Diet, microbiota, obesity, and NAFLD: A dangerous quartet. *Int. J. Mol. Sci.* **2016**, *17*. [CrossRef] [PubMed]

190. Fuchs, M. Non-alcoholic fatty liver disease: The bile acid-activated farnesoid x receptor as an emerging treatment target. *J. Lipids* **2012**, *2012*, 934396. [CrossRef] [PubMed]

# 12

# Correlations of Hepatic Hemodynamics, Liver Function and Fibrosis Markers in Nonalcoholic Fatty Liver Disease: Comparison with Chronic Hepatitis Related to Hepatitis C Virus

Ryuta Shigefuku [1,*,†], Hideaki Takahashi [1,2,†], Hiroyasu Nakano [1], Tsunamasa Watanabe [1], Kotaro Matsunaga [1], Nobuyuki Matsumoto [1], Masaki Kato [1], Ryo Morita [1], Yousuke Michikawa [1], Tomohiro Tamura [1,2], Tetsuya Hiraishi [1,3], Nobuhiro Hattori [1], Yohei Noguchi [1,2], Kazunari Nakahara [1], Hiroki Ikeda [1], Toshiya Ishii [1,3], Chiaki Okuse [1,3], Shigeru Sase [4], Fumio Itoh [1] and Michihiro Suzuki [1,3]

[1] Division of Gastroenterology and Hepatology, St. Marianna University School of Medicine, Kanagawa, Kawasaki 216-8511, Japan; hide-bo@marianna-u.ac.jp (H.T.); h-nakano@marianna-u.ac.jp (H.N.); twatanab@marianna-u.ac.jp (T.W.); kotarom@marianna-u.ac.jp (K.M.); nobu1020@marianna-u.ac.jp (N.M.); masaki0801_3@marianna-u.ac.jp (M.K.); r2morita@marianna-u.ac.jp (R.M.); y2michikawa@marianna-u.ac.jp (Y.M.); t2tamura@marianna-u.ac.jp (T.T.); t2hiraishi@marianna-u.ac.jp (T.H.); hattyorina.224@gmail.com (N.H.); y2noguchi@marianna-u.ac.jp (Y.N.); nakahara@marianna-u.ac.jp (K.N.); ikedahi@marianna-u.ac.jp (H.I.); t2ishii@marianna-u.ac.jp (T.I.); c2okuse@marianna-u.ac.jp (C.O.); fitoh@marianna-u.ac.jp (F.I.); michstmu@marianna-u.ac.jp (M.S.)
[2] Division of Gastroenterology, St. Marianna University School of Medicine, Yokohama City Seibu Hospital, Kanagawa, Yokohama 241-0811, Japan
[3] Division of Gastroenterology and Hepatology, Department of Internal Medicine, Kawasaki Municipal Tama Hospital, Kanagawa, Kawasaki 214-8525, Japan
[4] Anzai Medical Company, Ltd., Tokyo 141-0033, Japan; sase@anzai-med.co.jp
* Correspondence: r2shigefuku@marianna-u.ac.jp
† These authors contributed equally to this work.

Academic Editors: Amedeo Lonardo and Giovanni Targher

**Abstract:** The progression of chronic liver disease differs by etiology. The aim of this study was to elucidate the difference in disease progression between chronic hepatitis C (CHC) and nonalcoholic fatty liver disease (NAFLD) by means of fibrosis markers, liver function, and hepatic tissue blood flow (TBF). Xenon computed tomography (Xe-CT) was performed in 139 patients with NAFLD and 152 patients with CHC (including liver cirrhosis (LC)). The cutoff values for fibrosis markers were compared between NAFLD and CHC, and correlations between hepatic TBF and liver function tests were examined at each fibrosis stage. The cutoff values for detection of the advanced fibrosis stage were lower in NAFLD than in CHC. Although portal venous TBF (PVTBF) correlated with liver function tests, PVTBF in initial LC caused by nonalcoholic steatohepatitis (NASH-LC) was significantly lower than that in hepatitis C virus (C-LC) ($p = 0.014$). Conversely, the liver function tests in NASH-LC were higher than those in C-LC ($p < 0.05$). It is important to recognize the difference between NAFLD and CHC. We concluded that changes in hepatic blood flow occurred during the earliest stage of hepatic fibrosis in patients with NAFLD; therefore, patients with NAFLD need to be followed carefully.

**Keywords:** nonalcoholic steatohepatitis; chronic hepatitis C; liver function; hepatic hemodynamics; WFA$^+$-M2BP

## 1. Introduction

Nonalcoholic fatty liver disease (NAFLD) and nonalcoholic steatohepatitis (NASH) are increasingly recognized as common clinicopathological entities that occur in individuals without significant alcohol use [1]. The former is believed to have a benign clinical course, whereas the latter represents a form of liver injury that carries a risk for progressive fibrosis, liver cirrhosis (LC), and hepatocellular carcinoma (HCC) [2,3]. Due to the obesity epidemic and the increasing prevalence of metabolic syndrome, NAFLD and its progressive form, NASH, are seen more commonly in different parts of the world [4,5]. NAFLD has become a serious public health issue not only in Western countries, but also in many Asian countries, including Japan [6–8]. NASH is characterized by parenchymal injuries, including macrovesicular steatosis, ballooning degeneration, Mallory-Denk bodies, and inflammation in hepatic lobes [9]. On the other hand, chronic hepatitis C (CHC) is characterized by portal tract infiltration of dense aggregates of lymphocytes with follicle formation, and mild macrovesicular steatosis can be seen in lobules, particular in periportal hepatocytes [10,11]. Thus, the manner of fibrosis progression in NASH is different from that in CHC. Although there is currently no validated test involving serum biomarkers available to diagnose NASH, and histologic evaluation with a liver biopsy remains the gold standard, and screening for fibrosis is recommended in patients with suspected NASH. However, liver biopsy has some clinical problems related to its invasiveness and complications. On the other hand, there are validated tests with serum biomarkers available to diagnose the stage of hepatic fibrosis (e.g., Wisteria floribunda agglutinin positive Mac-2-binding protein (WFA$^+$-M2BP), hyaluronic acid (HA), 7S domain of type IV collagen, tissue inhibitor of metalloproteinase-1 (TIMP-1), type III procollagen N peptide (PIIIP), FIB4-index, etc.). Recently, WFA$^+$-M2BP has been reported to be a useful marker for staging in patients with NAFLD [12] and CHC [13,14]. Especially in CHC patients, WFA$^+$-M2BP can be a useful surrogate marker not only as a fibrotic marker, but also for the risk of HCC development [13,14]. However, there are few reports about WFA$^+$-M2BP on the basis of the etiology of chronic liver disease (CLD).

Since the liver receives blood flow from both the portal vein and hepatic artery, which account for 70% and 30%, respectively, this double blood supply mechanism is a specific characteristic of the liver. The portal vein receives the blood supply from the intestine, which engages in metabolism as a functional vessel. Xenon-CT has been established as a non-invasive technique to visualize tissue blood flow (TBF) in the neurosurgical field [15,16]. Xe-CT can also be applied to obtain separate measurements of hepatic arterial and venous blood flow to detect changes in hepatic blood flow (HBF). We previously reported that PVTBF and total hepatic TBF (THTBF) decrease with the progression of liver fibrosis in patients with CHC [17,18] and NAFLD [19,20]. However, few reports have addressed the association between HBF and liver function; no report has examined the progression of liver function according to the etiology of CLD. Moreover we previously reported that hepatic TBF in patients with liver cirrhosis varied according to the etiology of the disease and there is a close correlation between liver function and hepatic blood flow in patients with alcoholic liver cirrhosis [21,22]. In the present study, we investigated the difference in the fibrosis markers between patients with initial chronic hepatitis and those with advanced chronic hepatitis in NASH and CH-C. Furthermore, we attempted to clarify the relationship between hepatic TBF and liver function. It is extremely important to understand the characteristics of CLD progression for the management and treatment of CLD. The aim of this study was to elucidate the difference in disease progression between CHC and NAFLD in CLD by comparing the cutoff values for fibrosis markers and the associations of liver function and HBF.

## 2. Results

### 2.1. The Cutoff Value and Diagnostic Ability of Each Fibrosis Marker in NAFLD Patients

The receiver operating characteristic (ROC) curve and the area under the ROC (AUC) for each fibrosis marker predict definitive advanced fibrosis. The AUC values of WFA$^+$-M2BP, TIMP-1, HA,

PIIIP, platelet count (Plt), FIB4-index, aspartate aminotransferase-platelet index (APRI), AST/ALT ratio, and ICG-$R_{15}$ were 0.70, 0.50, 0.87, 0.58, 0.74, 0.77, 0.62, 0.75, and 0.74, respectively (Table 1).

**Table 1.** The cutoff value and diagnostic ability of each fibrosis marker in NAFLD patients.

| Fibrosis Markers | | Cutoff | AUROC | Sensitivity | Specificity |
|---|---|---|---|---|---|
| | | NAFLD ($n = 58$) | | | |
| WFA$^+$-M2BP | C.O.I | 1.06 | 0.70 | 75 | 67 |
| TIMP-1 | ng/mL | 242.0 | 0.50 | 50 | 68 |
| HA | ng/mL | 58.9 | 0.87 | 80 | 86 |
| PIIIP | ng/mL | 11.4 | 0.58 | 50 | 74 |
| Platelet count | $\times 10^4/\mu L$ | 17.7 | 0.74 | 67 | 80 |
| FIB-4 Index | – | 1.95 | 0.77 | 67 | 78 |
| APRI | – | 3.25 | 0.62 | 50 | 70 |
| AST/ALT ratio | – | 0.82 | 0.75 | 75 | 78 |
| ICG-$R_{15}$ | % | 10.5 | 0.74 | 67 | 64 |

Stage 0–2 ($n = 46$) vs. Stage 3–4 ($n = 12$). AUROC, area under the receiver operating characteristic curve; NAFLD: nonalcoholic fatty liver disease.

## 2.2. The Cutoff Value and Diagnostic Ability of Each Fibrosis Marker in CHC Patients

The ROC curve and the area under the ROC (AUC) for each fibrosis marker predict definitive advanced fibrosis. The AUC values of WFA$^+$-M2BP, TIMP-1, HA, PIIIP, Plt, FIB4-index, APRI, AST/ALT ratio, and ICG-$R_{15}$ were 0.89, 0.84, 0.87, 0.71, 0.82, 0.87, 0.82, 0.62, and 0.86, respectively (Table 2).

**Table 2.** The cutoff value and diagnostic ability of each fibrosis marker in CHC patients.

| Fibrosis Markers | | Cutoff | AUROC | Sensitivity | Specificity |
|---|---|---|---|---|---|
| | | CHC ($n = 72$) | | | |
| WFA$^+$-M2BP | C.O.I | 3.28 | 0.89 | 84 | 85 |
| TIMP-1 | ng/mL | 297.6 | 0.84 | 88 | 72 |
| HA | ng/mL | 116.5 | 0.87 | 79 | 79 |
| PIIIP | ng/mL | 10.6 | 0.71 | 74 | 64 |
| Platelet count | $\times 10^4/\mu L$ | 13.9 | 0.82 | 74 | 75 |
| FIB-4 Index | – | 3.19 | 0.87 | 89 | 79 |
| APRI | – | 5.41 | 0.82 | 79 | 79 |
| AST/ALT ratio | – | 0.76 | 0.62 | 63 | 53 |
| ICG-$R_{15}$ | % | 11.5 | 0.86 | 84 | 76 |

Stage 0–2 ($n = 53$) vs. Stage 3–4 ($n = 19$). AUROC, area under the receiver operating characteristic curve; CHC: chronic hepatitis related to hepatitis C virus.

## 2.3. Liver Function and Hepatic TBF in Each Stage of NAFLD Patients

Liver function and hepatic TBF in each stage of NAFLD patients are shown in Table 3. With fibrosis progression, Alb, ChE, TC, PT, Plt, PVTBF, and THTBF decreased significantly ($p < 0.001$, $r = -0.47$; $p < 0.001$, $r = -0.52$; $p < 0.01$, $r = -0.26$; $p < 0.001$, $r = -0.69$; $p < 0.001$, $r = -0.66$; $p < 0.001$, $r = -0.32$; $p < 0.01$, $r = -0.22$, respectively). On the other hand, with fibrosis progression, ICG-$R_{15}$, HA, and WFA$^+$-M2BP increased significantly ($p < 0.001$, $r = 0.58$; $p < 0.001$, $r = 0.78$; $p < 0.001$, $r = 0.50$, respectively).

**Table 3.** Liver function and hepatic tissue blood flow in each fibrosis stage in NAFLD.

| Fibrosis Stage | NAFL $n = 15$ | Stage 1 $n = 47$ | Stage 2 $n = 30$ | Stage 3 $n = 15$ | Initial LC $n = 25$ | Advanced LC $n = 7$ | p-Value * | r |
|---|---|---|---|---|---|---|---|---|
| Alb (g/dL) | 4.5 ± 0.3 | 4.5 ± 0.3 | 4.4 ± 0.3 | 4.4 ± 0.3 | 4.0 ± 0.3 | 3.1 ± 0.4 | <0.001 | −0.47 |
| ChE (IU/L) | 390.1 ± 107.2 | 372.8 ± 104.3 | 346.3 ± 96.0 | 260.5 ± 149.3 | 254.8 ± 63.2 | 155.4 ± 95.7 | <0.001 | −0.52 |
| TC (mg/dL) | 200.8 ± 40.9 | 200.4 ± 33.5 | 180.3 ± 62.0 | 170.3 ± 73.9 | 179.5 ± 36.3 | 119.7 ± 39.0 | <0.01 | −0.26 |
| PT (%) | 100.8 ± 5.4 | 98.9 ± 9.0 | 96.4 ± 6.5 | 87.0 ± 10.1 | 76.4 ± 16.2 | 57.0 ± 7.7 | <0.001 | −0.69 |
| ICG-$R_{15}$ (%) | 5.9 ± 2.9 | 9.8 ± 13.0 | 11.6 ± 6.6 | 17.7 ± 18.1 | 21.9 ± 12.5 | 26.0 ± 8.4 | <0.001 | 0.58 |
| HA (ng/mL) | 20.4 ± 16.5 | 53.4 ± 98.0 | 63.4 ± 51.3 | 151.4 ± 98.7 | 268.9 ± 193.9 | 347.3 ± 181.9 | <0.001 | 0.78 |
| $WFA^+$-M2BP (C.O.I) | 0.7 ± 0.3 | 0.8 ± 0.4 | 1.2 ± 0.7 | 1.3 ± 0.6 | 1.8 ± 1.5 | 4.4 ± 0.2 | <0.001 | 0.50 |
| Plt ($\times 10^4/\mu$L) | 24.2 ± 4.5 | 23.7 ± 6.5 | 20.1 ± 5.2 | 18.3 ± 7.3 | 11.5 ± 3.5 | 5.3 ± 3.0 | <0.001 | −0.66 |
| PVTBF (mL/100 mL/min) | 41.0 ± 6.3 | 34.3 ± 7.2 | 33.8 ± 7.0 | 29.9 ± 6.7 | 29.3 ± 7.9 | 29.9 ± 2.4 | <0.001 | −0.32 |
| HATBF (mL/100 mL/min) | 23.8 ± 9.0 | 21.30 ± 10.2 | 19.6 ± 10.1 | 20.5 ± 8.3 | 18.8 ± 8.6 | 24.2 ± 6.2 | NS | −0.09 |
| THTBF (mL/100 mL/min) | 64.9 ± 13.4 | 55.6 ± 14.0 | 53.4 ± 14.2 | 48.1 ± 10.1 | 46.5 ± 10.9 | 54.9 ± 9.4 | <0.01 | −0.22 |
| P/A ratio Fibro | 1.9 ± 0.7 | 1.9 ± 0.7 | 2.0 ± 0.6 | 1.6 ± 0.5 | 1.6 ± 0.5 | 1.4 ± 0.4 | NS | −0.15 |

* Spearman's rank correlation coefficient was used to examine correlations of TBF with the progression of fibrosis; NS: not significant; P/A ratio: portal flow/hepatic arterial flow ratio.

Table 4. Liver function and hepatic tissue blood flow in each fibrosis stage in CHC.

| Fibrosis Stage | Stage 1 n = 45 | Stage 2 n = 29 | Stage 3 n = 21 | Initial LC n = 30 | Advanced LC n = 27 | p-Value* | r |
|---|---|---|---|---|---|---|---|
| Alb (g/dL) | 4.3 ± 0.3 | 4.3 ± 0.3 | 4.1 ± 0.3 | 3.8 ± 0.8 | 3.1 ± 0.3 | <0.001 | −0.67 |
| ChE (IU/L) | 329.0 ± 81.4 | 268.2 ± 74.7 | 226.0 ± 54.8 | 202.9 ± 75.4 | 113.0 ± 40.7 | <0.001 | −0.65 |
| TC (mg/dL) | 182.8 ± 31.0 | 167.4 ± 34.7 | 150.7 ± 28.4 | 149.3 ± 33.9 | 120.8 ± 36.0 | <0.001 | −0.64 |
| PT (%) | 96.2 ± 8.7 | 88.0 ± 8.8 | 81.5 ± 10.9 | 86.4 ± 10.9 | 64.0 ± 9.7 | <0.001 | −0.69 |
| ICG-R15 (%) | 7.4 ± 3.7 | 13.5 ± 9.6 | 14.1 ± 5.1 | 21.7 ± 10.0 | 34.2 ± 11.2 | <0.001 | 0.39 |
| HA (ng/mL) | 54.8 ± 60.3 | 156.1 ± 203.4 | 275.8 ± 202.2 | 425.1 ± 362.7 | 565.2 ± 370.7 | <0.001 | 0.76 |
| WFA$^+$-M2BP (C.O.I) | 1.5 ± 1.5 | 1.9 ± 1.9 | 4.5 ± 4.5 | 4.0 ± 4.2 | 5.6 ± 5.8 | <0.001 | 0.62 |
| Plt ($\times 10^4$/μL) | 18.4 ± 4.8 | 15.1 ± 5.0 | 12.1 ± 3.6 | 9.3 ± 3.6 | 7.3 ± 2.7 | <0.001 | −0.74 |
| PVTBF (mL/100 mL/min) | 48.8 ± 13.9 | 40.4 ± 13.5 | 36.3 ± 7.9 | 36.3 ± 11.2 | 26.6 ± 7.5 | <0.001 | −0.56 |
| HATBF (mL/100 mL/min) | 26.1 ± 14.2 | 21.9 ± 8.6 | 20.5 ± 11.7 | 21.6 ± 15.0 | 21.5 ± 13.1 | NS | −0.18 |
| THTBF (mL/100 mL/min) | 74.9 ± 21.8 | 62.4 ± 16.9 | 56.8 ± 12.7 | 54.6 ± 15.1 | 48.3 ± 14.2 | <0.001 | −0.48 |
| P/A ratio | 2.1 ± 1.0 | 1.9 ± 0.9 | 1.9 ± 1.0 | 1.9 ± 0.8 | 1.6 ± 0.9 | NS | −0.17 |

* Spearman's rank correlation coefficient was used to examine correlations of TBF with the progression of fibrosis; NS: not significant; P/A ratio: portal flow/hepatic arterial flow ratio.

*2.4. Liver Function and Hepatic TBF in Each Stage of CHC Patients*

Liver function and hepatic TBF in each stage of CHC patients are shown in Table 4. With fibrosis progression, Alb, Ch-E, TC, PT, Plt, PVTBF, and THTBF decreased significantly ($p < 0.001$, $r = -0.67$; $p < 0.001$, $r = -0.65$; $p < 0.001$, $r = -0.64$; $p < 0.001$, $r = -0.69$; $p < 0.001$, $r = -0.74$; $p < 0.001$, $r = -0.56$; $p < 0.001$, $r = -0.48$, respectively). On the other hand, with fibrosis progression, ICG-$R_{15}$, HA, and WFA$^+$-M2BP increased significantly ($p < 0.001$, $r = 0.39$; $p < 0.001$, $r = 0.76$; $p < 0.001$, $r = 0.62$, respectively).

*2.5. Correlation between Hepatic TBF and Liver Function in NAFLD Patients*

Correlations between hepatic TBF, as measured by Xe-CT and liver function in NAFLD patients, are shown in Table 5. There were significant correlations between PVTBF and Alb, ChE, TC, PT, ICG-$R_{15}$, HA, and Plt ($p < 0.001$, $r = 0.53$; $p < 0.001$, $r = 0.46$; $p < 0.001$, $r = 0.29$; $p < 0.001$, $r = 0.40$; $p < 0.001$, $r = -0.25$; $p < 0.05$, $r = -0.17$; $p < 0.01$, $r = 0.25$, respectively). There were also significant correlations between HATBF and ChE and HA ($p < 0.05$, $r = 0.21$; $p < 0.05$, $r = 0.21$, respectively). There were significant correlations between THTBF and ChE, TC, and ICG-$R_{15}$ ($p < 0.001$, $r = 0.39$; $p < 0.001$, $r = 0.34$; $p < 0.05$, $r = 0.21$, respectively). There were significant correlations between the P/A ratio and ChE, TC, and PT ($p < 0.001$, $r = 0.37$; $p < 0.001$, $r = 0.42$; $p < 0.05$, $r = 0.17$, respectively) (Table 5).

**Table 5.** Correlations of liver function and hepatic tissue blood flow in NAFLD.

| TBF | PVTBF | | HATBF | | THTBF | | P/A Ratio | |
|---|---|---|---|---|---|---|---|---|
| | *p*-Value * | *r* | *p*-Value * | *r* | *p*-Value * | *r* | *p*-Value * | *r* |
| Alb (g/dL) | <0.001 | 0.53 | NS | −0.04 | NS | 0.02 | NS | 0.14 |
| ChE (IU/L) | <0.001 | 0.46 | <0.05 | 0.21 | <0.001 | 0.39 | <0.001 | 0.37 |
| TC (mg/dL) | <0.001 | 0.29 | NS | 0.16 | <0.001 | 0.34 | <0.001 | 0.42 |
| PT (%) | <0.001 | 0.40 | NS | −0.06 | NS | 0.02 | <0.05 | 0.17 |
| ICG-$R_{15}$ (%) | <0.01 | −0.25 | NS | 0.09 | <0.05 | 0.21 | NS | −0.01 |
| HA (ng/mL) | <0.05 | −0.17 | <0.05 | 0.21 | NS | 0.03 | NS | 0.06 |
| Plt ($\times 10^4$/μL) | <0.01 | 0.25 | NS | −0.02 | NS | 0.07 | NS | 0.05 |

* The Pearson product-moment correlation coefficient was used to examine correlations between TBF parameters and liver function tests. TBF: tissue blood flow; NS: not significant; P/A ratio: portal flow/hepatic arterial flow ratio.

*2.6. Correlation between Hepatic Blood Flow and Liver Function in CHC Patients*

Correlations between hepatic blood flow and liver function in CHC patients are shown in Table 6. There were significant correlations between PVTBF and Alb, ChE, TC, PT, ICG-$R_{15}$, HA, and Plt ($p < 0.001$, $r = 0.50$; $p < 0.001$, $r = 0.66$; $p < 0.001$, $r = 0.66$; $p < 0.001$, $r = 0.70$; $p < 0.001$, $r = -0.36$; $p < 0.001$, $r = 0.37$; $p < 0.001$, $r = 0.37$, respectively). There was also a significant correlation between HATBF and PT ($p < 0.05$, $r = 0.18$). There were significant correlations between THTBF and Alb, ChE, TC, PT, and Plt ($p < 0.001$, $r = 0.42$; $p < 0.001$, $r = 0.55$; $p < 0.001$, $r = 0.67$; $p < 0.001$, $r = 0.37$; $p < 0.001$, $r = 0.35$, respectively). There were significant correlations between the P/A ratio and Alb and ChE ($p < 0.01$, $r = 0.21$; $p < 0.001$, $r = 0.34$; $p < 0.01$, $r = 0.27$, respectively) (Table 6).

**Table 6.** Correlations of liver function and hepatic tissue blood flow in CHC.

| TBF | PVTBF | | HATBF | | THTBF | | P/A Ratio | |
|---|---|---|---|---|---|---|---|---|
| | *p*-Value * | *r* | *p*-Value * | *r* | *p*-Value * | *r* | *p*-Value * | *r* |
| Alb (g/dL) | <0.001 | 0.50 | NS | −0.05 | <0.001 | 0.42 | <0.01 | 0.21 |
| ChE (IU/L) | <0.001 | 0.66 | NS | 0.12 | <0.001 | 0.55 | <0.001 | 0.34 |
| TC (mg/dL) | <0.001 | 0.66 | NS | 0.10 | <0.001 | 0.67 | <0.01 | 0.27 |
| PT (%) | <0.001 | 0.70 | <0.05 | 0.18 | <0.001 | 0.37 | NS | 0.09 |
| ICG-$R_{15}$ (%) | <0.001 | −0.36 | NS | 0.07 | NS | 0.10 | NS | 0.05 |
| HA (ng/mL) | <0.001 | 0.37 | NS | −0.13 | NS | −0.10 | NS | 0.06 |
| Plt ($\times 10^4$/µL) | <0.001 | 0.37 | NS | 0.07 | <0.001 | 0.35 | NS | 0.07 |

* The Pearson product-moment correlation coefficient was used to examine correlations between TBF parameters and liver function tests; TBF: tissue blood flow; NS: not significant; P/A ratio: portal flow/hepatic arterial flow ratio.

## 2.7. Comparison of Each TBF at Initial LC (Child-Pugh A) in NASH-LC and C-LC

PVTBF and THTBF were significantly lower in NASH-LC than in C-LC ($p = 0.014$, $p = 0.048$, respectively). Hepatic arterial TBF (HATBF) did not differ significantly between the groups (Figure 1).

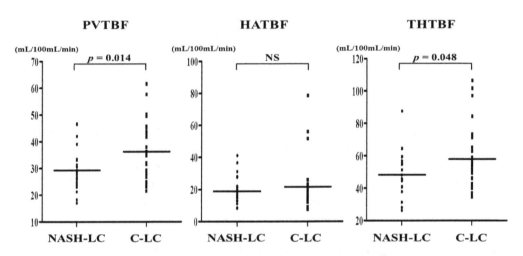

**Figure 1.** Comparison of each TBF at initial LC (Child-Pugh A) in NASH-LC and C-LC. PVTBF and THTBF are significantly lower in NASH-LC than in C-LC ($p = 0.014$, $p = 0.048$, respectively). HATBF is not significantly different between the LC groups. NS: not significant; PVTBF: portal venous tissue blood flow; HATBF: hepatic arterial tissue blood flow; THTBF: total hepatic tissue blood flow; NASH-LC: liver cirrhosis related to nonalcoholic steatohepatitis; C-LC: liver cirrhosis related to hepatitis C virus.

## 2.8. Comparison of Each Liver Function Test at Initial LC (Child-Pugh A) in NASH-LC and C-LC

Alb, Ch-E, TC, and Plt were significantly higher in NASH-LC than in C-LC ($p = 0.016$, $p = 0.016$, $p = 0.004$, $p = 0.021$, respectively). PT and ICG-$R_{15}$ were not significantly different between the groups (Figure 2).

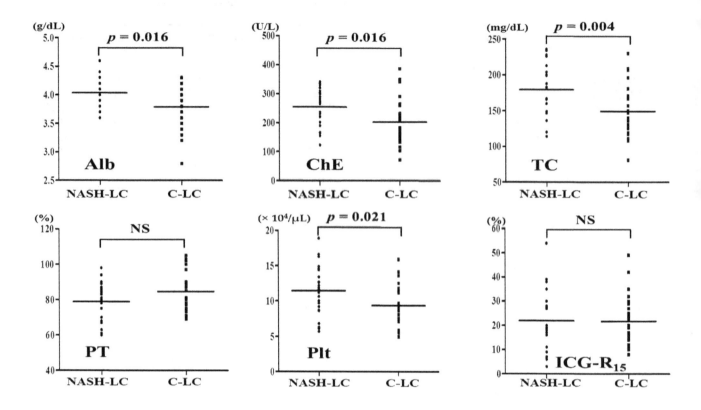

**Figure 2.** Comparison of each liver function test at initial LC (Child-Pugh A) in NASH-LC and C-LC. Albumin, cholinesterase, total cholesterol, and platelet count are significantly higher in NASH-LC than in C-LC ($p = 0.016$, $p = 0.016$, $p = 0.004$, $p = 0.021$, respectively). NS: not significant; NASH-LC: liver cirrhosis related to nonalcoholic steatohepatitis; C-LC: liver cirrhosis related to hepatitis C virus; Alb: albumin; ChE: cholinesterase; TC: total cholesterol; PT: prothrombin time; Plt: platelet count; ICG-R$_{15}$: retention rate of indocyanine green 15 min after administration.

## 2.9. Comparison of Typical Cases at Initial LC (Child-Pugh A) in NASH-LC and C-LC

Figure 3 shows cases of the advanced fibrosis stage in NASH and CHC. An 85-year-old Japanese man (case 1) was pathologically diagnosed with Stage 4 NASH (Brunt's classification [23]). His clinical features were also obviously LC-like (e.g., thrombocytopenia, HCC, and esophagogastric varices). His fibrosis markers were increased, reflecting advanced liver fibrosis. A 75-year-old Japanese man (case 2) was pathologically diagnosed with stage 3 CHC (Desmet's classification [24]). The WFA$^+$-M2BP was significantly lower in NASH-LC than in CHC (Figure 3). In this way, the cutoff values of fibrosis markers, including WFA$^+$-M2BP, might differ by the etiology of liver disease. The present results showed that the cutoff values (WFA$^+$-M2BP, TIMP-1, HA, and FIB-4 index) to detect the advanced fibrosis stage were lower in NAFLD than in CHC (Tables 1 and 2). Furthermore, the diagnostic reliability to detect the advanced fibrosis stage was lower in NAFLD than in CHC (Tables 1 and 2). The reason for this is that the manner of fibrosis progression differs between NASH and CHC. With fibrosis progression, PVTBF gradually decreases in both CHC and NASH. However, PVTBF decreases at an earlier stage in NAFLD than in CHC. This might be attributed to the different manner of fibrosis between NASH and CHC.

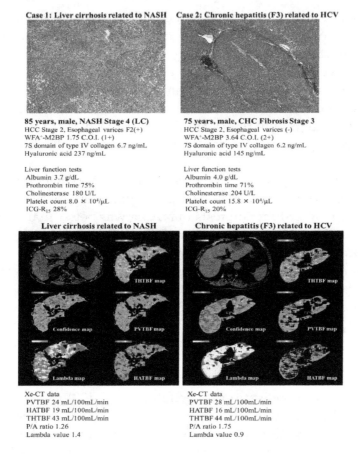

Case 1: Liver cirrhosis related to NASH    Case 2: Chronic hepatitis (F3) related to HCV

**85 years, male, NASH Stage 4 (LC)**
HCC Stage 2, Esophageal varices F2(+)
WFA⁺-M2BP 1.75 C.O.I. (1+)
7S domain of type IV collagen 6.7 ng/mL
Hyaluronic acid 237 ng/mL

Liver function tests
Albumin 3.7 g/dL
Prothrombin time 75%
Cholinesterase 180 U/L
Platelet count 8.0 × 10⁴/μL
ICG-R₁₅ 28%

**75 years, male, CHC Fibrosis Stage 3**
HCC Stage 2, Esophageal varices (-)
WFA⁺-M2BP 3.64 C.O.I. (2+)
7S domain of type IV collagen 6.2 ng/mL
Hyaluronic acid 145 ng/mL

Liver function tests
Albumin 4.0 g/dL
Prothrombin time 71%
Cholinesterase 204 U/L
Platelet count 15.8 × 10⁴/μL
ICG-R₁₅ 20%

**Liver cirrhosis related to NASH**        **Chronic hepatitis (F3) related to HCV**

Xe-CT data
PVTBF 24 mL/100mL/min
HATBF 19 mL/100mL/min
THTBF 43 mL/100mL/min
P/A ratio 1.26
Lambda value 1.4

Xe-CT data
PVTBF 28 mL/100mL/min
HATBF 16 mL/100mL/min
THTBF 44 mL/100mL/min
P/A ratio 1.75
Lambda value 0.9

**Figure 3.** Cases of advanced fibrosis stage in NASH and CHC. Figure 3 shows cases of the advanced fibrosis stage in NASH and CHC. An 85-year-old Japanese man (case 1) was pathologically diagnosed with Stage 4 NASH (Brunt's classification [23]). His clinical features were also obviously LC-like (e.g., thrombocytopenia, hepatocellular carcinoma, and esophagogastric varices). His fibrosis markers were increased to reflect advanced liver fibrosis. A 75-year-old Japanese man (case 2) was pathologically diagnosed with stage 3 CHC (Desmet's classification [24]). In case 2, TBF was evaluated in the whole liver excluding the region of hepatocellular carcinoma. The WFA⁺-M2BP of the NASH-LC case was significantly lower than that of the CHC case. TBF was evaluated in both cases. PVTBF and the P/A ratio are lower in NASH-LC (case 1) than in CHC (case 2).

## 3. Discussion

A definite diagnosis of NASH requires liver biopsy, though various non-invasive measures are under development [6]. NASH is characterized by parenchymal injury, including macrovesicular steatosis, ballooning degeneration, Mallory-Denk bodies, and inflammation in hepatic lobes [9]. Fibrosis begins in zone 3 or the centrilobular area of the hepatic lobule. Periportal and bridging fibrosis develop with progression of the disease, and once cirrhosis is established, features of steatohepatitis and perisinusoidal fibrosis may be obscured. It is well known that exercise, itself, is an important factor to treat NASH and, therefore, the role of exercise should be emphasized. Exercise, in fact, improves NASH-related fibrosis markers (collagen 1α1 mRNA, $p < 0.05$ and fibrosis score, $p < 0.01$) and the inflammation score; exercise increases the hepatic stellate cell senescence marker CCN1 [25,26].

On the other hand, fibrosis begins in zone 1 or the periportal area of the hepatic lobule in patients with CHC. CHC is characterized by a portal tract that is infiltrated by dense aggregates of lymphocytes with follicle formation, and mild macrovesicular steatosis can be seen in lobules, particularly in periportal hepatocytes [10,11]. Moreover, it has been reported that daily use of recreational drugs, in particular cannabis, has a deleterious effect on the speed of progression of fibrosis and steatosis in patients suffering from chronic hepatitis C [27]. There are other differences between NAFLD and CHC. Previous reports indicated that at the early stages of CLD the numbers of liver monocytes/macrophages were elevated without the evidence of local proliferation, supporting a role for infiltrating monocyte-derived macrophages in disease progression in patients with both CHC and NAFLD. However, CHC and NAFLD differentially affected the circulating monocyte phenotype, suggesting that unique injury-induced signals may contribute to the intrahepatic monocyte recruitment and the systemic activation state. Moreover, it was also shown that monocyte function was similarly impaired in patients with both CHC and NAFLD, particularly in advanced disease [28]. Thus, the manner of fibrosis progression resulting from inflammation could be different between NASH and CHC.

The results of present study showed the relationship between liver function and PVTBF (Tables 5 and 6). PVTBF was well correlated with hepatic synthesis capacity, which included Alb, ChE, TC, and PT. The reason why liver function tests in NASH was better than that in CHC is suggested the excess energy intake and lipid hypermetabolism [29]. $ICG\text{-}R_{15}$ is the indicator which reflects liver function [30] and the presence of portal hypertension. Furthermore $ICG\text{-}R_{15}$ is well correlated to the hepatic tissue blood flow [31]. Lisotti et al. reported that the $ICG\text{-}R_{15}$ test is an effective tool for assessment of portal hypertension in patients with compensated cirrhosis [30]. We confirmed that the hemodynamic changes occurred earlier in NAFLD relative to CHC. For example, 15% of $ICG\text{-}R_{15}$ correspond to the stage 3 in NASH and LC in CHC (Tables 3 and 4). Yamazaki reported that the average of $ICG\text{-}R_{15}$ was 15.4% in which the presence of esophageal varices cases [32], and their data, supported our results.

Alteration in hepatic microcirculation in human donor livers with steatosis was first reported during organ retrieval before mobilization by Seifalian et al. [33] using laser Doppler flowmetry. A significant decrease in hepatic microcirculation in liver donors with steatosis was observed in comparison with that in normal liver donors [34]. Experimental studies in animal models with fatty liver showed that steatosis led to reduce hepatic blood flow and microcirculation, and that there was an inverse correlation between the degree of steatosis and both total hepatic blood flow and flow in the microcirculation [30]. The severity of fatty infiltration has a greater effect on the microcirculation than on total hepatic blood flow [35,36]. In spite of steatosis alone, hepatic blood flow reduced. Moreover, hepatic blood flow reduced with fibrosis development, in addition to steatosis [37]. Fat-laden hepatocytes are swollen, and in steatohepatitis, further swelling occurs due to the ballooning of hepatocytes, causing sinusoidal distortion, as visualized by in vivo microscopy, reducing intrasinusoidal volume and microcirculation [38].

In addition to steatosis, a mechanism of decreasing portal blood flow other than steatosis has been reported in NAFLD. In livers with perfusion from cafeteria diet-fed rats, there was increased portal pressure and decreased endothelium-dependent vasodilation. This was associated with decreased Akt-dependent endothelial nitric-oxide synthase (eNOS) phosphorylation and NOS activity. They demonstrated in a rat model of the metabolic syndrome that hepatic endothelial dysfunction occurs before the development of fibrosis and inflammation [39]. Ying-Ying Yang et al. reported that hyperleptinemia increases hepatic endocannabinoid production, promotes hepatic fibrogenesis, enhances the hepatic vasoconstrictive response to endothelin-1, and aggravates hepatic microcirculatory dysfunction. These events subsequently increase intrahepatic resistance and portal hypertension in NASH cirrhotic rats [40].

The present data show that the liver function was better in initial NASH-LC than in C-LC. However, because PVTBF was lower in NASH than in C-LC, portal hypertension might occur at an earlier stage in NASH than in CHC. In fact, portal hypertension occurs without LC in NASH [41–43]. Mendes et al. investigated the prevalence of portal hypertension in NAFLD patients, and found that clinical signs of portal hypertension, including esophageal varices, splenomegaly, portosystemic encephalopathy, and ascites, were present in 25% of patients at the time of diagnosis. Furthermore, portal hypertension can occur in a small proportion of patients with mild or no fibrosis and is associated with the extent of steatosis [44]. Brunt et al. reported that hepatic fibrosis in

NAFLD patients was found in the pericellular space around the central vein and in the presinusoidal region in zone 3 in the early stage [23]. The pericellular fibrosis in the early stage of NAFLD patients may lead to an elevated portal vascular resistance and result in a change of hepatic blood flow [45]. Therefore, we considered that the hemodynamic changes occurred earlier in NAFLD relative to CHC.

In this study, there are two limitations, such as sampling error during liver biopsy and by permeation of Xe gas. Xe-CT cannot monitor the exact result in the patients with chronic lung disease (e.g., chronic obstructive pulmonary disease, lung cancer) and heart failure, because Xe gas is taken up by the lung via the respiratory tract. On the contrary, we believe that there are also many strong points of Xe-CT which objectively and repeatedly measure hepatic blood flow with reproducibility. Moreover, we have safely performed a Xe-CT for patients with acute or chronic renal failure because there are no complications associated with the contrast agent, such as allergic reactions and radiocontrast nephropathy.

Thus, in the present study, the difference between NAFLD and CHC was investigated based on TBF, fibrosis markers, and liver function. In conclusion, compared to C-LC, PVTBF decreased significantly in the Child-Pugh A stage of NASH-LC, indicating that portal hemodynamic changes could occur earlier in NASH-LC without impaired liver function. Therefore, patients with NASH should be monitored carefully for portal hypertensive complications in the early fibrosis stage.

## 4. Materials and Methods

### 4.1. Patients

Between October 2001 and March 2016, 730 patients underwent Xe-CT at the St. Marianna University School of Medicine Hospital. Of the 730 patients, 291 with NAFLD and CHC were enrolled in this study. Liver biopsy was performed for 118 of the 139 NAFLD patients and 106 of the 152 CHC patients. During hospitalization for three days, Xe-CT was performed before or after each liver biopsy. The NAFLD patients included 80 men and 59 women, with a mean age of $53.2 \pm 11.2$ years and a mean body mass index (BMI) of $28.5 \pm 4.9 \text{ kg/m}^2$. The CHC patients included 75 men and 77 women, with a mean age of $59.9 \pm 11.2$ years and a mean BMI of $23.2 \pm 3.7 \text{ kg/m}^2$ (Table 7).

**Table 7.** Characteristics of patients.

| Group | NAFLD | CHC |
|---|---|---|
| Number of cases | 139 | 152 |
| Sex (Male/Female) | 80/59 | 75/77 |
| Age (years) | $53.2 \pm 11.2$ | $59.9 \pm 11.2$ * |
| BMI (kg/m$^2$) | $28.5 \pm 4.9$ | $23.2 \pm 3.7$ * |
| Staging for fibrosis | NAFL/NASH Stage 1/2/3/4 + Child A/Child B,C | Stage 0,1/2/3/4 + Child A/Child B,C |
| | (Brunt's classification) 15/47/30/15/25/7 | (Desmet's classification) 45/29/21/30/27 |
| Number of cases ** | 58 | 72 |
| Mild fibrosis group (Stage 0–2) | 46 | 53 |
| Advanced fibrosis group (Stage 3–4) | 12 | 19 |

* $p < 0.05$ (unpaired $t$-test); ** In this study, 58 samples of NAFLD and 72 samples of CH-C were enrolled. The blood sample was taken on the day of the liver biopsy.

The diagnosis of NAFLD was based on: (1) substantial alcohol consumption (>20 g/day for women or >30 g/day for men); (2) pathological findings showing characteristics of NAFLD (large-droplet fat deposits, hepatocyte ballooning, inflammatory cell infiltration, and fibrosis around the central vein); and (3) the exclusion of other liver diseases, such as viral hepatitis, autoimmune liver disease, and drug-induced liver injury. The diagnosis of CHC was based on anti-HCV antibodies and HCV-RNA. Patients were excluded for the presence of other causes of liver disease, acute illness, acute or chronic inflammatory or infective diseases, an end-stage malignant disease, or other confounding conditions. Liver biopsy was performed through the right intercostal space under ultrasonography-guided liver biopsy using a 16-gauge needle biopsy kit (Quick-Core® biopsy needle set; Cook Medical, Bloomington, IN, USA). The aims of liver biopsy were to assess fibrosis and steatosis and to exclude other liver disease. Histological diagnosis was confirmed by two experienced pathologists who were blinded to the clinical data. There were 15 patients with nonalcoholic fatty liver (NAFL) who had no fibrosis and inflammatory cell infiltration. The patients with NASH were evaluated on the basis of Brunt's classification [21,46,47], while those with CHC were evaluated on the basis of Desmet's classification [22]. Staging fibrosis in NASH based on Brunt's classification: Stage 1: zone 3 perivenular perisinusoidal/pericellular fibrosis, focal or extensive; Stage 2: as above with focal or extensive periportal fibrosis; Stage 3: bridging fibrosis, focal or extensive; and Stage 4: cirrhosis. Staging fibrosis in CHC based on Desmet's classification: Stage 0: lack of fibrosis; Stage 1: fibrosis confined to portal tract; Stage 2: bridging fibrosis; Stage 3: bridging fibrosis with structural distortion; and Stage 4: cirrhosis. Clinical liver cirrhosis was defined by the presence of a portosystemic shunt or ascites.

### 4.2. Xe-CT Theory and Imaging Protocol

As described in previous publications, 25% stable Xe gas was used in conjunction with an AZ-726 Xe gas inhalation system (Anzai Medical, Tokyo, Japan) [48,49]. The wash-in and wash-out periods were both 4 min. The entire liver was CT-scanned at 1-min intervals at four levels, including the porta hepatis (nine scans in total, including the baseline scan). Using an AZ-7000W image processing system (Anzai Medical), PVTBF and HATBF were calculated, and PVTBF and HATBF maps were created. THTBF was calculated as the sum of PVTBF and HATBF, and THTBF maps were also created. The time course change rate for the arterial Xe concentration, which was needed to calculate PVTBF and HATBF, was derived using the time course of the Xe concentration in splenic tissue. An Aquilion CT scanner (Toshiba Medical Systems, Tokyo, Japan) was used, with exposure factors of 120 kV, 150 mA, and 13.8 mGy. All examinations were performed with the patients in the fasting state. Informed consent was obtained from each patient. All study protocols were reviewed and approved by the ethics committee at our institution (approval No. 480, 18 September 2001), and conformed to the ethics guidelines of the 1975 Declaration of Helsinki (Allen, 1991).

### 4.3. Liver Function Tests and Fibrosis Markers

Liver function tests were measured on admission. Liver function tests included the following parameters: albumin (Alb) (g/dL), cholinesterase (ChE) (IU/L), total cholesterol (TC) (mg/dL), prothrombin time (PT) (%), Plt ($\times 10^4$ $\mu L^{-1}$), hyaluronic acid (HA) (ng/mL), Wisteria floribunda agglutinin positive Mac-2-binding protein (WFA$^+$-M2BP) (C.O.I.), and the retention rate of indocyanine green 15 min after administration (ICG-R$_{15}$) (%). ICG (Diagnogreen®, Daiichisankyo Pharmaceutical Co., Tokyo, Japan; 0.5 mg/kg body weight) was administered via a peripheral vein, and venous blood was sampled before and 15 min after injection. Specimens were analyzed for ICG concentrations on a spectrophotometer (HITACHI, Tokyo, Japan) at 805 nm.

### 4.4. Measurements of TIMP-1, HA, PIIIP, and WFA$^+$-M2BP

For all patients in the cohort, the blood sample was taken on the day of the liver biopsy at the St. Marianna University School of Medicine Hospital. All samples were processed to separate serum and stored at $-80$ °C. At the time of blood withdrawal, all patients underwent liver biopsy. In this study, 58 samples of NAFLD and 72 samples of CHC were enrolled (Table 7). TIMP-1, HA, and PIIIP were measured using a fully automatic immunoanalyzer (Sysmex Co., Hyogo, Japan). WFA$^+$-M2BP quantification was measured based on a lectin-Ab sandwich immunoassay using a fully automatic immunoanalyzer, HISCL-2000i (Sysmex Co., Hyogo, Japan) [50].

*4.5. Statistical Analysis*

Each parameter is expressed as the mean ± standard deviation (SD). Spearman's rank correlation coefficient was used to examine correlations of TBF with progression of fibrosis. The Pearson product-moment correlation coefficient was used to examine correlations between TBF parameters and liver function tests. To assess the utility of each fibrosis marker to distinguish the advanced fibrosis stage, the sensitivity and specificity were calculated for each value, and then ROC curves were constructed by plotting the sensitivity against the reverse specificity (1-the specificity) for each value. We used Student's *t*-test, which was two-tailed and performed by the statistical software GraphPad Prism (GraphPad Software, San Diego, CA, USA). *p*-Values of <0.05 were considered significant.

## 5. Conclusions

It is important to recognize the difference between NAFLD and CHC. We concluded that changes in hepatic blood flow occurred during the earliest stage of hepatic fibrosis in patients with NAFLD and, therefore, patients with NAFLD need to be followed carefully.

**Acknowledgments:** The authors wish to thank the technical assistants at the Imaging Center of St. Marianna University School of Medicine Hospital for their assistance. This study was supported in part by JSPS KAKENHI Grant Number 16K19371.

**Author Contributions:** Ryuta Shigefuku, Hideaki Takahashi and Tunamasa Watanabe conceived and designed the experiments; Ryuta Shigefuku and Kotaro Matsunaga performed the experiments; Ryuta Shigefuku, Hideaki Takahashi, Hiroki Ikeda and Shigeru Sase analyzed the data; Ryuta Shigefuku, Hiroyasu Nakano, Masaki Kato, Ryo Morita, Yousuke Michikawa, Tomohiro Tamura, Tetsuya Hiraishi, Nobuhiro Hattori, Yohei Noguchi, Kazunari Nakahara, Toshiya Ishii, Nobuyuki Matsumoto, Chiaki Okuse, Fumio Itoh and Michihiro Suzuki contributed reagents/materials/analysis tools; Ryuta Shigefuku wrote the paper.

## Abbreviations

| | |
|---|---|
| Alb | albumin |
| APRI | aspartate aminotransferase-platelet index |
| CHC | chronic hepatitis related to hepatitis C virus |
| ChE | cholinesterase |
| CLD | chronic liver disease |
| CT | computed tomography |
| HA | hyaluronic acid |
| HATBF | hepatic arterial tissue blood flow |
| HBF | hepatic blood flow |
| HCV | hepatitis C virus |
| ICG-R$_{15}$ | retention rate of indocyanine green 15 min after administration |
| LC | liver cirrhosis |
| MRI | magnetic resonance imaging |
| NAFLD | nonalcoholic fatty liver disease |
| NASH | nonalcoholic steatohepatitis |
| Plt | platelet count |
| PT | prothrombin time |
| P/A | portal flow / hepatic arterial flow ratio |
| PVTBF | portal venous tissue blood flow |
| PIIIP | type III procollagen N peptide |
| ROI | region of interest |
| TC | total cholesterol |
| TBF | tissue blood flow |
| THTBF | total hepatic tissue blood flow |
| TIMP-1 | tissue inhibitor of metalloproteinase-1 |
| US | ultrasonography |
| WFA$^+$-M2BP | Wisteria floribunda agglutinin positive Mac-2-binding protein |
| Xe-CT | Xenon computed tomography |

## References

1.  Ludwig, J.; Viggiano, T.R.; McGill, D.B.; Oh, B.J. Nonalcoholic steatohepatitis: Mayo clinic experiences with a hitherto unnamed disease. *Mayo Clin. Proc.* **1980**, *55*, 434–438. [PubMed]
2.  Matteoni, C.A.; Younossi, Z.M.; Gramlich, T.; Boparai, N.; Liu, Y.C.; Mc Cullough, A.J. Nonalcoholic fatty liver disease: A spectrum of clinical and pathological severity. *Gastroenterology* **1999**, *116*, 1413–1419. [CrossRef]
3.  Farrell, G.C.; Larter, C.Z. Nonalcoholic fatty liver disease: From steatosis to cirrhosis. *Hepatology* **2006**, *43*, S99–S112. [CrossRef] [PubMed]
4.  Sayiner, M.; Koenig, A.; Henry, L.; Younossi, Z.M. Epidemiology of nonalcoholic fatty liver disease and nonalcoholic steatohepatitis in the United States and the rest of the world. *Clin. Liver Dis.* **2016**, *20*, 205–214. [CrossRef] [PubMed]
5.  Sherif, Z.A.; Saeed, A.; Ghavimi, A.; Nouraie, S.-M.; Laiyemo, A.O.; Brim, H.; Ashktorab, H. Global epidemiology of nonalcoholic fatty liver disease and perspectives on US minority populations. *Dig. Dis. Sci.* **2016**, *61*, 1214–1225. [CrossRef] [PubMed]
6.  Watanabe, S.; Hashimoto, E.; Ikejima, K.; Uto, H.; Ono, M.; Sumida, Y.; Seike, M.; Takei, Y.; Takehara, T.; Tokushige, K.; et al. Evidence-based clinical practice guidelines for nonalcoholic fatty liver disease/nonalcoholic steatohepatitis. *J. Gastroenterol.* **2015**, *50*, 364–377. [CrossRef] [PubMed]
7.  Eguchi, Y.; Hyogo, H.; Ono, M.; Mizuta, T.; Ono, N.; Fujimoto, K.; Chayama, K.; Saibara, T. JSG-NAFLD. Prevalence and associated metabolic factors of nonalcoholic fatty liver disease in the general population from 2009 to 2010 in Japan: A multicenter large retrospective study. *J. Gastroenterol.* **2012**, *47*, 586–595. [CrossRef] [PubMed]
8.  Farrell, G.C.; Wong, V.W.; Chitturi, S. NAFLD in Asia—As common and important as in the West. *Nat. Rev. Gastroenterol. Hepatol.* **2013**, *10*, 307–318. [CrossRef] [PubMed]
9.  Brunt, E.M. Nonalcoholic steatohepatitis. *Semin. Liver Dis.* **2004**, *24*, 3–20. [PubMed]
10. Freni, M.A.; Artuso, D.; Gerken, G.; Spanti, C.; Marafioti, T.; Alessi, N.; Spadaro, A.; Ajello, A.; Ferraù, O. Focal lymphocytic aggregates in chronic hepatitis C: Occurrence, immunohistochemical characterization, and relation to markers of autoimmunity. *Hepatology* **1995**, *22*, 389–394. [CrossRef] [PubMed]
11. Wong, V.S.; Wight, D.G.; Palmer, C.R.; Alexander, G.J. Fibrosis and other histological features in chronic hepatitis C virus infection: A statistical model. *J. Clin. Pathol.* **1996**, *49*, 465–469. [CrossRef] [PubMed]
12. Abe, M.; Miyake, T.; Kuno, A.; Imai, Y.; Sawai, Y.; Hino, K.; Hara, Y.; Hige, S.; Sakamoto, M.; Yamada, G.; et al. Association between *Wisteria floribunda* agglutinin-positive Mac-2 binding protein and the fibrosis stage of non-alcoholic fatty liver disease. *J. Gastroenterol.* **2015**, *50*, 776–784. [CrossRef] [PubMed]
13. Yamasaki, K.; Tateyama, M.; Abiru, S.; Komori, A.; Nagaoka, S.; Saeki, A.; Hashimoto, S.; Sasaki, R.; Bekki, S.; Kugiyama, Y.; et al. Elevated serum levels of *Wisteria floribunda* agglutinin-positive human Mac-2 binding protein predict the development of hepatocellular carcinoma in hepatitis C patients. *Hepatology* **2014**, *60*, 1563–1570. [CrossRef] [PubMed]
14. Tamaki, N.; Kurosaki, M.; Kuno, A.; Korenaga, M.; Togayachi, A.; Gotoh, M.; Nakakuki, N.; Takada, H.; Matsuda, S.; Hattori, N.; et al. *Wisteria floribunda* agglutinin positive human Mac-2-binding protein as a predictor of hepatocellular carcinoma development in chronic hepatitis C patients. *Hepatol. Res.* **2015**, *45*, E82–E88. [CrossRef] [PubMed]
15. Johnson, D.W.; Stringer, W.A.; Marks, M.P.; Yonas, H.; Good, W.F.; Gur, D. Stable xenon CT cerebral blood flow imaging: Rationale for and role in clinical decision making. *Am. J. Neuroradiol.* **1991**, *12*, 201–213. [PubMed]
16. Gur, D.; Good, W.F.; Wolfson, S.K., Jr.; Yonas, H.; Shabason, L. In vivo mapping of local cerebral blood flow by xenonenhanced computed tomography. *Science* **1982**, *215*, 1267–1268. [CrossRef] [PubMed]
17. Ikeda, H.; Suzuki, M.; Kobayashi, M.; Takahashi, H.; Matsumoto, N.; Maeyama, S.; Iino, S.; Sase, S.; Itoh, F. Xenon computed tomography shows hemodynamic change during the progression of chronic hepatitis C. *Hepatol. Res.* **2007**, *37*, 104–112. [CrossRef] [PubMed]
18. Shigefuku, R.; Takahashi, H.; Kato, M.; Yoshida, Y.; Suetani, K.; Noguchi, Y.; Hatsugai, M.; Nakahara, K.; Ikeda, H.; Kobayashi, M.; et al. Evaluation of hepatic tissue blood flow using xenon computed tomography with fibrosis progression in nonalcoholic fatty liver disease: Comparison with chronic hepatitis C. *Int. J. Mol. Sci.* **2014**, *15*, 1026–1039. [CrossRef] [PubMed]

19. Shigefuku, R.; Takahashi, H.; Kobayashi, M.; Ikeda, H.; Matsunaga, K.; Okuse, C.; Matsumoto, N.; Maeyama, S.; Sase, S.; Suzuki, M.; et al. Pathophysiological analysis of nonalcoholic fatty liver disease by evaluation of fatty liver changes and blood flow using xenon computed tomography: Can early-stage nonalcoholic steatohepatitis be distinguished from simple steatosis? *J. Gastroenterol.* **2012**, *47*, 1238–1247. [CrossRef] [PubMed]

20. Kobayashi, M.; Suzuki, M.; Ikeda, H.; Takahashi, H.; Matsumoto, N.; Maeyama, S.; Sase, S.; Iino, S.; Itoh, F. Assessment of hepatic steatosis and hepatic tissue blood flow by xenon computed tomography in nonalcoholic steatohepatitis. *Hepatol. Res.* **2009**, *39*, 31–39. [CrossRef] [PubMed]

21. Takahashi, H.; Suzuki, M.; Ikeda, H.; Kobayashi, M.; Sase, S.; Yotsuyanagi, H.; Maeyama, S.; Iino, S.; Itoh, F. Evaluation of quantitative portal venous, hepatic arterial, and total hepatic tissue blood flow using xenon CT in alcoholic liver cirrhosis—Comparison with liver cirrhosis related to hepatitis C virus and nonalcoholic steatohepatitis. *Alcohol. Clin. Exp. Res.* **2010**, *34*, S7–S13. [CrossRef] [PubMed]

22. Takahashi, H.; Shigefuku, R.; Yoshida, Y.; Ikeda, H.; Matsunaga, K.; Matsumoto, N.; Okuse, C.; Sase, S.; Itoh, F.; Suzuki, M. Correlation between hepatic blood flow and liver function in alcoholic liver cirrhosis. *World J. Gastroenterol.* **2014**, *20*, 17065–17074. [CrossRef] [PubMed]

23. Brunt, E.M.; Janney, C.G.; di Bisceglie, A.M.; Neuschwander-Tetri, B.A.; Bacon, B.R. Non-alcoholic steatohepatitis: A proposal for grading and staging the histological lesions. *Am. J. Gastroenterol.* **1999**, *94*, 2467–2474. [CrossRef] [PubMed]

24. Desmet, V.J.; Gerber, M.; Hoofnagle, J.H.; Manns, M.; Scheuer, P.J. Classification of chronic hepatitis: Diagnosis, grading and staging. *Hepatology* **1994**, *19*, 1513–1520. [CrossRef] [PubMed]

25. Linden, M.A.; Sheldon, R.D.; Meers, G.M.; Ortinau, L.C.; Morris, E.M.; Booth, F.W.; Kanaley, J.A.; Vieira-Potter, V.J.; Sowers, J.R.; Ibdah, J.A.; et al. Aerobic exercise training in the treatment of NAFLD related fibrosis. *J. Physiol.* **2016**. [CrossRef] [PubMed]

26. Finelli, C.; Tarantino, G. Have guidelines addressing physical activity been established in nonalcoholic fatty liver disease? *World J. Gastroenterol.* **2012**, *18*, 6790–6800. [CrossRef] [PubMed]

27. Tarantino, G.; Citro, V.; Finelli, C. Recreational drugs: A new health hazard for patients with concomitant chronic liver diseases. *J. Gastrointest. Liver Dis.* **2014**, *23*, 79–84.

28. Gadd, V.L.; Patel, P.J.; Jose, S.; Horsfall, L.; Powell, E.E.; Irvine, K.M. Altered peripheral blood monocyte phenotype and function in chronic liver disease: Implications for hepatic recruitment and systemic inflammation. *PLoS ONE* **2016**, *11*, e0157771. [CrossRef] [PubMed]

29. Neuschwander-Tetri, B.A. Hepatic lipotoxicity and the pathogenesis of nonalcoholic steatohepatitis: The central role of nontriglyceride fatty acid metabolites. *Hepatology* **2010**, *52*, 774–788. [CrossRef] [PubMed]

30. Makuuchi, M.; Kosuge, T.; Takayama, T.; Yamazaki, S.; Kakazu, T.; Miyagawa, S.; Kawasaki, S. Surgery for small liver cancers. *Semin. Surg. Oncol.* **1993**, *9*, 298–304. [CrossRef] [PubMed]

31. Lisotti, A.; Azzaroli, F.; Buonfiglioli, F.; Montagnani, M.; Cecinato, P.; Turco, L.; Calvanese, C.; Simoni, P.; Guardigli, M.; Arena, R.; et al. Indocyanine Green retention test as a noninvasive marker of portal hypertension and esophageal varices in compensated liver cirrhosis. *Hepatology* **2014**, *59*, 643–650. [CrossRef] [PubMed]

32. Yamazaki, S.; Takayama, N.; Nakamura, M.; Higaki, T.; Matsuoka, S.; Mizuno, S.; Moriyama, M. Prophylactic impact of endoscopic treatment for esophageal varices in liver resection: A prospective study. *J. Gastroenterol.* **2014**, *49*, 917–922. [CrossRef] [PubMed]

33. Seifalian, A.M.; Mallet, S.V.; Rolles, K.; Davidson, B.R. Hepatic microcirculation during human orthotopic liver transplantation. *Br. J. Surg.* **1997**, *84*, 1391–1395. [CrossRef] [PubMed]

34. Seifalian, A.M.; Chidambaram, V.; Rolles, K.; Davidson, B.R. In vivo demonstration of impaired microcirculation in steatotic human liver grafts. *Liver Transplant. Surg.* **1998**, *4*, 71–77. [CrossRef]

35. Seifalian, A.M.; Piasecki, C.; Agarwal, A.; Davidson, B.R. The effect of graded steatosis on flow in the hepatic parenchymal microcirculation. *Transplantation* **1999**, *68*, 780–784. [CrossRef] [PubMed]

36. Samia, I.; Wenxuan, Y.; Winslet, M.C.; Alexander, M.; Seifalian, A.M. Impairment of hepatic microcirculation in fatty liver. *Microcirculation* **2003**, *10*, 447–456.

37. Hayashi, N.; Kasahara, A.; Kurosawa, K.; Sasaki, Y.; Fusamoto, H.; Sato, N.; Kamada, T. Oxygen supply to the liver in patients with alcoholic liver disease assessed by organ-reflectance spectrophotometry. *Gastroenterology* **1985**, *88*, 881–886. [CrossRef]

38. Farrell, G.C.; Teoh, N.C.; McCuskey, R.S. Hepatic microcirculation in fatty liver disease. *Anat. Rec. (Hoboken)* **2008**, *291*, 684–692. [CrossRef] [PubMed]

39. Pasarín, M.; La Mura, V.; Gracia-Sancho, J.; García-Calderó, H.; Rodríguez-Vilarrupla, A.; García-Pagán, J.C.; Bosch, J.; Abraldes, J.G. Sinusoidal endothelial dysfunction precedes inflammation and fibrosis in a model of NAFLD. *PLoS ONE* **2012**, *7*, e32785. [CrossRef] [PubMed]

40. Yang, Y.-Y.; Tsai, T.-H.; Huang, Y.-T.; Lee, T.-Y.; Chan, C.-C.; Lee, K.-C.; Lin, H.-C. Hepatic endothelin-1 and endocannabinoids-dependent effects of hyperleptinemia in nonalcoholic steatohepatitis-cirrhotic Rats. *Hepatology* **2012**, *55*, 1540–1550. [CrossRef] [PubMed]

41. Francque, S.; Verrijken, A.; Mertens, I.; Hubens, G.; van Marck, E.; Pelckmans, P.; van Gaal, L.; Michielsen, P. Noncirrhotic human nonalcoholic fatty liver disease induces portal hypertension in relation to the histological degree of steatosis. *Eur. J. Gastroenterol. Hepatol.* **2010**, *22*, 1449–1457. [CrossRef] [PubMed]

42. Hashimoto, E.; Yatsuji, S.; Kaneda, H.; Yoshioka, Y.; Taniai, M.; Tokushige, K.; Shiratori, K. The characteristics and natural history of Japanese patients with nonalcoholic fatty liver disease. *Hepatol. Res.* **2005**, *33*, 72–76. [CrossRef] [PubMed]

43. Nakamura, S.; Konishi, H.; Kishino, M.; Yatsuji, S.; Tokushige, K.; Hashimoto, E.; Shiratori, K. Prevalence of esophagogastric varices in patients with nonalcoholic steatohepatitis. *Hepatol. Res.* **2008**, *38*, 572–579. [CrossRef] [PubMed]

44. Mendes, F.D.; Suzuki, A.; Sanderson, S.O.; Lindor, K.D.; Angulo, P. Prevalence and indicators of portal hypertension in patients with nonalcoholic fatty liver disease. *Clin. Gastroenterol. Hepatol.* **2012**, *10*, 1028–1033. [CrossRef] [PubMed]

45. Hirooka, M.; Koizumi, Y.; Miyake, T.; Ochi, H.; Tokumoto, Y.; Tada, F.; Matsuura, B.; Abe, M.; Hiasa, Y. Nonalcoholic fatty liver disease: Portal hypertension due to outflow block in patients without cirrhosis. *Radiology* **2015**, *274*, 597–604. [CrossRef] [PubMed]

46. Yeh, M.M.; Brunt, E.M. Pathological features of fatty liver disease. *Gastroenterology* **2014**, *147*, 754–764. [CrossRef] [PubMed]

47. Brunt, E.M. Nonalcoholic fatty liver disease: Pros and cons of histologic systems of evaluation. *Int. J. Mol. Sci.* **2016**, *17*, 97. [CrossRef] [PubMed]

48. Sase, S.; Monden, M.; Oka, H.; Dono, K.; Fukuta, T.; Shibata, I. Hepatic blood flow measurements with arterial and portal blood flow mapping in the human liver by means of xenon CT. *J. Comput. Assist. Tomogr.* **2002**, *26*, 243–249. [CrossRef] [PubMed]

49. Sase, S.; Takahashi, H.; Ikeda, H.; Kobayashi, M.; Matsumoto, N.; Suzuki, M. Determination of time-course change rate for arterial xenon using the time course of tissue xenon concentration in xenonenhanced computed tomography. *Med. Phys.* **2008**, *35*, 2331–2338. [CrossRef] [PubMed]

50. Kuno, A.; Ikehara, Y.; Tanaka, Y.; Ito, K.; Matsuda, A.; Sekiya, S.; Hige, S.; Sakamoto, M.; Kage, M.; Mizokami, M.; et al. A serum "sweet-doughnut" 272 protein facilitates fibrosis evaluation and therapy assessment in patients 273 with viral hepatitis. *Sci. Rep.* **2013**, *3*, 1065. [CrossRef] [PubMed]

# 13

# Weekly Treatment of 2-Hydroxypropyl-β-cyclodextrin Improves Intracellular Cholesterol Levels in LDL Receptor Knockout Mice

Sofie M. A. Walenbergh [1], Tom Houben [1], Tim Hendrikx [1], Mike L. J. Jeurissen [1],
Patrick J. van Gorp [1], Nathalie Vaes [1], Steven W. M. Olde Damink [2,3], Fons Verheyen [4],
Ger H. Koek [5], Dieter Lütjohann [6], Alena Grebe [7], Eicke Latz [7,8,9] and Ronit Shiri-Sverdlov [1,*]

[1] Department of Molecular Genetics, School of Nutrition and Translational Research in
Metabolism (NUTRIM), Maastricht University, Maastricht 6229ER, The Netherlands;
s.walenbergh@maastrichtuniversity.nl (S.M.A.W.); tom.houben@maastrichtuniversity.nl (To.H.);
t.hendrikx@maastrichtuniversity.nl (Ti.H.); m.jeurissen@maastrichtuniversity.nl (M.L.J.J.);
p.vangorp@maastrichtuniversity.nl (P.J.G.); n.vaes@maastrichtuniversity.nl (N.V.)

[2] Department of General Surgery, Maastricht University, Maastricht 6229ER, The Netherlands;
steven.oldedamink@maastrichtuniversity.nl

[3] Department of HPB and Liver Transplantation Surgery, Royal Free Hospital, University College London,
London NW3 2PF, UK

[4] Department of Molecular Cell Biology and Electron Microscopy, Maastricht University,
Maastricht 6229ER, The Netherlands; f.verheyen@maastrichtuniversity.nl

[5] Department of Internal Medicine, Division of Gastroenterology and Hepatology, Maastricht University
Medical Center (MUMC), Maastricht 6202AZ, The Netherlands; gh.koek@mumc.nl

[6] Institute of Clinical Chemistry and Clinical Pharmacology, University of Bonn, Bonn D-53105, Germany;
dieter.luetjohann@ukb.uni-bonn.de

[7] Institute of Innate Immunity, University Hospital, University of Bonn, Bonn D-53127, Germany;
alena.grebe@uni-bonn.de (A.G.); eicke.latz@umassmed.edu (E.L.)

[8] German Center for Neurodegenerative Diseases (DZNE), Bonn D-53127, Germany

[9] Division of Infectious Diseases and Immunology, University of Massachusetts Medical School,
Worcester, MA 01605, USA

* Author to whom correspondence should be addressed; r.sverdlov@maastrichtuniversity.nl

Academic Editors: Amedeo Lonardo and Giovanni Targher

**Abstract:** Recently, the importance of lysosomes in the context of the metabolic syndrome has received increased attention. Increased lysosomal cholesterol storage and cholesterol crystallization inside macrophages have been linked to several metabolic diseases, such as atherosclerosis and non-alcoholic fatty liver disease (NAFLD). Two-hydroxypropyl-β-cyclodextrin (HP-B-CD) is able to redirect lysosomal cholesterol to the cytoplasm in Niemann-Pick type C1 disease, a lysosomal storage disorder. We hypothesize that HP-B-CD ameliorates liver cholesterol and intracellular cholesterol levels inside Kupffer cells (KCs). Hyperlipidemic low-density lipoprotein receptor knockout ($Ldlr^{-/-}$) mice were given weekly, subcutaneous injections with HP-B-CD or control PBS. In contrast to control injections, hyperlipidemic mice treated with HP-B-CD demonstrated a shift in intracellular cholesterol distribution towards cytoplasmic cholesteryl ester (CE) storage and a decrease in cholesterol crystallization inside KCs. Compared to untreated hyperlipidemic mice, the foamy KC appearance and liver cholesterol remained similar upon HP-B-CD administration, while hepatic campesterol and 7α-hydroxycholesterol levels were back increased. Thus, HP-B-CD could be a useful tool to improve intracellular cholesterol levels in the context of the metabolic syndrome, possibly through modulation of phyto- and oxysterols, and should be tested in the future. Additionally, these data underline the existence of a shared etiology between lysosomal storage diseases and NAFLD.

**Keywords:** NAFLD; metabolic syndrome; cyclodextrin; electron microscopy; lysosomes

## 1. Introduction

Non-alcoholic fatty liver disease (NAFLD) describes several stages of liver disease characterized by no or little alcohol use, and is currently viewed as the precursor of the metabolic syndrome [1]. Initially, the excessive buildup of fat inside the liver, also referred to as steatosis, is a benign and reversible condition. However, later stages of NAFLD are characterized by liver inflammation, the formation of irreversible scar tissue (fibrosis-cirrhosis) and severe end-stage liver disease [2]. Currently, the prevalence of NAFLD is estimated to grow as a direct result of the global obesity epidemic [3]. Better insights into the mechanisms that cause NAFLD are required in order to develop novel therapeutic interventions.

Under healthy circumstances, lipoproteins are endocytosed by macrophages and initially directed to the endolysosomal compartment where further processing will take place. Subsequently, cholesterol is transferred from the lysosomes to the cytoplasm. Interestingly, previous studies from our group revealed that during hyperlipidemic conditions in mice, such as NAFLD, cholesterol is not transported into the cytoplasm, but rather accumulates inside lysosomes of the Kupffer cells (KCs). In addition to a resistance of cholesterol efflux from the lysosome, we observed increased cholesterol crystals in the livers of these mice [4,5]. These cholesterol crystals are so-called cholesterol deposits, formed upon excessive cholesterol uptake. Similar to our data, lysosomal cholesterol storage and cholesterol crystallization inside macrophages was also observed during atherosclerosis [6]. Therefore, the suggestion was raised that both these metabolic diseases share disease mechanisms and could be referred to as acquired lysosomal storage disorders [7,8]. A classical lysosomal storage disorder, such as Niemann-Pick type C (NPC) disease, is caused by a mutation in either the $Npc1$ or $Npc2$ gene, which encodes for a key protein that is responsible for cholesterol transport from the lysosomes to the cytoplasm. As a result, NPC disease patients demonstrate progressive accumulation of cholesterol inside lysosomes that severely damages almost all organs, leading to neurological disease, liver dysfunction and eventually premature death [9]. Notably, increased lysosomal cholesterol accumulation in $Npc1^{-/-}$ mice could be reversed by the administration of two-hydroxypropyl-β-cyclodextrin (HP-B-CD) and normalized the cholesterol metabolism in nearly every organ of the body [10–14]. Thus far, the effect of HP-B-CD on the cholesterol metabolism during NAFLD has never been studied.

The aim of the current study was to investigate whether HP-B-CD treatment is able to modify the cholesterol metabolism in the liver, as well as inside the KCs, in an established hyperlipidemic low-density lipoprotein receptor knockout ($Ldlr^{-/-}$) mouse model. Unlike wildtype mice, the $Ldlr^{-/-}$ mice demonstrate a human-like lipoprotein profile characterized by mildly elevated cholesterol levels which is mostly carried in the intermediate-density lipoprotein (IDL)/LDL fractions [15]. Additionally, recent research demonstrated that the presence of steatosis and hepatic inflammation is persisted for a long period of time, and even progressed into liver fibrosis [16]. The resemblance with a human-like lipoprotein profile, the sustained hepatic inflammatory response and the development of fibrosis makes hyperlipidemic $Ldlr^{-/-}$ mice an excellent mouse model to study the onset and progression of NAFLD. We hypothesized that HP-B-CD ameliorates liver cholesterol and intracellular cholesterol levels inside KCs. Once a week, we administered HP-B-CD to $Ldlr^{-/-}$ mice fed a high-fat, high-cholesterol (HFC) diet. Mice receiving phosphate-buffered saline (PBS) were used as a control. After HP-B-CD treatment, we found that lysosomal cholesterol levels and cholesterol crystallization were decreased inside KCs compared to control-treated hyperlipidemic mice. In contrast, no changes in the total level of liver cholesterol and KC area were seen. These data indicate for the first time that HP-B-CD could be a useful tool to improve intracellular cholesterol levels in the context of the metabolic syndrome.

## 2. Results

### 2.1. No Difference in Liver and Plasma Cholesterol Levels upon HP-B-CD Treatment

The mean spleen and liver weight in the HFC group was increased compared to chow, but remained similar upon weekly HP-B-CD treatment for a 12-week time period (Figure 1A). In line with these data, liver and plasma cholesterol levels were significantly higher upon HFC feeding than after 12 weeks of regular chow. However, no differences in cholesterol concentrations were found between PBS and HP-B-CD-treated mice on an HFC diet (Figure 1B). Thus, these data indicate that HP-B-CD has no effect on organ weight and cholesterol concentrations in plasma and liver.

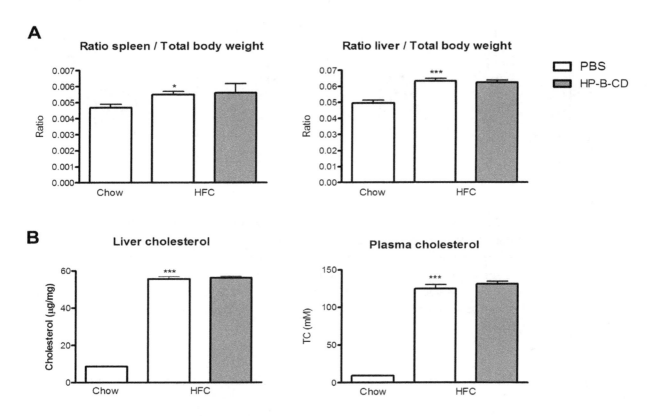

**Figure 1.** Relative spleen, liver weights and cholesterol levels. (**A**) Relative spleen and liver weights after 12-weeks of regular chow or HFC diet in $Ldlr^{-/-}$ mice with and without HP-B-CD treatment; and (**B**) Cholesterol levels were analyzed in liver as well as plasma of $Ldlr^{-/-}$ mice after 12 weeks of regular chow or HFC diet. TC: total cholesterol. Data are expressed as mean ± SEM ($n$ = 10 for the chow-fed mice; $n$ = 12 for the mice fed an HFC diet without treatment; $n$ = 12 for the HFC-fed mice receiving HP-B-CD treatment). * Significantly different from chow. * and *** indicate $p < 0.05$, and 0.001, respectively.

### 2.2. Foamy KC Appearance Is Similar between Control- and HP-B-CD-Injected Mice

To determine whether HP-B-CD affects the foamy appearance of KCs, liver sections were stained against CD68, a marker specifically for macrophages. As expected, HFC feeding increased the area of the KCs, compared to mice fed regular chow. No difference in CD68-positive area was observed between PBS- and HP-B-CD-injected mice on an HFC diet (Figure 2A). These data were confirmed upon quantification of the CD68-positive area of these livers (Figure 2B) and gene expression analysis of *Cd68* (Figure 2C), which both demonstrated no difference in the CD68 expression after HP-B-CD. To summarize, the HFC diet leads to a foamy KC appearance and was not affected upon HP-B-CD treatment.

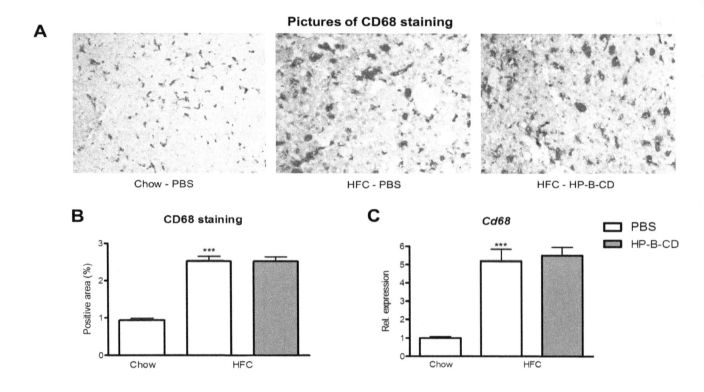

**Figure 2.** Hepatic CD68 expression. (**A**) Representative histological pictures of the CD68 staining (original magnification, 200×) performed on liver sections of chow, PBS-injected and HP-B-CD-injected HFC-fed mice; (**B**) Quantification of the percentage CD68-positive area; (**C**) Hepatic gene expression analysis of *Cd68*. Gene expression data are shown relative to chow. Data are expressed as mean ± SEM ($n$ = 10 for the chow-fed mice; $n$ = 12 for the mice fed an HFC diet without treatment; $n$ = 12 for the HFC-fed mice receiving HP-B-CD treatment). * Significantly different from chow. *** indicates $p < 0.001$.

## 2.3. HP-B-CD-Treated Mice Demonstrate Decreased Lysosomal Cholesterol Accumulation and Cholesterol Crystallization

Electron microscopy was performed to investigate the effect of HP-B-CD on redirecting lysosomal cholesterol to the cytoplasm and cholesterol crystallization. Livers were fixed and stained for acid phosphatase (ACPase), a marker for lysosomes. As demonstrated in Figure 3A, KCs of the non-treated HFC group displayed increased lysosomal cholesterol accumulation and cholesterol crystals compared to KCs of HP-B-CD-treated mice upon HFC feeding (Figure 3B). In the latter group, cholesterol droplets were mainly observed inside the cytoplasm. Scoring electron microscopy pictures of approximately 50 KCs from both HFC groups confirmed that lysosomal cholesterol was significantly decreased, while cytoplasmic cholesteryl ester (CE) droplets were increased upon HP-B-CD treatment. Moreover, mice administered HP-B-CD had less cholesterol crystals inside their KCs compared to control PBS-injected mice after a 12-week HFC diet (Figure 3C). These results suggest that HP-B-CD is able to redirect cholesterol from the lysosomes to the cytoplasm.

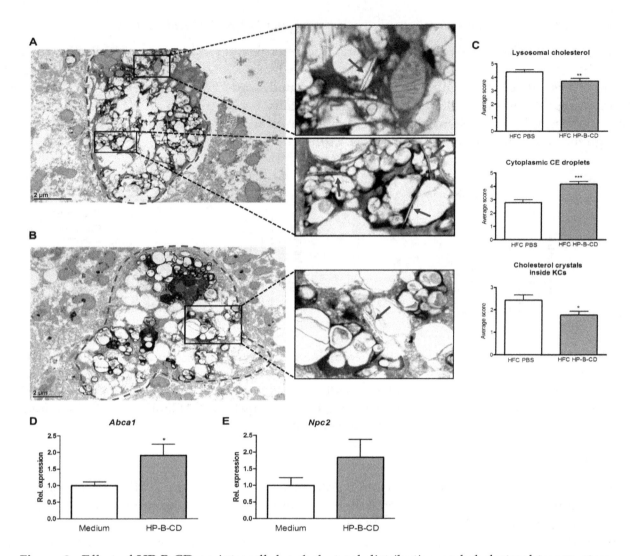

**Figure 3.** Effect of HP-B-CD on intracellular cholesterol distribution and cholesterol transporters. Representative electron microscopy pictures of Kupffer cells (KCs) of HFC-fed $Ldlr^{-/-}$ mice without (**A**) and with HP-B-CD treatment (**B**). Lysosomes are indicated in black by ACPase staining. KCs are depicted by the dashed line. Arrows point to cholesterol crystals; (**C**) Scoring of lysosomal cholesterol, cytoplasmic cholesteryl ester (CE) droplets and cholesterol crystals after 12 weeks of HFC diet. In total, 40 to 50 KCs were scored per HFC group and an average score was calculated. Gene expression levels of the cholesterol transporters $Abca1$ (**D**) and $Npc2$ (**E**) in oxLDL-loaded BMDM with or without HP-B-CD treatment. The *in vitro* results are the mean ± SEM from two separate experiments performed in triplicate. * Significantly different from control. *, ** and *** indicate $p < 0.05$, 0.01 and 0.001, respectively.

Previous studies found that it is mainly oxidized LDL (oxLDL) that tends to accumulate inside the lysosomes of $Ldlr^{-/-}$ mice and in cultured macrophages [5,17]. To show that HP-B-CD is able to modify lysosomal oxLDL, we isolated bone marrow-derived macrophages (BMDM) from wildtype mice and stimulated these with oxLDL. Subsequently, BMDM were treated with HP-B-CD (0.3%) or with control medium. Upon HP-B-CD treatment, gene expression of ATP-binding cassette transporter A1 ($Abca1$), a key regulator of cholesterol efflux, was elevated compared to control treatment (Figure 3D). Additionally, the gene expression of Niemann-Pick type C2 ($Npc2$), an intracellular lysosomal cholesterol transporter responsible for cholesterol transport out of the lysosome, was also elevated after HP-B-CD treatment compared to control (Figure 3E). These data demonstrate the ability of HP-B-CD to lower lysosomal oxLDL levels.

*2.4. Campesterol and 7α-Hydroxycholesterol Are Increased after HP-B-CD Treatment*

To obtain a better understanding in the cholesterol metabolism after HP-B-CD treatment, we analyzed campesterol, a phytosterol, and 7α-hydroxycholesterol (7aOH), an oxysterol, in the livers of control chow-fed and non-treated and HP-B-CD-treated HFC-fed mice. Hepatic campesterol and 7aOH levels were dramatically reduced upon an HFC diet compared to chow. Interestingly, campesterol and 7aOH were significantly increased after HP-B-CD treatment, although the elevation was minimal (Figure 4A,B).

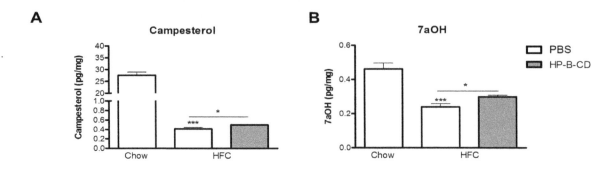

**Figure 4.** Hepatic levels of campesterol and 7α-hydroxycholesterol (7aOH). Campesterol (**A**) and 7aOH (**B**) were analyzed in liver pieces of $Ldlr^{-/-}$ mice after 12 weeks of regular chow or HFC diet. Data are expressed as mean ± SEM ($n$ = 10 for the chow-fed mice; $n$ = 12 for the mice fed an HFC diet without treatment; $n$ = 12 for the HFC-fed mice receiving HP-B-CD treatment). * Significantly different from chow. * and *** indicate $p$ < 0.05 and 0.001, respectively.

## 3. Discussion

Currently, no registered therapeutic interventions against NAFLD are available. Previous studies from our group suggest that lysosomal cholesterol accumulation can be considered as a key mechanism for the pathogenesis of NAFLD in mice. As such, we tested HP-B-CD, a compound known to redirect cholesterol from the lysosomes to the cytoplasm in the context of lysosomal storage diseases, to improve the cholesterol metabolism in an established hyperlipidemic mouse model to study NAFLD [16]. Unlike total hepatic cholesterol levels, we now show that it is the intracellular localization of cholesterol in hyperlipidemic mice that is improved after HP-B-CD treatment. Our novel data demonstrate that HP-B-CD reduces lysosomal cholesterol accumulation and cholesterol crystallization in KCs during hyperlipidemic conditions. Moreover, these data underline the shared etiology between lysosomal storage diseases and NAFLD.

Lysosomal cholesterol accumulation could be efficiently overcome by the administration of HP-B-CD to $Npc1^{-/-}$ mice and cells deficient for the $Npc1$ gene [10,13]. In the current study, a similar dosage (20% $w/v$, 4000 mg per kg body weight) and product (H107, Sigma-Aldrich) of HP-B-CD was administered subcutaneously as described in previous *in vivo* studies [11–14,18] and showed to decrease lysosomal cholesterol storage and increase cytoplasmic CE droplets inside KCs. Thus, HP-B-CD was able to reduce lysosomal cholesterol in a lysosomal storage disease and fatty liver disease and suggests a shared disease mechanism. Lysosomal cholesterol accumulation in macrophages is an underlying mechanism in diseases associated with the metabolic syndrome, such as atherosclerosis and NAFLD [4,7,8]. Unlike non-oxidized LDL that accumulates in lysosomes of NPC mice, recent evidence points toward the specific lysosomal trapping of oxLDL in $Ldlr^{-/-}$ mice and in cultured macrophages [5,17,19,20]. Besides NAFLD, increasing attention has been directed to the crucial role of oxLDL in the pathogenesis of various metabolic diseases, including atherosclerosis [7] and diabetes [21]. However, thus far, oxLDL has been shown to be highly resistant to removal from the lysosome [22] and to intracellular degradation [23]. As such, the ability of HP-B-CD to liberate lysosomal cholesterol in $Ldlr^{-/-}$ mice is an exciting opportunity for the amelioration of various metabolic diseases underlying lysosomal oxLDL accumulation.

HP-B-CD has cholesterol-binding capacities and normalizes cholesterol homeostasis in $Npc1$ deficient cells [24]. Upon absorption, HP-B-CD has been shown to be distributed over several tissues including the liver [25]. In line, numerous studies demonstrated a clear improvement in liver function of $Npc1^{-/-}$ mice after subcutaneous administration of HP-B-CD [11–14,26]. Much to our surprise, no changes in plasma and liver cholesterol levels and the foamy KC appearance were found in HP-B-CD-treated mice compared to their control. A possible explanation for these data is that cholesterol storage inside lysosomes is much less extreme in the $Ldlr^{-/-}$ model compared to the $Npc1^{-/-}$ mice fed an HFC diet. Therefore, the effect of HP-B-CD on total cholesterol levels, and also liver weight, in the $Ldlr^{-/-}$ model is not significant. In line with our observations, Taylor et al. demonstrated that HP-B-CD treatment does not lead to increased cholesterol levels in urine and plasma, leaving HP-B-CD to liberate lysosomal cholesterol for further processing within the cytosolic compartment only [27]. However, these results may be related to the fact that HP-B-CD was injected only one single time in the latter study.

In line with the unaffected plasma and liver cholesterol levels between HP-B-CD- and control-treated mice, we could not detect any differences in the foamy KC appearance. This is a striking result, since the amount of cholesterol crystals were lowered in mice treated with HP-B-CD compared to PBS and suggest that foamy KCs do not correlate with cholesterol crystallization. This is contrary to the current view that foamy macrophages are strongly associated with cholesterol crystallization [5,28–30]. Of note, cholesterol crystallization occurs within lipid-loaded lysosomes and not in the cytoplasm, hereby confirming that the actual formation of cholesterol crystals is dependent on lysosomal cholesterol levels [31]. Indeed, in line with a decreased level of lysosomal cholesterol, we observed less cholesterol crystallization. Altogether, these data indicate that there is dissociation between foam cell formation and cholesterol crystallization.

Despite much effort, the exact mechanism by which HP-B-CD normalizes cholesterol homeostasis is still under debate. After injection, HP-B-CD has the ability to be internalized into the lysosomes of cells via bulk phase endocytosis and release sequestered cholesterol from the lysosome into the cytosol [32]. Due to the unique structure of HP-B-CD, it can serve as a cholesterol sink, extract cholesterol and trap cholesterol in the presence of high cholesterol concentrations. However, during low cholesterol levels, HP-B-CD rather acts as a cholesterol shuttle, transporting cholesterol between membranes. Other evidence points towards HP-B-CD as a compound that extracts cholesterol from cell membranes by which the resulting HP-B-CD-cholesterol complex is then cleared via the kidneys.

In the current study, we have found that the HFC diet leads to a dramatic reduction of liver campesterol compared to chow. In the plasma, campesterol can be considered as a surrogate marker for intestinal cholesterol absorption, and likely has the same function when found in the liver [33]. Intestinal cholesterol absorption, and thus campesterol, is likely to be inhibited during consumption of a high fat diet, as a protective mechanism to prevent excess plasma cholesterol levels. Our data are in line with other studies pointing towards an inverse correlation between campesterol and BMI/obesity [34,35]. Likewise, elimination of overweight by lifestyle interventions normalized intestinal cholesterol absorption [33]. Campesterol and 7aOH in the liver were elevated upon HP-B-CD administration. While the molecular mechanisms behind this observation are not clear, it is known that both campesterol and 7aOH are liver X receptor (LXR) agonists which serve as an intracellular sensor of cholesterol content and mobilize cholesterol to the plasma membrane upon activation [36]. Thus, the upregulation of campesterol and 7aOH levels upon HP-B-CD could possibly contribute to the improved intracellular cholesterol trafficking observed upon administration of HP-B-CD. Despite the upregulation of campesterol and 7aOH upon HP-B-CD treatment, we did not observe a decrease in plasma and liver cholesterol. This observation can be explained by the fact that dietary phytosterols, including campesterol, have been shown to increase the affinity and efficiency of the LDLR for adequate cholesterol removal [37]. Since our study was performed in *Ldlr*$^{-/-}$ mice, campesterol was not able to enhance efficiency of the LDLR. Moreover, these results indicate that lysosomal cholesterol levels were reduced independent of the LDLR and support the view of campesterol and 7aOH being an LXR-agonist. Thus, campesterol and 7aOH levels were upregulated upon HP-B-CD and possibly improved intracellular cholesterol trafficking via LXR signaling.

## 4. Experimental Section

### 4.1. Mice, Diet and Injections

The mice were housed under standard conditions and given free access to food and water. All experiments were approved by the Committee for Animal Welfare of Maastricht University and performed according to Dutch regulations. Eleven to twelve-week old female *Ldlr*$^{-/-}$ mice on a C57/Bl6 background were either fed regular chow (*n* = 10) or an HFC diet (*n* = 12 per HFC group with and without HP-B-CD treatment) for 12 weeks. The effects of HP-B-CD were investigated by giving weekly subcutaneous injections at the start of the HFC diet with 4000 mg per kg of body weight of 20% *w/v* HP-B-CD (H107, Sigma-Aldrich GmbH, St. Louis, MO, USA) (*n* = 12). PBS was used for control injections. The HFC diet contained 21% milk butter, 0.2% cholesterol, 46% carbohydrates and 17% casein. Collection of blood and tissue specimens, biochemical determination of lipids in plasma, liver histology, electron microscopy, acid phosphatase (ACPase) enzyme cytochemistry, RNA isolation, complementary DNA synthesis and quantitative polymerase chain reaction were determined as described previously [4,5,38–41]. Pieces of liver were used for quantification of liver cholesterol and the hepatic levels of campesterol and 7α-hydroxycholesterol as described previously [42].

### 4.2. CD68 Staining

For the CD68 staining, six microscopical views (200× magnification) of each liver were obtained. Adobe Photoshop CS2 v.9.0 was used to analyze CD68-positive (red) pixels as well as total unstained tissue pixels of each microscopical picture. Subsequently, these data were used to calculate the percentage of CD68-positive area.

### 4.3. Scoring of Lysosomal Lipid Droplets, Cytoplasmic CE Droplets and Cholesterol Crystals

Electron microscopy was performed by an expert in the electron microscopical field of the liver. By using electron microscopy pictures, analysis of lysosomal cholesterol was performed by scoring the area of lysosomal lipid droplets, those that are inside ACPase-positive lysosomes indicated by the black membrane, and the area of cytoplasmic CE droplets in 40 to 50 KCs from each HFC group. Each KC was scored between 0 and 6; 0 indicated no lipid droplets inside lysosomes or no cytoplasmic CE droplets, whereas an extremely large area of lysosomal lipid droplets or cytoplasmic CE droplets was scored with a 6. Subsequently, the average lysosomal cholesterol and cytoplasmic CE area per KC was calculated. The scoring and the average calculation for cholesterol crystallization were performed similarly; the score 0 indicated no cholesterol crystals, while 5 indicated the highest area of cholesterol crystals and was performed as described previously [29].

### 4.4. Bone Marrow-Derived Macrophages

Bone marrow-derived macrophages (BMDM) were isolated from the tibiae and femurs of wildtype C57BL/6 mice. Cells were cultured in RPMI-1640 (GIBCO Invitrogen, Breda, The Netherlands) with 10% heat-inactivated fetal calf serum (Bodinco B.V. Alkmaar, The Netherlands), penicillin (100 U/mL), streptomycin (100 μg/mL) and L-glutamine 2 mM (all GIBCO Invitrogen), supplemented with 20% L929-conditioned medium (LCM) for 8–9 days to generate BMDM. After attachment, macrophages were seeded at 350,000 cells per well in 24-well plates and incubated for 72 h with oxLDL (25 μg/mL; Alfa Aesar: J65591, Wardhill, MA, USA), followed by a treatment with or without 0.3% HP-B-CD (H107, Sigma-Aldrich GmbH, St. Louis, MO, USA). Then cells were washed and stimulated with lipopolysaccharide (100 ng/mL) for 4 h. Finally, cells were lysed and further processed for gene expression analysis.

## 4.5. Statistical Analysis

Data were analyzed by two-tailed, unpaired, $t$-tests using GraphPad Prism, version 4.0 for Windows (GraphPad Software Inc., La Jolla, CA, USA). Data are represented as mean $\pm$ standard error of mean (SEM) and considered significant at $p < 0.05$ (* $p < 0.05$; ** $p < 0.01$ and *** $p < 0.001$, respectively).

## 5. Conclusions

Unlike total liver cholesterol, administration of HP-B-CD improves intracellular cholesterol localization inside KCs of NAFLD-susceptible $Ldlr^{-/-}$ mice. Therefore, HP-B-CD could be a useful tool to improve intracellular cholesterol levels and cholesterol crystals in the context of the metabolic syndrome and should be tested in the future. Further studies are necessary to determine the novel role of oxysterols and phytosterols in improving intracellular cholesterol trafficking. Additionally, these data underline the existence of a shared etiology between lysosomal storage diseases and NAFLD.

**Acknowledgments:** This research was supported by the Maag Lever Darm Stichting (MLDS) (WO 08-16 and WO 11-35), the Netherlands Organisation for Scientific Research (NWO) (Vidi grant number: 016.126.327), and by the Cardiovascular Research Netherlands (CVON) IN-CONTROL grant (CVON 2012-03).

**Author Contributions:** Sofie M. A. Walenbergh, Alena Grebe, Eicke Latz, Ronit Shiri-Sverdlov conceived and designed experiments; Sofie M. A. Walenbergh, Tom Houben, Tim Hendrikx, Mike L. J. Jeurissen, Patrick J. van Gorp, Nathalie Vaes, Fons Verheyen, Dieter Lütjohann, Ronit Shiri-Sverdlov performed the experiments; Sofie M. A. Walenbergh, Tom Houben, Nathalie Vaes, Ronit Shiri-Sverdlov analyzed data; Sofie M. A. Walenbergh, Steven W. M. Olde Damink, Ger H. Koek, Ronit Shiri-Sverdlov wrote the paper.

## Abbreviations

NAFLD: Non-alcoholic fatty liver disease; KCs: Kupffer cells; NPC: Niemann-Pick Type C; HP-B-CD: Two-hydroxypropyl-β-cyclodextrin; LDL(R): Low-density lipoprotein (receptor); IDL: Intermediate-density lipoprotein; HFC: High-fat, high-cholesterol; PBS: Phosphate-buffered saline; CE: Cholesteryl ester; ACPase: Acid phosphatase; 7aOH: 7α-Hydroxycholesterol; OxLDL: Oxidized LDL; LXR: Liver X receptor.

## References

1. Lonardo, A.; Ballestri, S.; Marchesini, G.; Angulo, P.; Loria, P. Nonalcoholic fatty liver disease: A precursor of the metabolic syndrome. *Dig. Liver Dis.* **2015**, *47*, 181–190. [CrossRef] [PubMed]
2. Angulo, P. Nonalcoholic fatty liver disease. *N. Engl. J. Med.* **2002**, *346*, 1221–1231. [CrossRef] [PubMed]
3. Starley, B.Q.; Calcagno, C.J.; Harrison, S.A. Nonalcoholic fatty liver disease and hepatocellular carcinoma: A weighty connection. *Hepatology* **2010**, *51*, 1820–1832. [CrossRef] [PubMed]
4. Bieghs, V.; Hendrikx, T.; van Gorp, P.J.; Verheyen, F.; Guichot, Y.D.; Walenbergh, S.M.; Jeurissen, M.L.; Gijbels, M.; Rensen, S.S.; Bast, A.; et al. The cholesterol derivative 27-hydroxycholesterol reduces steatohepatitis in mice. *Gastroenterology* **2013**, *144*, 167–178.e1. [CrossRef] [PubMed]
5. Bieghs, V.; van Gorp, P.J.; Walenbergh, S.M.; Gijbels, M.J.; Verheyen, F.; Buurman, W.A.; Briles, D.E.; Hofker, M.H.; Binder, C.J.; Shiri-Sverdlov, R. Specific immunization strategies against oxidized low-density lipoprotein: A novel way to reduce nonalcoholic steatohepatitis in mice. *Hepatology* **2012**, *56*, 894–903. [CrossRef] [PubMed]
6. Duewell, P.; Kono, H.; Rayner, K.J.; Sirois, C.M.; Vladimer, G.; Bauernfeind, F.G.; Abela, G.S.; Franchi, L.; Nunez, G.; Schnurr, M.; et al. NLRP3 inflammasomes are required for atherogenesis and activated by cholesterol crystals. *Nature* **2010**, *464*, 1357–1361. [CrossRef] [PubMed]
7. Hendrikx, T.; Walenbergh, S.M.; Hofker, M.H.; Shiri-Sverdlov, R. Lysosomal cholesterol accumulation: Driver on the road to inflammation during atherosclerosis and non-alcoholic steatohepatitis. *Obes. Rev.* **2014**, *15*, 424–433. [CrossRef] [PubMed]

8.   Jerome, W.G. Advanced atherosclerotic foam cell formation has features of an acquired lysosomal storage disorder. *Rejuv. Res.* **2006**, *9*, 245–255. [CrossRef] [PubMed]

9.   Vanier, M.T. Niemann-Pick disease type C. *Orphanet J. Rare Dis.* **2010**, *5*, 16. [CrossRef] [PubMed]

10.  Abi-Mosleh, L.; Infante, R.E.; Radhakrishnan, A.; Goldstein, J.L.; Brown, M.S. Cyclodextrin overcomes deficient lysosome-to-endoplasmic reticulum transport of cholesterol in Niemann-Pick type C cells. *Proc. Natl. Acad. Sci. USA* **2009**, *106*, 19316–19321. [CrossRef] [PubMed]

11.  Davidson, C.D.; Ali, N.F.; Micsenyi, M.C.; Stephney, G.; Renault, S.; Dobrenis, K.; Ory, D.S.; Vanier, M.T.; Walkley, S.U. Chronic cyclodextrin treatment of murine Niemann-Pick C disease ameliorates neuronal cholesterol and glycosphingolipid storage and disease progression. *PLoS ONE* **2009**, *4*, e6951. [CrossRef] [PubMed]

12.  Liu, B.; Ramirez, C.M.; Miller, A.M.; Repa, J.J.; Turley, S.D.; Dietschy, J.M. Cyclodextrin overcomes the transport defect in nearly every organ of NPC1 mice leading to excretion of sequestered cholesterol as bile acid. *J. Lipid Res.* **2010**, *51*, 933–944. [CrossRef] [PubMed]

13.  Liu, B.; Turley, S.D.; Burns, D.K.; Miller, A.M.; Repa, J.J.; Dietschy, J.M. Reversal of defective lysosomal transport in NPC disease ameliorates liver dysfunction and neurodegeneration in the $npc1^{-/-}$ mouse. *Proc. Natl. Acad. Sci. USA* **2009**, *106*, 2377–2382. [CrossRef] [PubMed]

14.  Ramirez, C.M.; Liu, B.; Taylor, A.M.; Repa, J.J.; Burns, D.K.; Weinberg, A.G.; Turley, S.D.; Dietschy, J.M. Weekly cyclodextrin administration normalizes cholesterol metabolism in nearly every organ of the Niemann-Pick type C1 mouse and markedly prolongs life. *Pediatr. Res.* **2010**, *68*, 309–315. [CrossRef] [PubMed]

15.  Ishibashi, S.; Brown, M.S.; Goldstein, J.L.; Gerard, R.D.; Hammer, R.E.; Herz, J. Hypercholesterolemia in low density lipoprotein receptor knockout mice and its reversal by adenovirus-mediated gene delivery. *J. Clin. Investig.* **1993**, *92*, 883–893. [CrossRef] [PubMed]

16.  Bieghs, V.; van Gorp, P.J.; Wouters, K.; Hendrikx, T.; Gijbels, M.J.; van Bilsen, M.; Bakker, J.; Binder, C.J.; Lutjohann, D.; Staels, B.; *et al.* LDL receptor knock-out mice are a physiological model particularly vulnerable to study the onset of inflammation in non-alcoholic fatty liver disease. *PLoS ONE* **2012**, *7*, e30668. [CrossRef] [PubMed]

17.  Bieghs, V.; Walenbergh, S.M.; Hendrikx, T.; van Gorp, P.J.; Verheyen, F.; Olde Damink, S.W.; Masclee, A.A.; Koek, G.H.; Hofker, M.H.; Binder, C.J.; *et al.* Trapping of oxidized LDL in lysosomes of Kupffer cells is a trigger for hepatic inflammation. *Liver Int.* **2013**, *33*, 1056–1061. [CrossRef] [PubMed]

18.  Ramirez, C.M.; Liu, B.; Aqul, A.; Taylor, A.M.; Repa, J.J.; Turley, S.D.; Dietschy, J.M. Quantitative role of LAL, NPC2, and NPC1 in lysosomal cholesterol processing defined by genetic and pharmacological manipulations. *J. Lipid Res.* **2011**, *52*, 688–698. [CrossRef] [PubMed]

19.  Jerome, W.G.; Cash, C.; Webber, R.; Horton, R.; Yancey, P.G. Lysosomal lipid accumulation from oxidized low density lipoprotein is correlated with hypertrophy of the Golgi apparatus and trans-Golgi network. *J. Lipid Res.* **1998**, *39*, 1362–1371. [PubMed]

20.  Schmitz, G.; Grandl, M. Endolysosomal phospholipidosis and cytosolic lipid droplet storage and release in macrophages. *Biochim. Biophys. Acta* **2009**, *1791*, 524–539. [CrossRef] [PubMed]

21.  Sims-Robinson, C.; Bakeman, A.; Rosko, A.; Glasser, R.; Feldman, E.L. The role of oxidized cholesterol in diabetes-induced lysosomal dysfunction in the brain. *Mol. Neurobiol.* **2015**. [CrossRef] [PubMed]

22.  Yancey, P.G.; Jerome, W.G. Lysosomal cholesterol derived from mildly oxidized low density lipoprotein is resistant to efflux. *J. Lipid Res.* **2001**, *42*, 317–327. [PubMed]

23.  Lougheed, M.; Zhang, H.F.; Steinbrecher, U.P. Oxidized low density lipoprotein is resistant to cathepsins and accumulates within macrophages. *J. Biol. Chem.* **1991**, *266*, 14519–14525. [PubMed]

24.  Peake, K.B.; Vance, J.E. Normalization of cholesterol homeostasis by 2-hydroxypropyl-β-cyclodextrin in neurons and glia from Niemann-Pick C1 (NPC1)-deficient mice. *J. Biol. Chem.* **2012**, *287*, 9290–9298. [CrossRef] [PubMed]

25.  Stella, V.J.; He, Q. Cyclodextrins. *Toxicol. Pathol.* **2008**, *36*, 30–42. [CrossRef] [PubMed]

26.  Lopez, A.M.; Terpack, S.J.; Posey, K.S.; Liu, B.; Ramirez, C.M.; Turley, S.D. Systemic administration of 2-hydroxypropyl-β-cyclodextrin to symptomatic NPC1-deficient mice slows cholesterol sequestration in the major organs and improves liver function. *Clin. Exp. Pharmacol. Physiol.* **2014**, *41*, 780–787. [CrossRef] [PubMed]

27. Taylor, A.M.; Liu, B.; Mari, Y.; Liu, B.; Repa, J.J. Cyclodextrin mediates rapid changes in lipid balance in $Npc1^{-/-}$ mice without carrying cholesterol through the bloodstream. *J. Lipid Res.* **2012**, *53*, 2331–2342. [CrossRef] [PubMed]

28. Grebe, A.; Latz, E. Cholesterol crystals and inflammation. *Curr. Rheumatol. Rep.* **2013**, *15*, 313. [CrossRef] [PubMed]

29. Hendrikx, T.; Bieghs, V.; Walenbergh, S.M.; van Gorp, P.J.; Verheyen, F.; Jeurissen, M.L.; Steinbusch, M.M.; Vaes, N.; Binder, C.J.; Koek, G.H.; *et al.* Macrophage specific caspase-1/11 deficiency protects against cholesterol crystallization and hepatic inflammation in hyperlipidemic mice. *PLoS ONE* **2013**, *8*, e78792. [CrossRef] [PubMed]

30. Ioannou, G.N.; Haigh, W.G.; Thorning, D.; Savard, C. Hepatic cholesterol crystals and crown-like structures distinguish nash from simple steatosis. *J. Lipid Res.* **2013**, *54*, 1326–1334. [CrossRef] [PubMed]

31. Tangirala, R.K.; Jerome, W.G.; Jones, N.L.; Small, D.M.; Johnson, W.J.; Glick, J.M.; Mahlberg, F.H.; Rothblat, G.H. Formation of cholesterol monohydrate crystals in macrophage-derived foam cells. *J. Lipid Res.* **1994**, *35*, 93–104. [PubMed]

32. Rosenbaum, A.I.; Zhang, G.; Warren, J.D.; Maxfield, F.R. Endocytosis of β-cyclodextrins is responsible for cholesterol reduction in Niemann-Pick type C mutant cells. *Proc. Natl. Acad. Sci. USA* **2010**, *107*, 5477–5482. [CrossRef] [PubMed]

33. Simonen, P.; Gylling, H.; Howard, A.N.; Miettinen, T.A. Introducing a new component of the metabolic syndrome: Low cholesterol absorption. *Am. J. Clin. Nutr.* **2000**, *72*, 82–88. [PubMed]

34. Pinedo, S.; Vissers, M.N.; von Bergmann, K.; Elharchaoui, K.; Lutjohann, D.; Luben, R.; Wareham, N.J.; Kastelein, J.J.; Khaw, K.T.; Boekholdt, S.M. Plasma levels of plant sterols and the risk of coronary artery disease: The prospective EPIC-Norfolk Population Study. *J. Lipid Res.* **2007**, *48*, 139–144. [CrossRef] [PubMed]

35. Chan, D.C.; Watts, G.F.; Barrett, P.H.; O'Neill, F.H.; Thompson, G.R. Plasma markers of cholesterol homeostasis and apolipoprotein B-100 kinetics in the metabolic syndrome. *Obes. Res.* **2003**, *11*, 591–596. [CrossRef] [PubMed]

36. Rigamonti, E.; Helin, L.; Lestavel, S.; Mutka, A.L.; Lepore, M.; Fontaine, C.; Bouhlel, M.A.; Bultel, S.; Fruchart, J.C.; Ikonen, E.; *et al.* Liver X receptor activation controls intracellular cholesterol trafficking and esterification in human macrophages. *Circ. Res.* **2005**, *97*, 682–689. [CrossRef] [PubMed]

37. Ruiu, G.; Pinach, S.; Veglia, F.; Gambino, R.; Marena, S.; Uberti, B.; Alemanno, N.; Burt, D.; Pagano, G.; Cassader, M. Phytosterol-enriched yogurt increases LDL affinity and reduces CD36 expression in polygenic hypercholesterolemia. *Lipids* **2009**, *44*, 153–160. [CrossRef] [PubMed]

38. Bieghs, V.; Verheyen, F.; van Gorp, P.J.; Hendrikx, T.; Wouters, K.; Lutjohann, D.; Gijbels, M.J.; Febbraio, M.; Binder, C.J.; Hofker, M.H.; *et al.* Internalization of modified lipids by CD36 and SR-A leads to hepatic inflammation and lysosomal cholesterol storage in kupffer cells. *PLoS ONE* **2012**, *7*, e34378. [CrossRef] [PubMed]

39. Bieghs, V.; Wouters, K.; van Gorp, P.J.; Gijbels, M.J.; de Winther, M.P.; Binder, C.J.; Lutjohann, D.; Febbraio, M.; Moore, K.J.; van Bilsen, M.; *et al.* Role of scavenger receptor A and CD36 in diet-induced nonalcoholic steatohepatitis in hyperlipidemic mice. *Gastroenterology* **2010**, *138*, 2477–2486.e3. [CrossRef] [PubMed]

40. Wisse, E.; Braet, F.; Duimel, H.; Vreuls, C.; Koek, G.; Olde Damink, S.W.; van den Broek, M.A.; de Geest, B.; Dejong, C.H.; Tateno, C.; *et al.* Fixation methods for electron microscopy of human and other liver. *World J. Gastroenterol.* **2010**, *16*, 2851–2866. [CrossRef] [PubMed]

41. Wouters, K.; van Gorp, P.J.; Bieghs, V.; Gijbels, M.J.; Duimel, H.; Lutjohann, D.; Kerksiek, A.; van Kruchten, R.; Maeda, N.; Staels, B.; *et al.* Dietary cholesterol, rather than liver steatosis, leads to hepatic inflammation in hyperlipidemic mouse models of nonalcoholic steatohepatitis. *Hepatology* **2008**, *48*, 474–486. [CrossRef] [PubMed]

42. Lutjohann, D.; Stroick, M.; Bertsch, T.; Kuhl, S.; Lindenthal, B.; Thelen, K.; Andersson, U.; Bjorkhem, I.; Bergmann Kv, K.; Fassbender, K. High doses of simvastatin, pravastatin, and cholesterol reduce brain cholesterol synthesis in guinea pigs. *Steroids* **2004**, *69*, 431–438. [CrossRef] [PubMed]

# Permissions

The contributors of this book come from diverse backgrounds, making this book a truly international effort. This book will bring forth new frontiers with its revolutionizing research information and detailed analysis of the nascent developments around the world.

We would like to thank all the contributing authors for lending their expertise to make the book truly unique. They have played a crucial role in the development of this book. Without their invaluable contributions this book wouldn't have been possible. They have made vital efforts to compile up to date information on the varied aspects of this subject to make this book a valuable addition to the collection of many professionals and students.

This book was conceptualized with the vision of imparting up-to-date information and advanced data in this field. To ensure the same, a matchless editorial board was set up. Every individual on the board went through rigorous rounds of assessment to prove their worth. After which they invested a large part of their time researching and compiling the most relevant data for our readers.

The editorial board has been involved in producing this book since its inception. They have spent rigorous hours researching and exploring the diverse topics which have resulted in the successful publishing of this book. They have passed on their knowledge of decades through this book. To expedite this challenging task, the publisher supported the team at every step. A small team of assistant editors was also appointed to further simplify the editing procedure and attain best results for the readers.

Apart from the editorial board, the designing team has also invested a significant amount of their time in understanding the subject and creating the most relevant covers. They scrutinized every image to scout for the most suitable representation of the subject and create an appropriate cover for the book.

The publishing team has been an ardent support to the editorial, designing and production team. Their endless efforts to recruit the best for this project, has resulted in the accomplishment of this book. They are a veteran in the field of academics and their pool of knowledge is as vast as their experience in printing. Their expertise and guidance has proved useful at every step. Their uncompromising quality standards have made this book an exceptional effort. Their encouragement from time to time has been an inspiration for everyone.

The publisher and the editorial board hope that this book will prove to be a valuable piece of knowledge for researchers, students, practitioners and scholars across the globe.

# List of Contributors

**Katrine D. Galsgaard**
Department of Biomedical Sciences, Faculty of Health and Medical Sciences, University of Copenhagen, 2200 Copenhagen, Denmark
Novo Nordisk Foundation Center for Basic Metabolic Research, Faculty of Health and Sciences, University of Copenhagen, 2200 Copenhagen, Denmark

**Wim Verlinden, Thomas Vanwolleghem, Luisa Vonghia, Jonas Weyler and Sven Francque**
Laboratory of Experimental Medicine and Pediatrics, Division of Gastroenterology and Hepatology, University of Antwerp, 2610 Antwerp, Belgium
Department of Gastroenterology and Hepatology, Antwerp University Hospital, 2650 Antwerp, Belgium

**Eugénie Van Mieghem and Laura Depauw**
Laboratory of Experimental Medicine and Pediatrics, Division of Gastroenterology and Hepatology, University of Antwerp, 2610 Antwerp, Belgium

**Ann Driessen**
Department of Pathology, Antwerp University Hospital, 2650 Antwerp, Belgium

**Dirk Callens and Laurence Roosens**
Department of Clinical Biology, Antwerp University Hospital, 2650 Antwerp, Belgium

**Eveline Dirinck, An Verrijken and Luc Van Gaal**
Department of Endocrinology, Diabetology and Metabolism, Antwerp University Hospital, 2650 Antwerp, Belgium

**Alexandre Losekann, Angelo A. de Mattos, Cristiane V. Tovo and Gabriela P. Coral**
Post-Graduation Program, Hepatology at Universidade Federal de Ciências da Saúde de Porto Alegre (UFCSPA), Porto Alegre 90.050-170, Brasil

**Antonio C. Weston, Luis A. de Carli, Marilia B. Espindola and Sergio R. Pioner**
Centro de Tratamento da Obesidade (CTO), Hospital Santa Casa de Misericórdia de Porto Alegre, Porto Alegre 92.010-300, Brasil

**Eyal Shteyer**
The Liver Unit, Gastroenterology Institute, Hadassah Medical Center, Hadassah Medical School, The Hebrew University, Jerusalem 9112001, Israel
Pediatric Gastroenterology Institute, Shaare Zedek Medical Center, Hadassah Medical School, The Hebrew University, Jerusalem 9103102, Israel

**Rivka Villenchik and Nidaa Nator**
The Liver Unit, Gastroenterology Institute, Hadassah Medical Center, Hadassah Medical School, The Hebrew University, Jerusalem 9112001, Israel

**Mahmud Mahamid**
Liver Unit, Gastroenterology Institute, Shaare Zedek Medical Center, Hadassah Medical School, The Hebrew University, Jerusalem 9112001, Israel
Liver Unit, Holy Family Hospital; Safed Medical School, Bar Ilan University, Nazareth 1641110, Israel

**Rifaat Safadi**
The Liver Unit, Gastroenterology Institute, Hadassah Medical Center, Hadassah Medical School, The Hebrew University, Jerusalem 9112001, Israel
Liver Unit, Holy Family Hospital; Safed Medical School, Bar Ilan University, Nazareth 1641110, Israel

**Linda A. Ban and Susan V. McLennan**
Greg Brown Diabetes and Endocrine Laboratory, Charles Perkins Centre, University of Sydney, NSW 2006, Australia

**Nicholas A. Shackel**
Liver Cell Biology Laboratory, Centenary Institute of Cancer Medicine and Cell Biology, Camperdown, NSW 2006, Australia

**David Houghton and Michael Trenell**
Institute of Cellular Medicine, Newcastle University, Newcastle upon Tyne NE4 6BE, UK

**Christopher J. Stewart**
Alkek Center for Metagenomics and Microbiome Research, Department of Molecular Virology and Microbiology, Baylor College of Medicine, Houston, TX 77030, USA

**Christopher P. Day**
Institute of Cellular Medicine, Newcastle University, Newcastle upon Tyne NE4 6BE, UK
Liver Unit, Newcastle upon Tyne Hospitals NHS Trust, Freeman Hospital, Newcastle upon Tyne NE7 7DN, UK

**Elina M. Petäjä and Hannele Yki-Järvinen**
Minerva Foundation Institute for Medical Research, 00290 Helsinki, Finland
Department of Medicine, University of Helsinki and Helsinki University Central Hospital, 00290 Helsinki, Finland

**Alessandra Caligiuri, Alessandra Gentilini and Fabio Marra**
Dipartimento di Medicina Sperimentale e Clinica, Università degli Studi di Firenze, Firenze 50121, Italy

**Alessandro Mantovani and Giovanni Targher**
Section of Endocrinology, Diabetes and Metabolism, Department of Medicine, University and Azienda Ospedaliera Universitaria Integrata of Verona, Piazzale Stefani, 1, Verona 37126, Italy

**Paolo Gisondi**
Section of Dermatology, Department of Medicine, University and Azienda Ospedaliera Universitaria Integrata of Verona, Piazzale Stefani, 1, Verona 37126, Italy

**Amedeo Lonardo**
Outpatient Liver Clinic and Division of Internal Medicine—Department of Biomedical, Metabolic and Neural Sciences, NOCSAE, University of Modena and Reggio Emilia and Azienda USL Modena, Baggiovara, Modena 41126, Italy

**Maria Perticone**
Department of Experimental and Clinical Medicine, University Magna Græcia, Catanzaro 88100, Italy

**Antonio Cimellaro, Angela Sciacqua, Giorgio Sesti and Francesco Perticone**
Department of Medical and Surgical Sciences, University Magna Græcia, Catanzaro 88100, Italy

**Raffaele Maio and Benedetto Caroleo**
Unit of Cardiovascular Diseases, Azienda Ospedaliera Mater Domini, Catanzaro 88100, Italy

**Jonathan L. Temple, Paul Cordero, Jiawei Li and Vi Nguyen**
Faculty of Life Sciences and Medicine, King's College London, Strand, London WC2R 2LS, UK

**Jude A. Oben**
Faculty of Life Sciences and Medicine, King's College London, Strand, London WC2R 2LS, UK
Department of Gastroenterology and Hepatology, Guy's and St Thomas' Hospital, NHS Foundation Trust, Westminster Bridge Rd., London SE1 7EH, UK

**Ryuta Shigefuku, Hiroyasu Nakano, Tsunamasa Watanabe, Kotaro Matsunaga, Nobuyuki Matsumoto, Masaki Kato, Ryo Morita, Yousuke Michikawa, Nobuhiro Hattori, Kazunari Nakahara, Hiroki Ikeda and Fumio Itoh**
Division of Gastroenterology and Hepatology, St. Marianna University School of Medicine, Kanagawa, Kawasaki 216-8511, Japan

**Hideaki Takahashi, Tomohiro Tamura and Yohei Noguchi**
Division of Gastroenterology and Hepatology, St. Marianna University School of Medicine, Kanagawa, Kawasaki 216-8511, Japan
Division of Gastroenterology, St. Marianna University School of Medicine, Yokohama City Seibu Hospital, Kanagawa, Yokohama 241-0811, Japan

**Tetsuya Hiraishi, Toshiya Ishii, Chiaki Okuse and Michihiro Suzuki**
Division of Gastroenterology and Hepatology, St. Marianna University School of Medicine, Kanagawa, Kawasaki 216-8511, Japan
Division of Gastroenterology and Hepatology, Department of Internal Medicine, Kawasaki Municipal Tama Hospital, Kanagawa, Kawasaki 214-8525, Japan

**Shigeru Sase**
Anzai Medical Company, Ltd., Tokyo 141-0033, Japan

**Sofie M. A. Walenbergh, Tom Houben, Tim Hendrikx, Mike L. J. Jeurissen, Patrick J. van Gorp, Nathalie Vaes and Ronit Shiri-Sverdlov**
Department of Molecular Genetics, School of Nutrition and Translational Research in Metabolism (NUTRIM), Maastricht University, Maastricht 6229ER, The Netherlands

**Steven W. M. Olde Damink**
Department of General Surgery, Maastricht University, Maastricht 6229ER, The Netherlands
Department of HPB and Liver Transplantation Surgery, Royal Free Hospital, University College London, London NW3 2PF, UK

**Fons Verheyen**
Department of Molecular Cell Biology and Electron Microscopy, Maastricht University, Maastricht 6229ER, The Netherlands

**Ger H. Koek**
Department of Internal Medicine, Division of Gastroenterology and Hepatology, Maastricht University Medical Center (MUMC), Maastricht 6202AZ, The Netherlands

**Dieter Lütjohann**
Institute of Clinical Chemistry and Clinical Pharmacology, University of Bonn, Bonn D-53105, Germany

**Alena Grebe**
Institute of Innate Immunity, University Hospital, University of Bonn, Bonn D-53127, Germany

**Eicke Latz**
Institute of Innate Immunity, University Hospital, University of Bonn, Bonn D-53127, Germany
German Center for Neurodegenerative Diseases (DZNE), Bonn D-53127, Germany
Division of Infectious Diseases and Immunology, University of Massachusetts Medical School, Worcester, MA 01605, USA

# Index

Printed in the USA
CPSIA information can be obtained
at www.ICGtesting.com
JSHW051626061123
51533JS00005B/123